EXTRAORDINARY USES

FOR ORDINARY THINGS

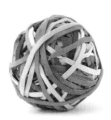
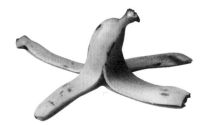

Reader's Digest

New York | Montreal

ISBN 978-1-62145-436-6 (paperback)
ISBN 978-1-62145-437-3 (e-pub)

Library of Congress catalogued the previous edition of this book as follows:
Library of Congress Cataloging-in-Publication Data
Extraordinary uses for ordinary things/Reader's Digest. – 1st ed.
p. cm.
Includes index.
1.   Home economics. I. Reader's Digest Association.
TX145.E95 2004
640—dc22

2004020058

Photo credits: All photographs and illustrations in this book are the copyright of Trusted Media Brands, Inc. except for the following: Katrina Leigh/Shutterstock, **back cover** *right;* Corel Corporation, **216** *center, both;* Photodisc, **43** *bottom right;* **58** *bottom right;* **94** *top;* **143** *bottom right;* **273** *top right;* **346** *bottom;* **348** *top left.*

We are committed to both the quality of our products and the service we provide to our customers. We value your comments, so please feel free to contact us.

Reader's Digest Adult Trade Publishing
44 South Broadway
White Plains, NY 10601

For more Reader's Digest products and information, visit our website:
www.rd.com (in the United States)

Printed in China

1 3 5 7 9 10 8 6 4 2

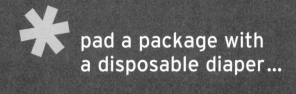 pad a package with
a disposable diaper...

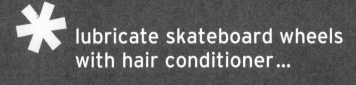 lubricate skateboard wheels
with hair conditioner...

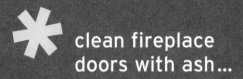 clean fireplace
doors with ash...

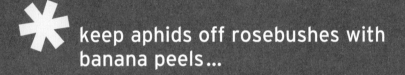 keep aphids off rosebushes with
banana peels...

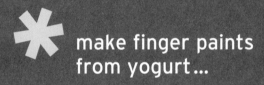 make finger paints
from yogurt...

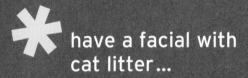 have a facial with
cat litter...

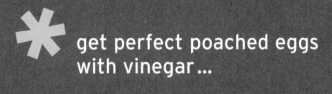 get perfect poached eggs
with vinegar...

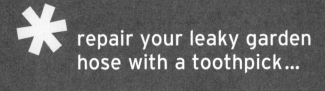 repair your leaky garden
hose with a toothpick...

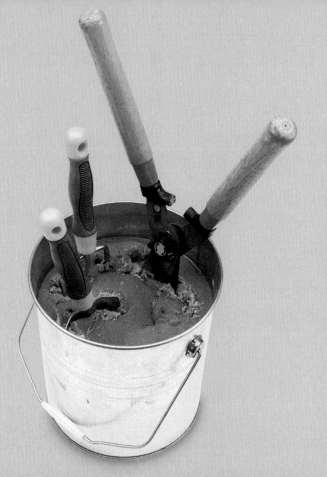

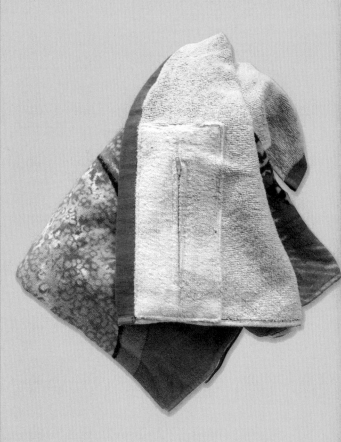

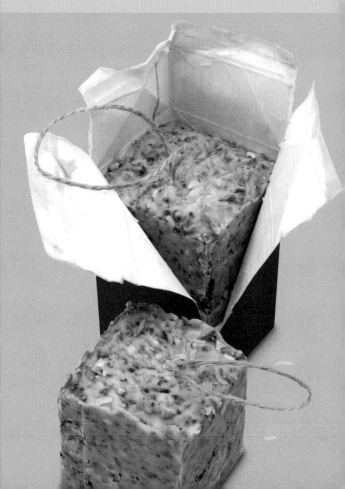

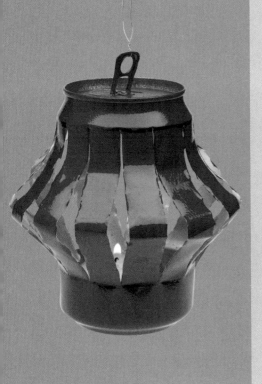

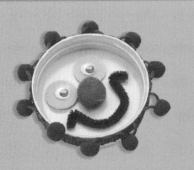

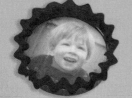

ABOUT THIS BOOK

Welcome to *Extraordinary Uses for Ordinary Things*. On the following pages we'll show you thousands of ingenious ways to use 205 ordinary household products to restore, replace, repair, or revive practically everything in and around your home or to pamper yourself or entertain your children. You'll save time and money—and you'll save shelf space because you won't need all of those commercial products. You'll even save on gas, because you won't need to run out to the store every time you need a staple such as air freshener, shampoo, oven cleaner, or wrapping paper.

The main part of this book is arranged like an encyclopedia, with the 205 product categories organized in A to Z fashion (from Address Labels to Zucchini), to provide instant access to information as well as entertaining reading. But before that, in Most Useful Items for Just About Anything, you'll find a guide that targets the most useful items for certain areas, such as the garden or for cooking, as well as a list of the Super Items (*page 14*) that everyone should have in their home.

Scattered throughout, you'll also find hundreds of fascinating anecdotes and helpful tips. Some highlight specific warnings and safety precautions, or offer advice about buying or using certain items. And others are just plain fun—providing quirky historical information about the invention or origins of products. We've also included dozens of engaging activities and simple science experiments you can do with children.

Whether you delight in discovering new ways to use commonplace household items, or if you simply hate to throw things away, you're bound to find the ideas in this book both entertaining and informative.

The Editors

CONTENTS

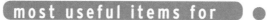

most useful items for • • •

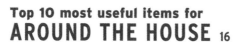
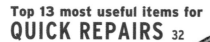

your complete ••• A-Z GUIDE 34

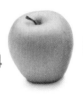

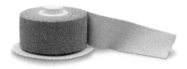

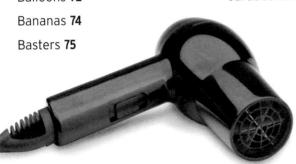

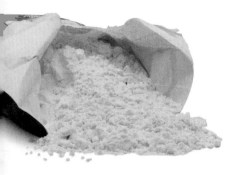

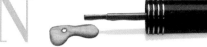

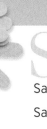

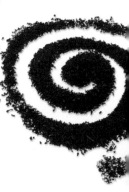

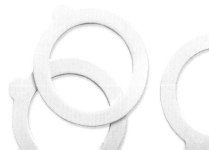

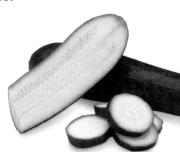

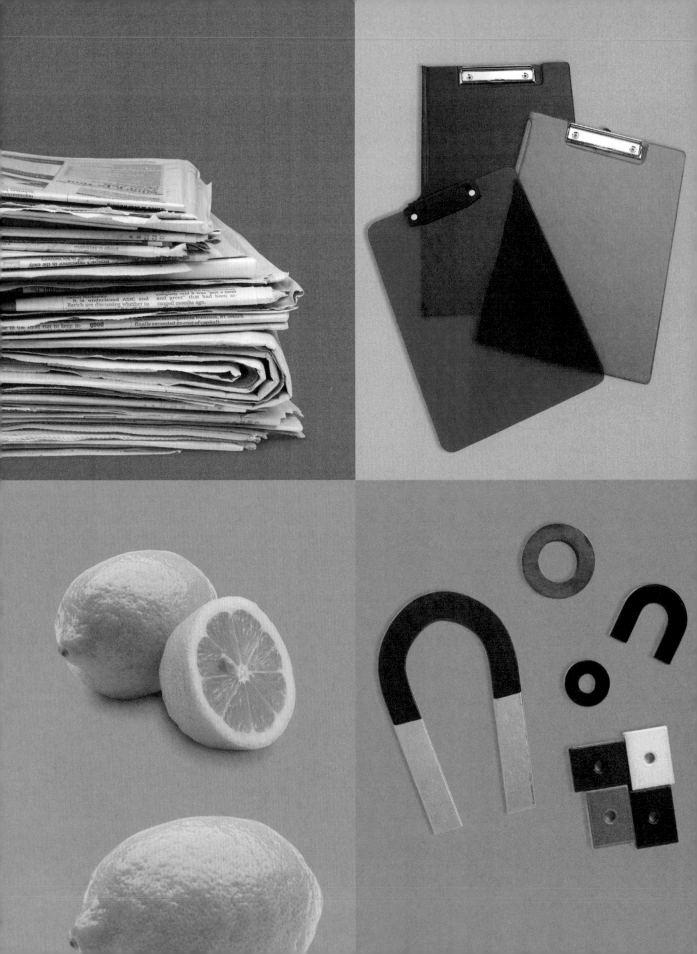

... JUST ABOUT ANYTHING

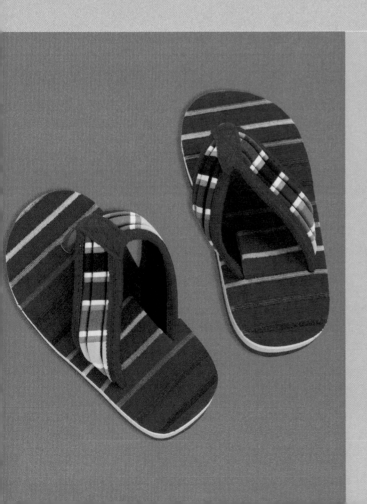

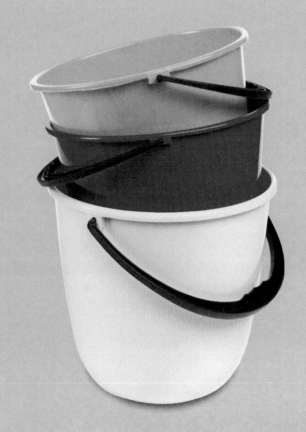

what's in your cupboard? what's in your cupboard?
what's in your cupboard?
WHAT'S IN YOUR CUPBOARD?

DISCOVER WHAT'S HIDING
IN YOUR CUPBOARD

The items featured throughout this book are not costly commercial products. Rather, they are everyday items that you're likely to find in your home—in your kitchen, medicine cabinet, desk, garage, and even the trash. And you'll be amazed by how much you can actually accomplish using just a few of the most versatile of these items, such as baking soda, duct tape, pantyhose, salt, vinegar, and WD-40.

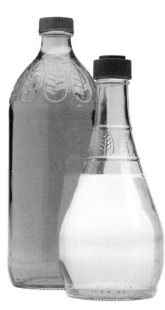

Some things, like washing windows, don't need to be complicated. But somehow, they have become more complicated. Today, supermarket shelves are filled with a dazzling array of cleaning products, each with a unique use, a special formula, and a million-dollar advertising campaign. Window cleaners alone take up plenty of space. The bottles are filled with colorful liquids and have labels boasting their orange power, berry bouquet, or lemon or apple–herbal scent. Ironically, many credit the added power of vinegar or ammonia as their 'secret' ingredient.

This is the way of the world today. Every problem, every mess, every hobby, every daily task seems to require special tools, unique products, and extensive know-how. Why use a knife to chop garlic when there are so many varieties of garlic presses available? Why use a rag for cleaning when you have specialized sponges, wipes, Swiffers, magnetically charged dusters, and HEPA-filter vacuums? The list of gadgets and gizmos goes on and on.

Which begs the question: Why not just use a solution of vinegar or ammonia like our grandparents did to clean the windows? It works just as well as those expensive, complicated products—if not better.

And it costs only about a quarter as much, and sometimes less than that.

LEARN HOW TO USE WHAT'S IN YOUR CUPBOARD

Making do with what you've already got. It's a smart, money-saving approach to life. And in fact, it can be easy and pleasurable. You can buy a fancy lint brush to remove cat hairs from clothing, but it's pretty amazing how a few cents' worth of tape does the job just as well. And you can use strong kitchen chemicals to clean the inside of a vase that held its flower water a bit too long, but isn't it easier, and more fun, to use a couple of Alka-Seltzer tablets instead to fizz away the stuck-on grime? On the following pages, the lists of most useful items will help you target specific areas, such as the house or garden, or interests, such as repairs and beauty, so that you can zoom in on the subject area that's of most interest to you. And in the list of 'super items', you'll find amazing examples of how you can use the more common items lurking inside your cupboard.

what's in your cupboard?
WHAT'S IN YOUR CUPBOARD?
what's in your cupboard?
what's in your cupboard?

LESS TOXIC AND MORE EARTH-FRIENDLY ITEMS

In addition to saving you time and money, there are other, less tangible advantages to using these everyday household products. For one thing, many of the items are safer to use and considerably more environmentally friendly than their off-the-shelf counterparts. Consider, for example, using vinegar and baking soda to clear a clogged bathroom or kitchen drain (*see page 22*). It's usually just as effective as a commercial drain cleaner. The only difference is that the baking soda-and-vinegar combination is far less caustic on your plumbing. Plus, you don't have to worry about getting it on your skin or in your eyes.

The hints scattered throughout this book will also help you reduce household waste by giving you hundreds of delightful and surprising suggestions for reusing many of the items that you would otherwise toss in the garbage or recycling bin. These include lemon rinds, milk cartons, egg cartons, used tea bags, worn-out pantyhose, plastic bags, empty bottles, aluminium cans, and newspapers, to name just a few.

At the end of the day, you'll experience the distinct pleasure that can only come from learning creative, new ways to use those familiar objects in and around your house that you always thought you knew so well. Even if you never used Alka-Seltzer tablets to clean your toilet bowl, or repair your glasses with a dab of nail polish, isn't it great to know you can?

Much of the advice you'll find in the following pages isn't really new—it's just new to us. After all, 'Waste not, want not' isn't merely a quaint adage from a bygone era. It actually defined a way of life for generations. In the days before mass manufacturing and mass marketing transformed us into a throwaway society, most people knew perfectly well that table salt and baking soda (or as it was referred to in the olden days as bicarbonate of soda) had dozens upon dozens of uses.

Now, as landfills swell and we realize that the earth's resources aren't really endless, there are signs of a shift back to the old-fashioned ways. From recycling programs to energy-efficient appliances to hybrid cars, we're constantly looking for new ways to apply the old, common sense values. And the good news is that while you're saving money and doing your bit to live in an earth-friendly way, you'll also be freeing your home and garage of clutter.

The lists of the most useful items for just about anything on the following pages will help you target your efforts, and give you specific examples of how to use those ordinary things in ways that are extraordinary and practical.

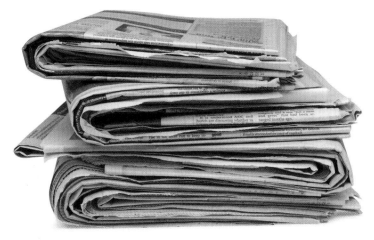

super items for everyone   super items for everyone
super items for everyone
SUPER ITEMS FOR EVERYONE

top 18 Super items FOR EVERYONE

ALUMINIUM FOIL

page 40

- Decorate a cake ■ Make a toasted cheese sandwich ■ Polish silverware ■ Sharpen scissors ■ Prevent paint from skinning over ■ Make a fishing lure

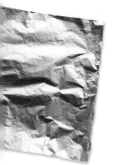

AMMONIA

page 48

- Repel moths ■ Stop mosquito bites from itching ■ Get rid of stains on concrete ■ Use as plant food ■ Keep stray animals out of the trash

BAKING SODA

page 60

- Make your own dishwashing detergent
- Get yellow stains off piano keys
- Control dandruff ■ Make deodorizing dog shampoo

CARDBOARD BOXES

page 97

- Make a breakfast-in-bed tray
- Repair a roof temporarily
- Use to protect fingers while hammering ■ Make a garage floor drip pan

DUCT TAPE

page 139

- Waterproof footwear ■ Catch flies ■ Replace garden-chair webbing ■ Make an emergency shoelace ■ Fix a toilet seat

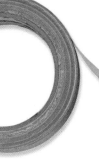

LEMONS

page 179

- Remove warts ■ Clean a microwave oven ■ Make soggy lettuce crisp again ■ Create blond highlights ■ Turn a lemon into a battery

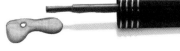

NAIL POLISH

page 198

- Tighten loose screws
- Tarnish-proof costume jewelry ■ Get rid of a wart
- Mend holes in window screens
- Plug a hole in a picnic cooler
- Fix torn blinds

PANTYHOSE

page 216

- Vacuum a fish tank ■ Stop a rolling pin from sticking ■ Make a ponytail scrunchy ■ Dust under the fridge ■ Clean your pool ■ Use to strain paint

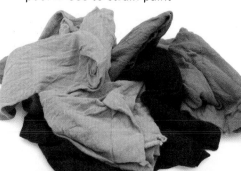

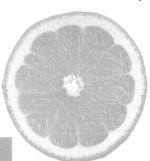

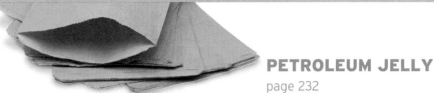

PAPER BAGS
page 221

■ Create a table decoration ■ Keep bread fresh
■ Clean artificial flowers ■ Add to compost
■ Make a kite ■ Make fire starters

PETROLEUM JELLY
page 232

■ Create emergency makeup
■ Remove lipstick stains ■ Shine
patent leather shoes ■ Prevent
unwanted hair dye runs ■ Keep
a bottle lid from sticking

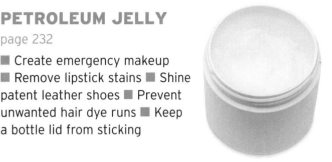

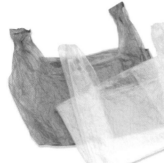

PLASTIC BAGS
page 239

■ Line a cracked flower
vase ■ Treat chapped
hands ■ Keep purses in
shape ■ Spin-dry salad
greens ■ Make a jump
rope ■ Ripen fruit

PLASTIC BOTTLES
page 246

■ Make a foot warmer ■ Save water when
flushing the toilet ■ Create a drip irrigator
for plants ■ Keep a cooler cold ■ Space
seeds in the garden

SANDWICH AND FREEZER BAGS
page 274

■ Soften hard marshmallows ■ Make a bath pillow
■ Use as a portable water dish ■ Make instant dessert treats

SALT
page 263

■ Give brooms a longer life
■ Make your own brass and
copper polish ■ Keep oven
spills from hardening ■ Revive
overcooked coffee ■ Condition
your skin

TAPE
page 307

■ Make flypaper ■ Prevent
jewelry tangles ■ Deter cats
from scratching furniture ■ Make
sewing easier ■ Mend a broken
plant stem

TEA
page 311

■ Tan your skin
■ Stop foot odor
■ Drain a boil ■ Feed
ferns ■ Tenderize
tough meat

WD-40
page 358

■ Relieve arthritis symptoms
■ Remove chewing gum
from hair ■ Protect a bird
feeder ■ Kill poison ivy and
prickly weeds ■ Remove
barnacles on boats

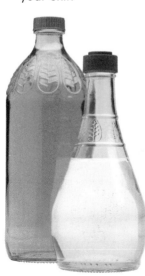

VINEGAR
page 329

■ Unclog drains ■ Clean and
deodorize just about anything
■ Unset old stains ■ Prevent
bruises ■ Repel insects ■ Speed
up seed germination

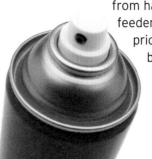

top 10 Most useful items for AROUND THE HOUSE

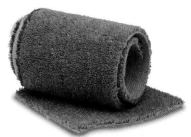

CARPET SCRAPS page 103
■ Make an exercise mat, car mat, or knee pad
■ Muffle appliance noise ■ Protect flooring
under plants ■ Cushion kitchen shelves
■ Give your car traction ■ Protect tools

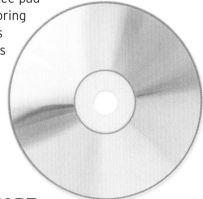

COMPACT DISCS page 126
■ Use as Christmas ornaments, driveway reflectors, or a
circle template ■ Catch candle drips ■ Make an artistic
bowl, decorative suncatcher, or a clock

DUCT TAPE AND ELECTRICAL TAPE
pages 139 and 147, respectively
■ Repair toilet seats, screens, vacuum hoses, and frames
■ Make a bandage or bumper sticker ■ Catch flies
■ Replace a grommet ■ Hem pants ■ Hang Christmas
lights ■ Make a Halloween costume ■ Cover a book,
wallet, or present ■ Reinforce book binding
■ Remove lint

FABRIC SOFTENER SHEETS page 153
■ Freshen air and deodorize cars, dogs, gym bags, suitcases, and
sneakers ■ Pick up pet hair ■ Repel mosquitoes ■ Stop static cling
■ Make bedsheets smell good ■ Stop sewing thread from tangling

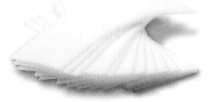

NAIL POLISH page 198
■ Mark hard-to-see items ■ Mark thermostat and shower settings
and levels in measuring cups and buckets ■ Label sports gear and
poison containers ■ Seal envelopes and labels ■ Stop shoe scuffs
and keep laces, ribbons, and fabric from unraveling ■ Make needle
threading easier ■ Keep buckles and jewelry shiny ■ Stop a stocking
run ■ Temporarily repair glasses ■ Fix nicks in floors and glass
■ Repair lacquered items ■ Fill bathtub nicks

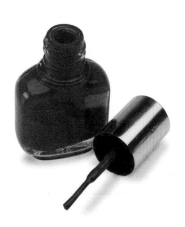

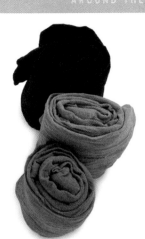

PANTYHOSE page 216
■ Find and pick up small objects
■ Buff shoes ■ Keep a hairbrush clean
■ Remove nail polish ■ Keep spray
bottles clog-free ■ Organize suitcases
■ Hang-dry sweaters ■ Secure garbage
bags ■ Dust under the fridge ■ Prevent
soil erosion in houseplants

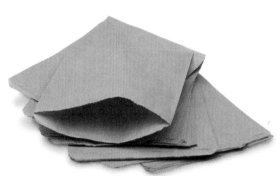

PAPER BAGS page 221
■ Bring on trips for souvenirs ■ Dust off mops ■ Carry laundry
■ Cover textbooks ■ Create a table decoration ■ Use as gift bags
and wrapping paper ■ Reshape knits after washing ■ Use as a
pressing cloth ■ Bag newspapers for recycling

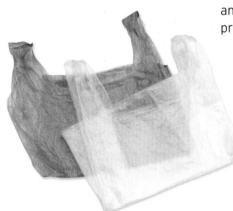

PLASTIC BAGS page 239
■ Keep mattresses dry ■ Stuff curtain
valances, pillows, and crafts ■ Drain bath
toys ■ Clean out pockets before doing
laundry ■ Make bibs and a highchair
drop cloth ■ Line a litter box ■ Dispose
of a Christmas tree

RUBBER BANDS page 258
■ Reshape a broom ■ Childproof cabinets ■ Keep thread from
tangling ■ Make a holder for car visors ■ Use to grip paper ■ Extend
a button ■ Use as a bookmark ■ Cushion a remote control ■ Secure
bed slats and tighten furniture casters

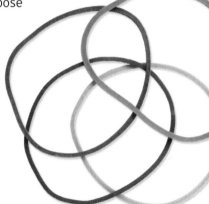

SANDWICH AND FREEZER BAGS page 274
■ Protect pictures and padlocks ■ Dispense fabric softener
■ Display baby teeth ■ Carry baby wipes ■ Mold soap
■ Starch craft items ■ Feed birds ■ Make a funnel

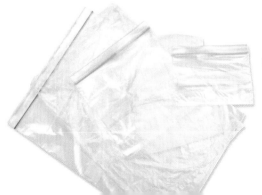

TIP pad a package with
a disposable diaper...
page 139

17

top 12

Most useful items for
THE COOK

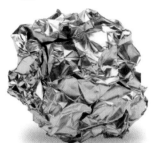

ALUMINIUM FOIL page 40
■ Bake a perfect piecrust ■ Soften brown sugar ■ Decorate a cake and create custom-shaped cake pans ■ Keep rolls and bread warm ■ Make an extra-large salad bowl

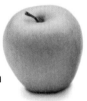

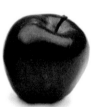

APPLES page 51
■ Keep a roast chicken moist and cakes fresh ■ Ripen green tomatoes ■ Soften hardened brown sugar ■ Absorb excess salt in soups

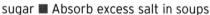

BAKING SODA page 60
■ Clean fruit and vegetables ■ Remove fish smells ■ Reduce the acidity of coffee and tomato-based sauces ■ Reduce gas-producing properties of beans ■ Make fluffy omelets ■ Replace yeast

COFFEE FILTERS page 121
■ Cover food in microwave ■ Filter cork crumbs from wine or food remnants from cooking oil ■ Hold a taco, ice-cream cone, or popsicle

ICE CUBE TRAYS page 171
■ Freeze eggs, pesto, chopped vegetables, and herbs, chicken soup–even leftover wine–for future use

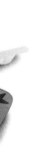

LEMONS page 179
■ Prevent potatoes from turning brown or rice from sticking ■ Keep guacamole green ■ Make soggy lettuce crisp again ■ Freshen the fridge and chopping boards

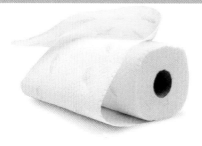

PAPER TOWELS page 227
■ Microwave bacon, clean corn, and strain stock ■ Keep vegetables crisp and vegetable crisper clean ■ Avoid soggy bread and rusty pots

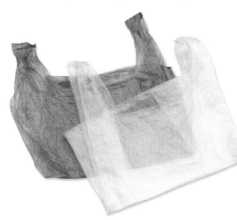

PLASTIC BAGS page 239
■ Cover a cookbook ■ Bag dirty hands to answer the phone ■ Make cookie crumbs ■ Use as a mixing bowl or salad spinner ■ Ripen fruit

RUBBER BANDS page 258
■ Keep spoons from sliding into bowls ■ Secure casserole lids for travel ■ Anchor a chopping board ■ Get a better grip on twist-off lids and glasses

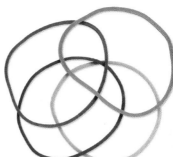

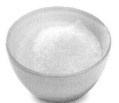

SALT page 263
■ Prevent grease from splattering ■ Speed up the cooking process ■ Shell hard-boiled eggs or pecans easier ■ Test eggs for freshness and poach eggs perfectly ■ Wash spinach more effectively ■ Keep salad crisp ■ Revive wrinkled apples and stop cut fruit from browning ■ Use to whip cream, beat eggs, and keep milk fresh ■ Prevent mold from forming on cheese

SANDWICH AND FREEZER BAGS page 274
■ Store grater with cheese ■ Make a pastry bag ■ Dispose of cooking oil ■ Color cookie dough ■ Keep ice cream from forming crystals ■ Soften marshmallows, melt chocolate, and keep soda from going flat ■ Grease cake pans

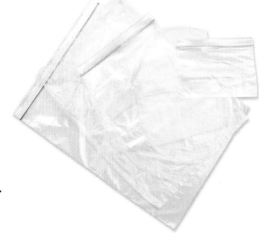

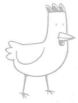

TIP

the secret to perfect poached eggs is vinegar ... page 338

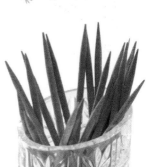

TOOTHPICKS page 320
■ Mark steaks for rare, medium, or well done ■ Retrieve garlic cloves from marinade ■ Prevent pots from boiling over ■ Microwave potatoes faster ■ Limit salad dressing ■ Make frying sausages easier

top 11

Most useful items for
HEALTH AND BEAUTY

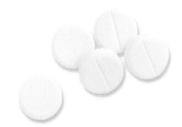

ASPIRIN page 53
■ Dry up pimples ■ Treat calluses ■ Control dandruff ■ Cut inflammation from bites and stings ■ Restore hair color after swimming in chlorinated water

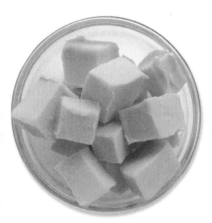

BABY OIL page 56
■ Remove a band-aid painlessly ■ Treat cradle cap ■ Make your own bath oil ■ Remove acrylic paint from skin without irritation

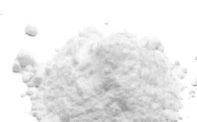

BAKING SODA page 60
■ Soothe minor burns, sunburn, poison ivy rash, bee stings, diaper rash, and other skin irritations ■ Combat cradle cap ■ Control dandruff ■ Use as a gargle or mouthwash ■ Scrub teeth and clean dentures ■ Alleviate itching in casts and athlete's foot ■ Soothe tired, stinky feet ■ Remove built-up hair gel, spray, or conditioner ■ Use as an antiperspirant

BUTTER page 91
■ Make pills easier to swallow ■ Soothe aching feet ■ Remove tree sap from skin ■ Smooth legs after shaving ■ Use as shaving cream ■ Moisturize dry hair

CHEST RUB page 110
■ Make calluses disappear ■ Soothe aching feet ■ Stop insect-bite itch ■ Treat toenail fungus ■ Repel ticks and biting insects

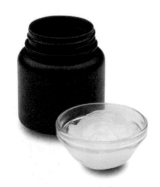

TIP 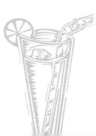 restore hair color with club soda ...
page 116

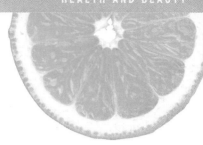

LEMONS page 179
■ Disinfect cuts and scrapes ■ Soothe poison ivy rash ■ Relieve rough hands and sore feet ■ Remove warts ■ Lighten age spots ■ Create blond highlights ■ Clean and whiten nails ■ Cleanse and exfoliate your face ■ Treat dandruff ■ Soften dry elbows

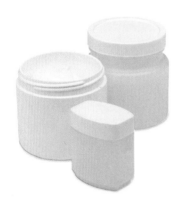

MAYONNAISE page 190
■ Relieve sunburn pain ■ Give yourself a facial ■ Condition hair ■ Remove dead skin cells ■ Strengthen fingernails

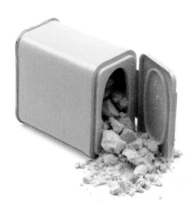

MUSTARD page 197
■ Soothe an aching back ■ Relax stiff muscles ■ Relieve congestion ■ Make a facial mask

PETROLEUM JELLY page 232
■ Heal windburn ■ Help prevent diaper rash ■ Protect baby's eyes from shampoo ■ Moisturize face and lips ■ Remove makeup ■ Create emergency makeup ■ Strengthen perfume ■ Soften hands ■ Do a professional manicure ■ Smooth wild eyebrow hairs ■ Stop hair-dye runs

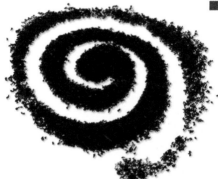

TEA page 311
■ Relieve tired eyes ■ Soothe bleeding gums ■ Cool sunburn ■ Relieve baby's pain from an injection ■ Reduce razor burn ■ Condition dry hair and get the gray out ■ Tan your skin ■ Drain a boil ■ Stop foot odor ■ Soothe mouth pain

VINEGAR page 329
■ Control dandruff and condition hair ■ Protect blond hair from chlorine ■ Apply as antiperspirant ■ Soak aching muscles ■ Freshen breath ■ Ease sunburn and itching ■ Banish bruises ■ Soothe sore throat ■ Clear congestion ■ Heal cold sores and athlete's foot ■ Pamper skin ■ Erase age or sun spots ■ Soften cuticles ■ Treat jellyfish or bee stings ■ Treat corns and calluses on feet

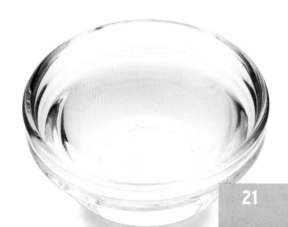

top 11

Most useful items for CLEANING

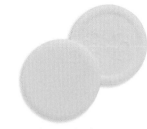

ALKA-SELTZER page 37
■ Clean residue off a narrow-necked vase ■ Unclog a drain
■ Clean your ovenproof glass cookware, coffeemaker, toilet
bowl, and gold and silver jewelry

AMMONIA page 48
■ Clean carpets, upholstery, ovens, fireplace doors,
windows, porcelain fixtures, crystal, jewelry, and
white shoes ■ Remove tarnish and stains ■ Fight
mildew ■ Strip floor wax

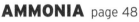

BAKING SODA page 60
■ Clean baby bottles, thermoses, chopping boards, appliances,
sponges and towels, coffeemakers, teapots, cookware, and fixtures
■ Clear clogged drains ■ Deodorize garbage cans ■ Boost dishwashing
liquid (or make your own) ■ Remove stains ■ Shine jewelry, stainless
steel, chrome, and marble ■ Wash wallpaper and remove crayon marks

BORAX page 85
■ Clear a clogged drain
■ Remove stains ■ Clean
windows and mirrors
■ Remove mildew from fabrics
■ Eliminate urine odor

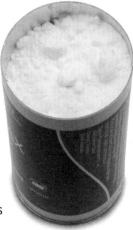

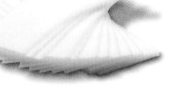

FABRIC SOFTENER SHEETS page 153
■ Lift burned-on food ■ Freshen drawers ■ Remove soap scum
■ Repel dust on TV and computer screens ■ Freshen laundry baskets
and wastebaskets ■ Buff chrome ■ Keep dust off blinds ■ Renew
grubby stuffed toys ■ Prevent musty odors in bags and suitcases

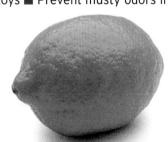

LEMONS page 179
■ Get rid of tough stains on marble ■ Polish
metals ■ Clean the microwave ■ Deodorize
chopping boards, fridge, and garbage cans

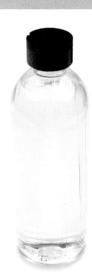

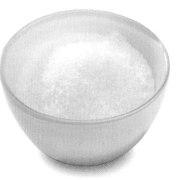

RUBBING ALCOHOL page 261
■ Clean bathroom fixtures, venetian blinds, windows, and phones ■ Remove hair spray from mirrors ■ Prevent ring around the collar ■ Remove ink stains

SALT page 263
■ Clean vases, discolored glass, flowerpots, artificial flowers, percolators, refrigerators, woks, and wicker ■ Make brooms last ■ Easy fireplace or flour clean-up ■ Make metal polish ■ Remove wine and grease from carpet, watermarks from wood, and lipstick from glasses ■ Restore a sponge ■ Remove baked-on food ■ Soak up oven spills ■ Remove stains from saucepans and clean cast iron

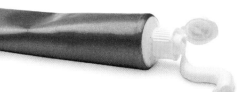

TOOTHPASTE page 318
■ Clean piano keys and sinks ■ Polish metal and jewelry ■ Deodorize baby bottles ■ Remove ink or lipstick from fabric, crayon from walls, and watermarks from furniture

VINEGAR page 329
■ Clean blinds, bricks, tiles, panelling, carpets, piano keys, computers, appliances, and chopping boards ■ Clean china, crystal, glassware, coffeemakers, cookware, and windows ■ Banish kitchen grease ■ Clean and deodorize drains ■ Polish metal ■ Erase ballpoint pen marks ■ Remove water rings and wax from furniture ■ Revitalize leather ■ Clean a variety of fixtures ■ Get rid of insects in the pantry

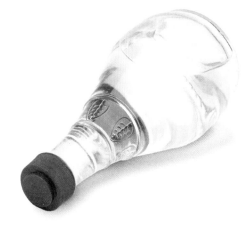

WD-40 page 358
■ Remove carpet stains and floor scuffs ■ Remove tea and tomato stains ■ Clean toilet bowls ■ Condition leather furniture ■ Clean a chalkboard ■ Remove felt pen and crayon from walls

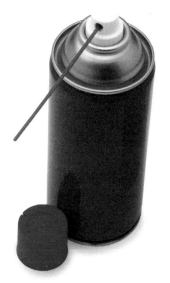

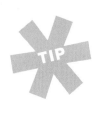

TIP clean fireplace doors with ash ... page 52

top **11**

Most useful items for
THE GARDEN

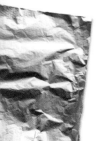

ALUMINIUM FOIL page 40

■ Create a window box for plants or an incubator for seedlings ■ Mix with mulch to deter insects ■ Hang strips to scare crows and other birds ■ Wrap tree trunks to prevent sunscald or to keep deer and rabbits away ■ Prevent cuttings from getting tangled

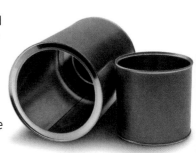

COFFEE CANS page 119

■ Make a sprinkler to spread seeds and fertilizer ■ Measure rain to ensure your garden is getting enough water ■ Make a bird feeder ■ Collect food scraps for compost

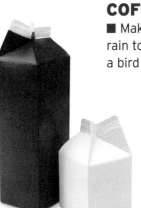

MILK CARTONS page 193

■ Make a bird feeder ■ Use as a seed starter ■ Make a collar to protect vegetables ■ Collect food scraps for compost

NEWSPAPER page 204

■ Protect and ripen end-of-season tomatoes ■ Use as mulch or add to compost to remove odor ■ Block weeds in flower and vegetable beds ■ Get rid of earwigs

PANTYHOSE page 216

■ Stake delicate plants ■ Fill with hair clippings to repel deer ■ Make a hammock for growing melons ■ Store onions and off-season bulbs ■ Prevent soil loss in houseplants ■ Fill with soap scraps for cleaning hands at a garden faucet

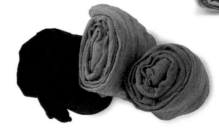

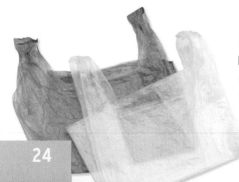

PLASTIC BAGS page 239

■ Protect plants from frost and shoes from mud ■ Speed budding of poinsettias ■ Keep insects off fruit ripening on trees ■ Store outdoor equipment manuals ■ Clean a barbecue easily

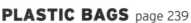

PLASTIC BOTTLES page 246

■ Make a bird feeder, an all-purpose scoop, a watering can, or an individual drip irrigator for a plant ■ Secure netting over flower beds ■ Isolate weeds when spraying ■ Cover seed-packet markers or make plant tags from cut strips ■ Use as a garbage can when you mow the lawn ■ Use to space seeds ■ Trap insects

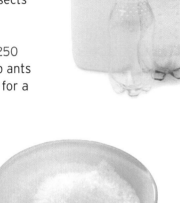

PLASTIC CONTAINERS page 250

■ Make traps for slugs and wasps ■ Stop ants from crawling up picnic table legs ■ Use for a dog's outdoor water bowl

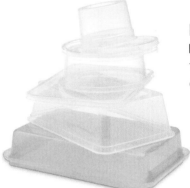

SALT page 263

■ Kill snails and slugs ■ Inhibit the growth of weeds in walkway cracks ■ Extend the life of cut flowers ■ Clean flowerpots

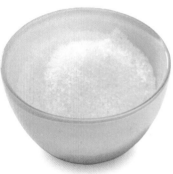

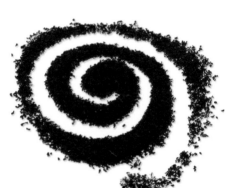

TEA page 311

■ Spur growth of rosebushes ■ Water acid-loving plants ■ Nourish houseplants ■ Prepare a planter for potting ■ Speed the decomposition of compost

WD-40 page 358

■ Keep animals out of flower beds and squirrels off bird feeders ■ Keep tool handles from splintering ■ Stop snow from sticking on a shovel ■ Prevent wasps from building nests and repel pigeons ■ Kill thistle plants ■ Protect a bird feeder

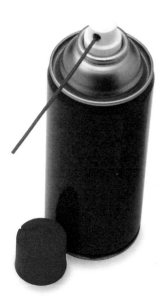

TIP keep aphids off rosebushes with banana peels ... page 75

top **11** Most useful items for **OUTDOORS**

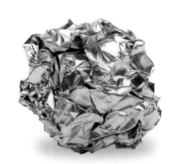

ALUMINIUM FOIL page 40
■ Improve outdoor lighting ■ Keep bees away from beverages
■ Make an impromptu picnic platter or improvise a frying pan
■ Make a drip pan for a barbecue and clean the grill ■ Warm your
toes when camping and keep a sleeping bag and matches dry

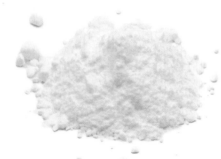

BAKING SODA page 60
■ Keep weeds out of concrete cracks ■ Clean resin garden furniture
■ Feed flowering plants ■ Maintain proper pool alkalinity ■ Scour
a barbecue grate to remove food residue

BUBBLE WRAP page 88
■ Keep soft drinks cold ■ Sleep on air while
camping ■ Cushion seats and benches

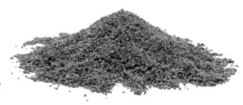

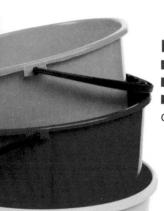

BUCKETS page 90
■ Boil lobster over a campfire
■ Use as a food-storage bin
■ Build a camp washing machine
or make a camp shower

CAT LITTER page 106
■ Give your car traction on ice ■ Prevent
barbecue grease fires ■ Keep tents and
sleeping bags free of musty odors
■ Remove grease spots from the driveway

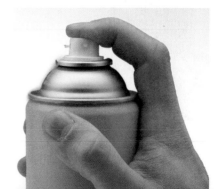

COOKING SPRAY page 128
■ Prevent grass from sticking to your
mower ■ Spray on fishing line for quicker
casting ■ Prevent snow from sticking to
your shovel ■ Lubricate a bicycle chain

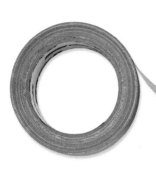

DUCT AND ELECTRICAL TAPE
pages 139 and 147, respectively

■ Make bike streamers ■ Seal out ticks ■ Create a clothesline ■ Stash a secret car key ■ Patch a canoe or a pool ■ Repair outdoor cushions and patio-chair webbing ■ Tighten hockey shin guards and revive a hockey stick ■ Preserve skateboarders' shoes ■ Repair ski gloves or a tent ■ Waterproof footwear

PLASTIC BOTTLES page 246
■ Make a scoop or bailer for a boat ■ Make a bottle into a weight for anchoring or lifting ■ Make a bird feeder ■ Fill a bottle with sand or cat litter for winter traction ■ Keep a picnic cooler cold

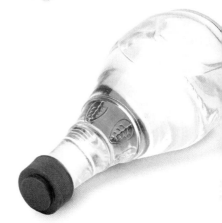

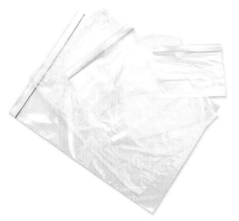

SANDWICH AND FREEZER BAGS page 274
■ Inflate to make valuables float when boating ■ Store hand cleaner for the beach ■ Use as a portable water dish ■ Apply insect repellent with ease

VINEGAR page 329
■ Keep water fresh ■ Clean outdoor furniture and decks ■ Repel insects ■ Trap flying insects ■ Get rid of ants ■ Clean off bird droppings

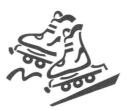

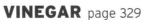

WD-40 page 358
■ Repel pigeons and wasps ■ Waterproof boots and shoes ■ Remove wax from skis and snowboards ■ Remove barnacles from a boat and protect it from corrosion ■ Untangle a fishing line and lure fish ■ Clean and protect golf clubs ■ Remove burrs from a horse's mane and protect hooves in winter ■ Keep flies off cows

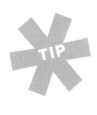

TIP lubricate skate wheels with hair conditioner ... page 165

top **12** **Most useful items for**
STORAGE

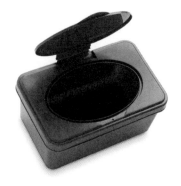

BABY WIPES CONTAINERS page 59

■ Organize sewing supplies, recipe cards, coupons, craft and office supplies, small tools, photos, receipts, bills, and more ■ Store plastic shopping bags
■ Store towels and rags

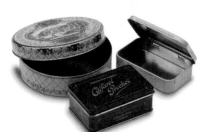

CANDY TINS page 95

■ Make an emergency sewing kit ■ Store broken jewelry
■ Make a birthday keepsake ■ Prevent jewelry-chain tangles ■ Store car fuses ■ Keep earrings together
■ Store workshop accessories

CANS page 95

■ Compartmentalize your tool pouch with juice cans ■ Make a desk organizer ■ Create pigeonholes to store silverware, nails, office supplies, and other odds and ends

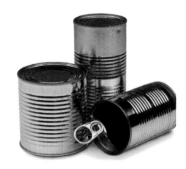

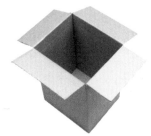

CARDBOARD BOXES page 97

■ Make magazine holders from detergent boxes ■ Make a home office in-a-box
■ Store hoes, rakes, and other long-handled garden tools and kids' sporting equipment ■ Protect glassware or lightbulbs ■ Store posters and artwork
■ Store Christmas decorations ■ Organize dowels, moldings, weather stripping, and metal rods

CARDBOARD TUBES page 100

■ Store knitting needles, fabric scraps, and string
■ Keep Christmas lights tidy ■ Preserve kids' artwork, important documents, and posters ■ Keep linens and pants crease-free and electrical cords tangle-free ■ Protect fluorescent light tubes

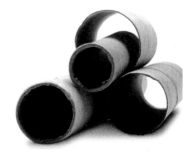

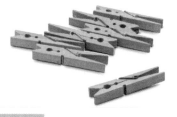

CLOTHESPINS page 113

■ Keep snacks fresh ■ Organize workshop, kitchen, bathroom, and wardrobes ■ Keep gloves together

COFFEE CANS page 119
■ Make a kids' piggy bank ■ Collect kitchen scraps ■ Carry toilet paper when camping ■ Store screws, nuts, and nails ■ Organize and store belts ■ Collect stuff from clothes' pockets before laundering

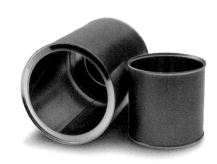

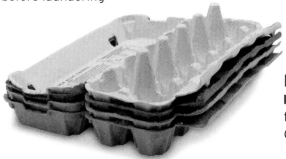

EGG CARTONS page 146
■ Store and sort coins ■ Organize buttons, safety pins, threads, bobbins and fasteners ■ Store golf balls or Christmas ornaments

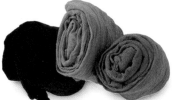

PANTYHOSE page 216
■ Store wrapping paper ■ Bundle blankets ■ Store onions or flower bulbs

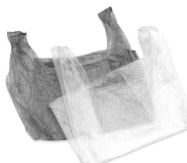

PLASTIC BAGS page 239
■ Store extra baby wipes ■ Collect used clothes ■ Protect clothes ■ Store skirts ■ Keep stored purses in shape

PLASTIC BOTTLES page 246
■ Store sugar ■ Store and organize small workshop items ■ Use as a boot tree ■ Make a bag or string dispenser

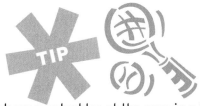

SANDWICH AND FREEZER BAGS page 274
■ Protect fragile breakables ■ Store seasonal sweaters ■ Add cedar to a closet ■ Make a pencil bag ■ De-clutter the bathroom

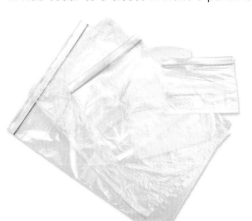

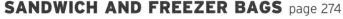

TIP

stash your valuables at the gym in a tennis ball ...
page 314

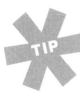

top **15** Most useful items for KIDS

TIP make finger paints from yogurt ... page 368

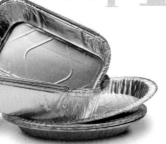

ALUMINIUM FOIL PANS page 46
■ Use as molds for ice ornaments ■ Minimize glitter mess and make trays for craft supplies

BAKING SODA page 60
■ Make watercolor paints or invisible ink ■ Produce gas to blow up a balloon ■ Clean crayon marks from walls and baby vomit from clothing ■ Combat cradle cap and diaper rash ■ Wash chemicals out of new baby clothes

BATHTUB APPLIQUÉS page 78
■ Stick to bottom of kiddy pool ■ Affix to toddler training cups and high-chair seats

CARDBOARD BOXES page 97
■ Make a medieval castle, a puppet theater or a sundial ■ Make a garage for toy vehicles ■ Store tennis racquets, baseball bats, fishing rods, and other sporting goods ■ Use as an impromptu sled ■ Make a liquor-box skee-ball game

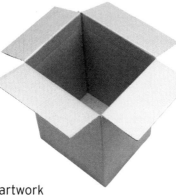

CARDBOARD TUBES page 100
■ Make a kazoo or a megaphone ■ Preserve kids' artwork ■ Build a toy log cabin ■ Make Christmas bonbons

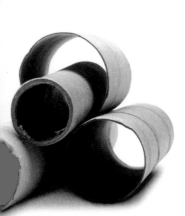

COMPACT DISCS page 126
■ Make a fun picture frame ■ Make wall art for a teenager's room ■ Create spinning tops ■ Use as Christmas ornaments

CORKS page 130
■ Use burnt cork as Halloween face paint ■ Create craft stamps ■ Make a cool bead curtain for a kid's room

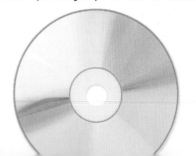

DUCT AND ELECTRICAL TAPE
pages 139 and 147, respectively
■ Make Halloween or dress-up costumes, a toy sword, or hand puppets ■ Create bicycle streamers

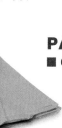

JARS page 175
■ Make a piggy bank ■ Dry kids' mittens ■ Bring along baby treats and store baby food portions ■ Collect insects ■ Create a miniature biosphere

MARGARINE TUBS page 187
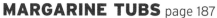
■ Make a baby footprint paperweight ■ Divide ice cream into individual portions ■ Bring ready-made food for baby ■ Make a piggy bank ■ Give kids some lunchbox variety

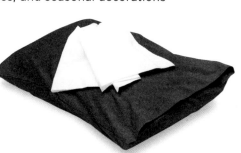

PAPER BAGS page 221
■ Cover textbooks ■ Make a kite ■ Create a life-sized body poster

PAPER PLATES page 226
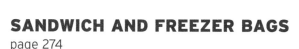
■ Make prompt cards and Frisbee flash cards ■ Make masks, mobiles, and seasonal decorations

PILLOWCASES page 236
■ Prepare travel pillows for kids ■ Make wall hangings for kids' rooms ■ Clean stuffed animals

SANDWICH AND FREEZER BAGS
page 274
■ Display baby teeth ■ Make cheap baby wipes ■ Dye pasta for crafts ■ Make kids' kitchen gloves ■ Make a pencil bag ■ Keep spare kids' clothes in the car for mishaps ■ Cure car sickness ■ Play football while making pudding

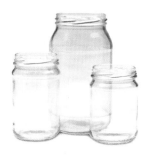

TAPE page 307
■ Secure a baby's bib ■ Create childproofing in a pinch ■ Make multicolored pen designs ■ Make an unpoppable balloon

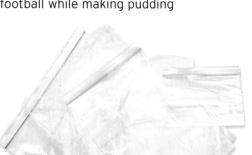

top 13 Most useful items for QUICK REPAIRS

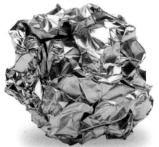

ALUMINIUM FOIL page 40

■ Make a flexible funnel for hard-to-reach places ■ Reflect light for photography ■ Reattach vinyl floor ■ Make an artist's palette ■ Prevent paint from skinning over ■ Line roller pans and keep paint off doorknobs ■ Keep a paintbrush wet

BAKING SODA page 60

■ Clean car-battery terminals and remove tar from car ■ Use as a footpath de-icer ■ Tighten cane chair seats ■ Give decks a weathered look ■ Clean air conditioner filters ■ Keep a humidifier odor-free

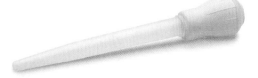

BASTERS page 75

■ Cure a musty air conditioner ■ Transfer paints and solvents ■ Fix a leaky refrigerator

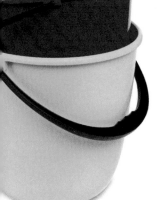

BUCKETS page 90

■ Hold paint and supplies when painting on a ladder and use lids to contain paint drips ■ Organize extension cords ■ Soak a saw to clean it ■ Use as a Christmas tree stand

TIP repair your leaky garden hose with a toothpick ... page 322

CARDBOARD BOXES page 97

■ Make a temporary roof repair ■ Protect fingers while hammering small nails ■ Make an oil drip pan ■ Identify fluid leaking from your car ■ Make a bed tray ■ Make an in-box ■ Organize your workshop ■ Keep upholstery tacks straight

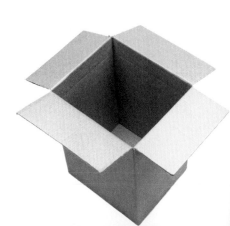

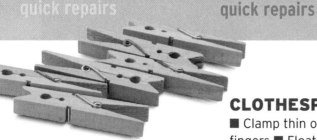

CLOTHESPINS page 113
■ Clamp thin objects ■ Make a clipboard ■ Grip a nail to protect fingers ■ Float paintbrushes in solvent

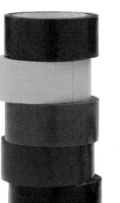

DUCT TAPE page 139
■ Repair siding ■ Make a temporary roof shingle
■ Create a clothesline
■ Stash a secret car key ■ Patch a canoe
■ Repair a garbage can

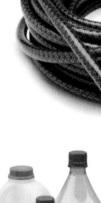

ELECTRICAL TAPE page 147
■ Temporarily fix a car taillight ■ Remove broken window glass safely ■ Hang glue and caulk tubes for storage ■ Repair outdoor cushions

GARDEN HOSE page 162
■ Protect handsaw and ice skate blades
■ Make a rounded sanding block ■ Make a paint-can grip

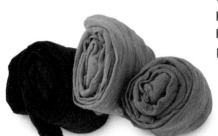

PANTYHOSE page 216
■ Test a sanding job ■ Apply stain in tight corners ■ Patch holes in screens
■ Strain paint

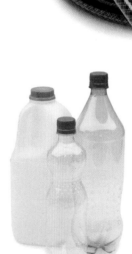

PLASTIC BAGS page 239
■ Protect a ceiling fan when painting a ceiling
■ Store paintbrushes ■ Contain paint overspray

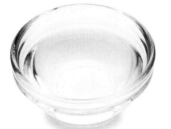

PLASTIC BOTTLES page 246
■ Make a neater paint bucket ■ Store paints ■ Make a workshop organizer
■ Use as a level ■ Make an anchor for weighting tarps and patio umbrellas

VINEGAR page 329
■ Wash concrete off skin ■ Remove paint fumes ■ Degrease grates, fans, and air conditioner grilles ■ Disinfect filters ■ Help paint adhere to concrete ■ Remove rust from tools ■ Peel off wallpaper
■ Slow plaster hardening ■ Revive hardened paintbrushes

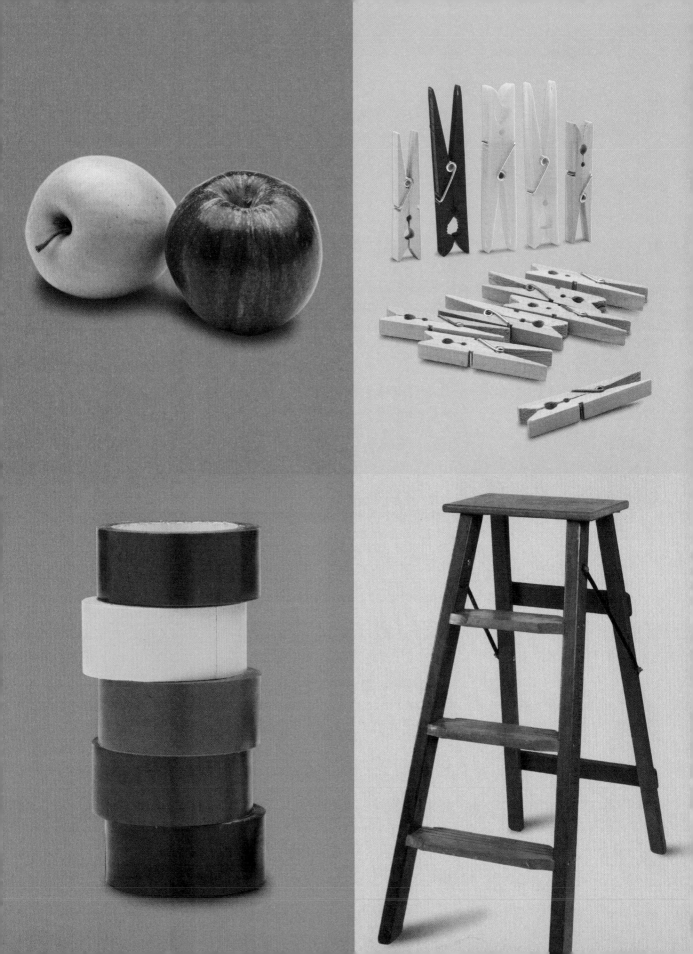

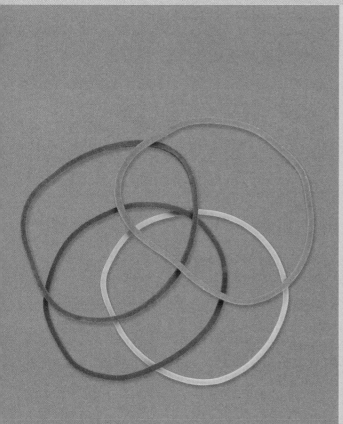
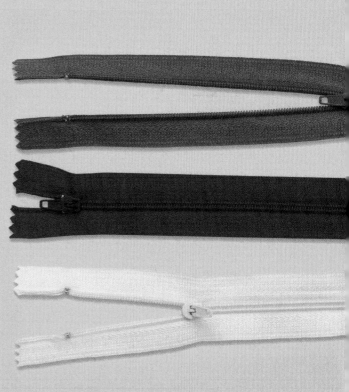

ADDRESS LABELS

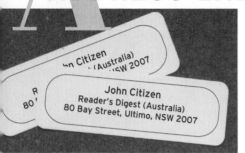

TAG YOUR BAGS • Address labels aren't only for sticking on envelopes. They can be an effective, inexpensive way of making sure your lost items stand a chance of finding their way home. Place an address label—covered with a small piece of sticky tape or clear packing tape to prevent wear—inside your laptop or iPad case, designer eyeglass case, gym bag, backpack, and all pieces of luggage—whether they are tagged or not.

LABEL YOUR STUFF • Few people bother to take out insurance on their collection of personal electronics equipment, but replacing an iPhone, digital camera, or MP3 player can run into some serious money. Still, a tape-covered address label conspicuously placed on your gear just may facilitate its safe return. Of course, there are no guarantees, but it's cheap enough.

SECURE SCHOOL SUPPLIES • It's one of the universal truths of parenthood—kids' pencil cases, folders, felt-tip pens, and other school supplies are forever disappearing. You may be able to lessen the losses, however, by affixing address labels with a piece of transparent tape to the contents of your child's desk and backpack.

HANG ON TO YOUR UMBRELLA •

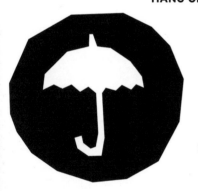

A well-made umbrella can last for years, but that won't help if you lose it. Minimize the risk of your loss becoming someone else's gain by sticking an address label on the umbrella handle, then covering it with clear packing tape. This protects the label from the elements, and makes it more difficult to remove.

TAG ITEMS OUT FOR REPAIRS

Do you suffer from separation anxiety when you take your laptop or stereo equipment to the repair store? You may feel better if you tag those valuables with an address label placed somewhere on the base or another unobtrusive, undamaged area. This practice is not recommended for all personal treasures—you probably wouldn't want to label things like documents, paintings, and photos.

ADHESIVE TAPE

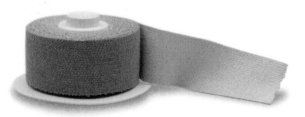

REMOVE A SPLINTER • Is a splinter too tiny or too deep to remove with tweezers? Avoid the agony of digging it out with a needle. Instead, cover the splinter with adhesive tape. After about three days, pull the tape off slowly, and the splinter should come out with it.

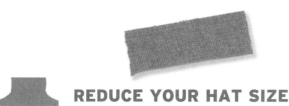

REDUCE YOUR HAT SIZE

Got a hat that's a bit too big for your head? Wrap adhesive tape around the sweatband—it might take two or three layers depending on the size discrepancy. As a bonus, the adhesive tape will absorb brow sweat on hot days.

GET A GRIP ON TOOLS • Adhesive tape has just the right texture for wrapping tool handles. It gives you a positive, comfortable grip, and it's highly absorbent so tools won't become slippery if your hand sweats. When you wrap tool handles, overlap each wrap of adhesive tape by half a tape width and use as many layers as needed to get the best grip. Here are some useful applications:

■ Screwdriver handles are sometimes too narrow and slippery to grip well when you drive or remove stubborn screws. Wrap layers of adhesive tape around the handle until it feels comfortable in your hand— useful if you have arthritis in your fingers.

■ Take a tip from carpenters who wrap wooden hammer handles that can get slippery with sweat. Wrap the whole gripping area of the tool. A few wraps just under the head will also protect the handle from damage caused by misdirected blows.

■ Plumbers also keep adhesive tape in their tool kits. When they want to cut a pipe in a spot that's too tight for their hacksaw frame, they make a mini-hacksaw by removing the blade and wrapping tape on one end to form a handle.

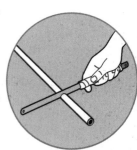

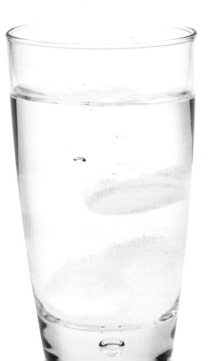

ALKA-SELTZER

CLEAN JEWELRY • Drop your dull-looking jewelry into a glass of fizzing Alka-Seltzer for a couple of minutes. It will sparkle and shine when you take it out.

CLEAN YOUR COFFEEMAKER • Fill the water reservoir of your drip coffeemaker with water and drop in four Alka-Seltzer tablets. When the tablets dissolve, run a brew cycle to clean the tubes. Rinse the chamber out thoroughly, and run a brew cycle again with plain water.

CLEAN A VASE • That residue at the bottom of narrow-necked vases is easy to clean if you bubble it away. Fill half the vase with water and add two Alka-Seltzer tablets. When the fizzing stops, rinse the vase clean.

more ALKA-SELTZER over →

CLEAN GLASS COOKWARE • Say goodbye to scouring those stubborn stains on ovenproof glass cookware. Just fill the container with water and add up to six Alka-Seltzer tablets. Let it soak for an hour and the stains should easily scrub away.

CLEAN YOUR TOILET • The citric acid in Alka-Seltzer when combined with its fizzing action makes an effective toilet bowl cleaner. Just drop a couple of tablets into the bowl and find something else to do for 20 minutes or so. When you return, a few swipes with a toilet brush will make your bowl gleam.

MAKE A LAVA LAMP

In a clear plastic bottle, add water until about one-quarter full. Pour in vegetable oil to the halfway mark and wait for the oil and water to separate. Add ten or twelve drops of food coloring which will fall through the oil and into the water. Cut an Alka-Seltzer tablet into four or five pieces and drop them in. When the fizzing starts, colorful bubbles will start floating around inside the bottle. Take your "lamp" into a dark room and shine a flashlight up through the bottom and watch it light up!

UNCLOG A DRAIN • Drain clogged again? Get almost instant relief by dropping a couple of Alka-Seltzer tablets down the opening, then pouring in a cup of vinegar. Wait a few minutes and run the hot water at full force to clear the clog. This is also a good way to get rid of kitchen drain odors.

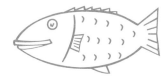

ATTRACT FISH • Anglers know fish are attracted to bubbles. If you use a hollow plastic tube jig on your line, break off a piece of Alka-Seltzer and slip it into the tube. The jig will produce a stream of bubbles as it sinks.

WHITEN CLOTHES • To get rid of yellow stains in white cotton clothes, fill a sink with a gallon of warm water and drop in two Alka-Seltzer tablets. When the water is fizzing, toss in your dirty whites, and let them soak for 20 or 30 minutes. Most stains will just disappear, but a little scrubbing will handle the tough ones. Hang dry (in the sun, if possible) and admire your bright whites.

SOOTHE INSECT BITES • Are mosquito or other insect bites driving you crazy? To ease the itch, drop two Alka-Seltzer tablets into half a glass of water. Dip a cotton ball in the glass and apply the solution to the bite. **CAUTION:** Do NOT do this if you are allergic to aspirin, which is a key ingredient in Alka-Seltzer.

SCIENCE WORKS!

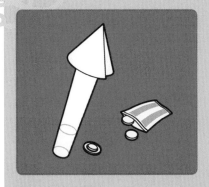

Turn 'plop, plop, fizz, fizz' into 'whoosh, whoosh, gee whiz' with this Alka-Seltzer rocket.

The rocket gets its thrust from the gas created when you drop a couple of Alka-Seltzer tablets into some water inside an empty film canister.

The type of film canister you use is important. A 35-mm plastic canister that has a lid that fits inside the canister is what you need. Canisters with lids that fit around an outside lip won't work. You'll also need a couple of pieces of thick paper, sticky tape, and a pair of scissors.

To form the body of the rocket, wrap a piece of thick paper around the canister with the canister's open end facing out the bottom end of the tube. Then tape the paper in place. Form a quarter-sheet of thick paper into a nose cone and trim it evenly on the bottom. Tape it onto the top of the rocket's body.

To launch the rocket, fill the canister about halfway with refrigerated water—cold water is vital to a successful lift-off. Drop in 2 Alka-Seltzer tablets, quickly pop on the lid, put the rocket on the ground, and stand back. The gas will quickly build up pressure in the canister, causing the canister lid to pop off and the rocket to launch a few feet into the air.

ALUMINIUM CANS

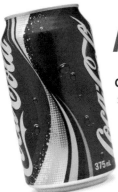

CREATE A DECORATIVE SNOWMAN • Wrap an old soda drink can with white paper and tape with transparent tape. For a head, use a polystyrene foam ball and tape it to the top of the can. Cover the body with cotton batting or cotton bandaging material and tape or glue it into place. Make a cone-shaped paper hat. Make eyes and a nose with buttons. To add arms, punch holes into the sides of the can and insert twigs. Use dots from a black marker pen to make buttons down the snowman's front and make a scarf from a scrap of wooly fabric.

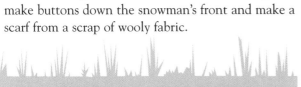

FOR THOSE WITH GREEN FINGERS ...

MAKE PLANTERS MORE PORTABLE • Don't strain your back moving a planter loaded with heavy soil. Reduce the amount of soil and lighten the load by first filling one-third to one-half of the bottom of the planter with empty, upside-down aluminium cans. Finish filling with soil and add your plants. In addition to making the planter lighter, the rustproof aluminium cans also help it to drain well.

PROTECT YOUNG PLANTS • Remove both ends of an aluminium can, then push it into the earth to serve as a collar to protect young garden plants from cutworms. You can also use a soup can or a coffee can, depending on the size you need. Remove any paper labels.

KEEP TRACK OF BULBS AND SEEDLINGS • After removing the top and bottom of a can, cut plant labels from the remaining aluminium sheet. Write on them with an old ballpoint pen and attach them to plant stakes or pots to identify the type and color of your plants, such as dahlias, orchids, bulbs, and newly-sown vegetable seeds.

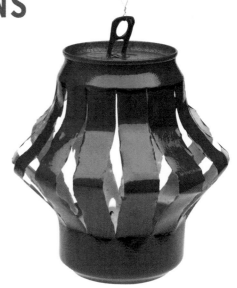

CREATE A SIMPLE CHINESE LANTERN

1 Mark two lines around a clean, empty can, about 1 inch (2.5 cm) from the top and bottom. With a sharp craft knife, make vertical cuts between the lines, about 1/2 inch (1.25 cm) apart.

2 Make a cut across the bottom of two adjacent strips to make an opening for a candle.

3 Gently press down on the can to make the strips bend in the middle. Insert a tea light through the opening, then tuck the cut ends of the opening strips inside the can.

4 Attach a hanging loop. You can also spray paint the can before cutting, if you like.

MAKE REPOUSSÉ CHRISTMAS DECORATIONS • Use a craft knife or old scissors to cut the top and bottom from empty cans, then slit the cylinder to create a flat piece. Cut simple shapes, such as stars or circles, and use a ballpoint pen to draw designs on the wrong side. Decorate with stick-on jewels or transparent glass paint, if desired, and add a wire for hanging.

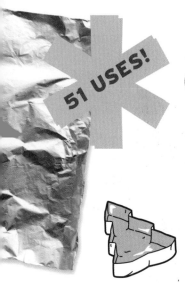

51 USES!

ALUMINIUM FOIL

in the kitchen

BAKE A PERFECT PIECRUST • To keep the edges of your homemade pies from burning, all you have to do is cover them with strips of aluminium foil. The foil prevents the edges from getting overdone while the rest of your pie gets perfectly browned.

CREATE CUSTOM-SHAPED CAKE PANS • You can make a teddy bear birthday cake, a Valentine's Day heart cake, a Christmas tree cake or whatever shaped cake the occasion may call for. All you have to do is form a double thickness of heavy-duty aluminium foil into the shape you want, then sit the cake pan inside a larger cake pan.

SOFTEN BROWN SUGAR • To restore your hardened brown sugar to its former powdery glory, chip off a piece, wrap it in aluminium foil and bake it in the oven at 300°F (150°C) for 5 minutes.

DECORATE A CAKE • No pastry bag handy? Just form a piece of heavy-duty aluminium foil into a tube shape and fill it with cake frosting. The real bonus is that there's no pastry bag to clean—simply toss out the foil when you're done.

MAKE AN EXTRA-LARGE SALAD BOWL • If you've invited a large group of friends over for dinner, but don't have a bowl big enough to toss that much salad, don't panic. Just line the kitchen sink with aluminium foil and toss away!

KEEP ROLLS AND BREADS WARM • Want to lock in the oven-fresh warmth of your homemade rolls or breads for a dinner party or picnic? Before you load up your basket, wrap the freshly baked goods in a napkin and place a layer of aluminium foil underneath. The foil will reflect the heat and keep your bread warm for quite some time.

SILVERWARE CARE

POLISH YOUR SILVER • If your silverware is looking a bit dull, try cleaning it using an ion exchange—a molecular reaction in which aluminium acts as a catalyst. Simply line a dish with a sheet of aluminium foil, fill it with cold water and add 2 teaspoons (10 ml) salt. Drop your tarnished silverware into the solution, let it sit for 2 to 3 minutes, then rinse off and dry.

KEEP SILVERWARE UNTARNISHED • Store freshly cleaned silverware on top of a sheet of aluminium foil to deter tarnishing. For long-term storage of silverware, first tightly cover each piece in plastic wrap—make sure you squeeze out as much air as possible—then wrap the bundle in aluminium foil and seal the ends.

CATCH ICE CREAM CONE DRIPS • Keep children from making a mess of their clothes or your house by wrapping the bottom of an ice cream cone (or a wedge of watermelon) with a piece of aluminium foil before handing it to them.

Foil-eating acidic foods

Think twice before ripping off a sheet of aluminium foil to wrap up your leftover meat loaf—particularly one that's dripping with a tomato-based sauce.

Highly acidic or salty foods such as lemons, grapefruit, tomato sauce, and pickles accelerate the oxidation of aluminium and can actually 'eat' through foil with prolonged exposure. This can also leach aluminium into the food, which can affect its flavor and may pose a health risk. If you want to use foil for that meat loaf, however, cover it first with a layer or two of plastic wrap or waxed paper to prevent the sauce from coming into contact with the foil.

KEEP THE OVEN CLEAN • When you're baking a bubbly lasagna or casserole, keep messy drips off the bottom of the oven by laying a sheet of aluminium foil over the rack below. However, do not line the bottom of the oven with foil, as it could cause a fire.

TOAST YOUR OWN CHEESE SANDWICH • Next time you're packing for a trip, include a couple of cheese sandwiches wrapped in aluminium foil. That way, if you book into a hotel after the kitchen has closed, you won't have to resort to the cold, overpriced snacks in the mini-bar. Instead, use the hotel room iron to press both sides of the wrapped sandwich and you'll have an instant, tasty, hot snack.

PRESERVE STEEL WOOL PADS • It's maddening. You use a steel wool pad once, put it in a dish by the sink and the next day you find a rusty mess fit only for the garbage can. To prevent rust and to get your money's worth from a pad, wrap it in foil and put it into the freezer. You can also lengthen the life of your steel wool soap pads by crumpling up a sheet of aluminium foil and placing it under the steel wool in its dish or container. (Don't forget to periodically drain off the water that collects at the bottom.)

SCRUB YOUR POTS • If you don't have a scrubbing pad handy at cleanup time, just crumple up a handful of aluminium foil and use it to scrub your pots.

around the house

IMPROVE RADIATOR EFFICIENCY • Here's a simple way to get more heat out of old cast-iron radiators without spending more money on your heating bill: Make a heat reflector to put behind them. Tape some heavy-duty aluminium foil to cardboard with the shiny side of the foil facing out. The radiant heat waves will bounce off the foil into the room instead of being absorbed by the wall behind the radiator. If your radiators have covers, it also helps to attach a piece of foil under the cover's top.

PROTECT A CHILD'S MATTRESS • As any parent of a toilet-trained small child knows, accidents happen. When they happen in bed, however, you can spare the mattress—even if you don't have a plastic protector available. Firstly, lay several sheets of aluminium foil across the width of the mattress. Then, cover them with a good-sized beach towel. Finally, attach the mattress pad and bottom sheet.

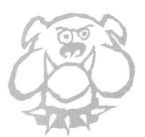

KEEP PETS OFF FURNITURE • Can't keep your pampered pet off your brand new couch? Place a piece of aluminium foil on the seat cushions, and after one try at settling down on the noisy surface, your pet will no longer consider it a comfy place to snooze.

more ALUMINIUM FOIL over →

aluminium foil aluminium foil
aluminium foil aluminium foil
aluminium foil
ALUMINIUM

Kids' Stuff

Mixing finger paints is a great way for kids to learn firsthand how colors combine while also expressing their creativity. Unfortunately, their early learning experiences can quickly turn into your worst nightmare.

To contain the mess, cut down the sides of a wide cardboard box so that they are about 3 inches (8 cm) high. Line the inside of the box with aluminium foil and let the kids pour in the paint. With any luck, the paint should stay within the confines of the box, keeping splatters off walls and the floor.

SHARPEN YOUR SCISSORS • What can you do with those clean pieces of leftover foil you have hanging around? Use them to sharpen up your dull scissors! Smooth them out if necessary, and then fold the strips into several layers and start cutting. Seven or eight passes should do the trick. Pretty simple, huh? (*See page 43 to find out how you can use the resulting scraps of aluminium foil for mulching or keeping birds off your fruit trees.*)

CLEAN JEWELRY • To clean your jewelry, simply line a small bowl with aluminium foil. Fill the bowl with hot water and mix in 1 tablespoon (15 ml) bleach-free powdered laundry detergent (not liquid). Put the jewelry into the solution and let it soak for a minute. Rinse well and air dry. This procedure makes use of the chemical process known as ion exchange, which can also be used to clean silverware (*see also page 40*).

MOVE FURNITURE WITH EASE • To slide big pieces of furniture over a smooth floor, place small pieces of aluminium foil under the legs of the furniture. Have the dull side of the foil facing downwards, as the dull side is actually more slippery than the shiny side.

FIX LOOSE BATTERIES • Is your flashlight, game console, or your kid's toy working intermittently? Check the battery compartment. Those springs that hold the batteries in place can lose their tension after a while, letting the batteries loosen. Fold a small piece of aluminium foil until you have a pad that's thick enough to take up the slack. Place the pad between the battery and the spring.

DON'T DYE YOUR GLASSES

You want to catch up on your reading during the time it takes to color your hair, but you can't read without your specs, and if you put them on, hair dye can stain them. What can you do? Simply wrap the arms of your glasses with aluminium foil to protect them from the dye.

CLEAN OUT YOUR FIREPLACE • An easy way to clean the ash out of your fireplace is to place a double layer of heavy-duty aluminium foil across the bottom of the fireplace or under the wood grate. The next day—or once you're sure all the ashes have cooled—simply fold it up and throw it away. (*See pages 52–53 to find out how you can use the ash.*)

DID YOU KNOW?

Have you ever wondered why aluminium foil has one side that's shinier than the other? The answer has to do with how it's manufactured. According to Alcoa (one of a number of manufacturers of aluminium foil), the different shades of silver result during the final rolling process, when two layers of foil pass through the rolling mill simultaneously. The sides that contact the mill's heavy, polished rollers come out shiny, while the inside layers retain a dull, or matte, finish. Of course, the shiny side is better for reflecting light and heat, but when it comes to wrapping foods or lining grills, both sides are equally good.

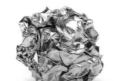

in the laundry

SPEED YOUR IRONING • When you iron clothing, a lot of the iron's heat is sucked up by the board itself—requiring you to make several passes with the iron to remove wrinkles. To speed things up, put a piece of aluminium foil under your ironing board cover. The foil will reflect the heat back through the clothing, smoothing the wrinkles more quickly.

ATTACH A PATCH • An iron-on patch is an easy way to fix small holes in clothing—but only if it doesn't get stuck on your ironing board. To avoid this happening, put a piece of aluminium foil under the hole. It won't stick to the patch, and you can just slip it out when you're finished.

CLEAN YOUR IRON • Is starch building up on your clothes iron and causing it to stick? To get rid of it, run your hot iron over a piece of aluminium foil.

in the garden

PUT SOME BITE IN YOUR MULCH • To keep hungry insects and slugs away from your cucumbers and other vegetables, mix strips of aluminium foil in with your garden mulch. As a bonus benefit, the foil will reflect light back up onto your plants.

PROTECT TREE TRUNKS • Deer, rabbits and other animals often feed on the bark of young trees during winter. A cheap and effective deterrent is to wrap the tree trunks with a double layer of heavy-duty aluminium foil in late autumn. But make sure you remove the foil in spring.

SCARE CROWS AND OTHER BIRDS • Are the birds eating the fruit on your trees? To trick them, dangle strips of aluminium foil from the branches using monofilament fishing line. Even better, hang some foil-wrapped seashells, which will add a bit of noise to further startle those fine-feathered thieves.

Prevent sunscald on trees   TIP

If you live in a cold climate, wrapping young tree trunks with a couple of layers of aluminium foil during the winter can help prevent sunscald, which is a condition of some young thin-barked trees—especially fruit trees, ashes, maples, oaks, and also willow trees.

The problem occurs on warm winter days when the sun's rays reactivate some dormant cells underneath the tree's bark. The subsequent drop in nighttime temperatures kills the cells and can injure the tree. You can remove the aluminium wrapping in early spring when the danger's passed.

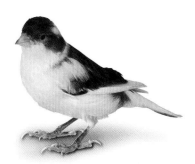

CREATE A WINDOW BOX FOR PLANTS • A sunny window is a great place to keep plants that love a lot of light. However, since the light always comes from the same direction, plants tend to bend towards it. To bathe your plants in light from all sides, make a window box. Remove the top and one side from a cardboard box and line the other three sides and bottom with aluminium foil, shiny side out, taping or gluing it in place. Place the plants in the box and put it near a window.

more ALUMINIUM FOIL over →

a **43**

BUILD A SEED INCUBATOR • To give plants grown from seed a healthy head start, line an old shoe box with aluminium foil, shiny side up, allowing about 2 inches (5 cm) of foil to extend out over the sides. Poke several drainage holes into the bottom penetrating the foil and fill the box slightly more than halfway with potting mix and plant the seeds. The aluminium foil inside the box will absorb heat to keep the seeds warm as they germinate, while the foil outside the box will reflect light onto the young sprouts. Place the box near a sunny window, keep the soil moist, then watch 'em grow!

GROW UNTANGLED CUTTINGS • Help plant cuttings grow strong and uncluttered by starting them in a container covered with a sheet of aluminium foil. Simply poke a few holes into the foil and insert the cuttings through the holes. There's even an added bonus—the foil slows water evaporation, so you'll need to add water less frequently.

in the great outdoors

KEEP BEES AWAY FROM BEVERAGES • You're about to relax in your backyard with a well-deserved glass of lemonade or soft drink. Suddenly bees start buzzing around your drink—which they view as sweet nectar. Keep them away by tightly covering the top of your glass with aluminium foil. Poke a straw through it and enjoy your drink in peace.

MAKE A BARBECUE DRIP TRAY • To keep meat drippings off your barbecue coals, create a disposable drip tray out of a couple of layers of heavy-duty aluminium foil. Shape it freehand, or use an inverted baking dish as a mold (remember to remove the dish once your creation is finished). Also, don't forget to make your drip tray slightly larger than the meat barbecuing on the grill.

CLEAN YOUR BARBECUE GRATE • After the last steak has been brought in, and while the coals are still red-hot, lay a sheet of aluminium foil over the barbecue grate to burn off any remaining foodstuffs. The next time you use your barbecue, crumple up the foil and use it to easily scrub off the burned food before you start cooking.

IMPROVE OUTDOOR LIGHTING • Brighten up the electrical lighting in your backyard or campsite by making a foil reflector to put behind the light. Attach the reflector to the fixture with a few strips of electrical tape or duct tape—do not apply tape directly to the bulb.

MAKE AN IMPROMPTU PICNIC PLATTER • When you need a convenient disposable platter for picnics or school fundraisers, just cover a piece of cardboard with heavy-duty aluminium foil.

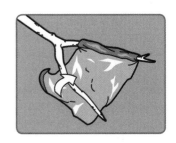

IMPROVISE A FRYING PAN • If you don't feel like lugging a frying pan along on a camping trip you can form your own by centering a forked stick over two layers of heavy-duty aluminium foil. Wrap the edges of the foil tightly around the forked branches, while leaving some slack in the foil between the forks. Invert the stick and depress the center to hold food for frying.

WARM YOUR TOES WHEN CAMPING • Keep your feet toasty at night while camping during periods of cold weather. Simply wrap some stones in aluminium foil and heat them by the campfire while you are toasting marshmallows. At bedtime, wrap the stones in towels and put them in the bottom of your sleeping bag.

KEEP YOUR SLEEPING BAG DRY • Place a piece of heavy-duty aluminium foil under your sleeping bag to insulate against moisture.

KEEP MATCHES DRY • It's a tried-and-true soldier's trick worth remembering: Wrap your kitchen matches in aluminium foil to keep them from getting damp or wet on camping trips.

DID YOU KNOW?

'Hand me the tinfoil, will ya?' To this day, it's not uncommon for people to ask for tinfoil when they want to wrap up leftover food. Household foil was made entirely of tin until 1947, when aluminium foil was introduced into the home, eventually replacing tinfoil in the kitchen drawer.

LURE A FISH • If none of your fancy fishing lures are working, you can make one in a jiffy that just might do the trick. Wrap some aluminium foil around a fishhook. Fringe the foil so that it covers the hook and wiggles invitingly when you reel in the line.

for the do-it-yourselfer

MAKE A FUNNEL • For those times that you can't find a funnel, try doubling up a length of heavy-duty aluminium foil and rolling it into the shape of a cone. This impromptu funnel has an advantage over a permanent funnel—you can bend the aluminium foil to reach awkward holes, like the oil filler hole tucked against the engine of a ride-on mower.

REATTACH A VINYL FLOOR TILE • Don't become unglued just because a vinyl floor tile does. Just re-position the tile on the floor, lay a piece of aluminium foil over it, and run a hot clothes iron over it a few times until you feel the glue melting underneath. Put a pile of books or bricks on top of the tile to weigh it down while the glue resets. This technique also works well to smooth out bulges and straighten curled seams in sheet-vinyl flooring.

PREVENT PAINT FROM SKINNING OVER • When you open a half-used can of paint, you'll typically find a skin of dried paint on the surface. Not only is this annoying to remove, but dried bits can wind up in the paint. You can prevent this by using a two-pronged attack when you close a used paint can. Firstly, put a piece of aluminium foil under the can

MAKE AN ARTIST'S PALETTE • Tear off a length of heavy-duty aluminium foil, crimp up the edges and you've got a ready-to-use palette for mixing paints. If you want to get a little fancier, cut a piece of cardboard into the shape of a palette, complete with thumb hole and cover it with foil. Or if you already have a wooden palette, cover it with foil before each use so you can just strip off the foil instead of cleaning the palette.

and trace around it. Cut out the circle and drop the aluminium foil disc onto the paint surface. Then take a deep breath, blow into the can and quickly put the top in place. The carbon dioxide in your breath replaces some of the oxygen in the can, and helps to prevent the paint from drying.

LINE ROLLER PANS • Cleaning out paint roller pans is a pain, which is why a lot of people buy disposable plastic pans or liners. But lining a metal roller pan with aluminium foil works just as well—and is not only cheaper, but can go in the recycling bin.

more ALUMINIUM FOIL over →

a 45

aluminium foil
aluminium foil pans
aluminium foil
aluminium foil pans
ALUMINIUM

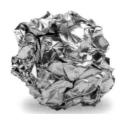

KEEP PAINT OFF DOORKNOBS • When you're painting a door, aluminium foil is great for wrapping doorknobs to keep paint off them. Overlap the foil onto the door when you wrap the knob, then run a sharp utility knife around the base of the knob to trim the foil. That way you can paint right up to the edge of the knob. In addition to wrapping knobs on the doors that you'll paint, wrap all the doorknobs that are along the route to where you will clean your hands and brushes.

KEEP A PAINTBRUSH WET • If you're going to continue painting tomorrow morning, don't clean the brush—just squeeze out the excess paint and wrap it tightly in aluminium foil (or plastic wrap). Use a rubber band to hold the foil tightly at the base of the handle. For extended wet-brush storage, toss the wrapped brush in the freezer. But don't forget to defrost it for an hour or so before you start painting again the next day.

LIGHT USES

REFLECT LIGHT FOR PHOTOGRAPHY • Professional photographers use reflectors to throw extra light on dark areas of their subject and to even out the overall lighting. To make a reflector, lightly coat a piece of matte board or heavy cardboard with rubber cement and cover it with aluminium foil, shiny side out. You can make one single reflector, as large as you want, but it's better to make three panels and join them together with duct tape so that they stand up by themselves, and fold up for handy storage and carrying.

SHINE YOUR CHROME • For sparkling chrome on a variety of appliances, strollers, golf club shafts, and older car bumpers, crumple up a handful of aluminium foil with the shiny side out and apply some elbow grease. If you rub really hard, the foil will even remove rust spots. But be warned that most 'chrome' on new cars is actually plastic—don't rub it with aluminium foil.

ALUMINIUM FOIL PANS

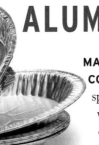

MAKE AN INSTANT COLANDER • The pot of spaghetti is almost done when you realize that the colander is broken. Instead of panicking, just grab a clean aluminium foil pan and a small nail and start poking holes. When you're done, bend the pan to fit comfortably over a deep bowl. Rinse your new colander clean, place it over the bowl and carefully pour in your spaghetti.

REIN IN SPLATTERS WHEN FRYING • Why risk burning yourself or anyone else with oil splatters from a hot frying pan? A safer way to fry is to poke a few holes in the bottom of an aluminium foil pan and place it upside down over the food in your frying pan. Use a pair of tongs or a fork to lift the foil pan and don't forget to wear an oven glove.

CREATE A CENTERPIECE • Here's how to make a quick centerpiece for your table. Secure a pillar candle or a few tea lights to an aluminium foil pan by melting some wax from the bottom of the candles onto the pan. Add a thin layer of water or sand and put in several rose petals or seashells to decorate.

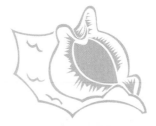

a

Kids' Stuff

Looking for a way to keep the kids busy indoors on a cold, wintry day? How about making an ice ornament that you can hang on a tree outside your house as a homemade winter decoration? All you'll need is an aluminium foil pan, some water, a piece of heavy string or a shoelace, and a mix of decorative—preferably biodegradable—materials, such as dried flowers, dried leaves, pinecones, seeds, shells, and twigs.

Let the children arrange the materials in the foil pan to their liking. Then fold the string or shoelace in half and place it in the pan. The fold should hang over the edges of the pan, while the two ends meet in the center. Slowly fill the pan with water, stopping just shy of the rim. You may have to place an object on the string to keep it from floating to the top.

If you live in an area where the temperatures outside your home are likely to be below freezing, you can simply put the pan on your doorstep to freeze. Otherwise just pop it into your freezer. Once the water has frozen solid, slide off the pan and let your children choose the optimal outdoor location to display their artwork in ice.

CONTAIN THE MESS FROM KIDS' PROJECTS • Glitter is notorious for turning up in the corners and crevices of your home long after your young artist's masterpiece has been mailed to Grandma. But you can minimize some of those inevitable messes by using an aluminium foil pan to encase projects that involve glitter, beads, spray paint, feathers, and all sorts of things.

MAKE TRAYS FOR CRAFT SUPPLIES • Bring some order to your children's—or your own—inventory of crayons, beads, buttons, sequins, pipe cleaners, and other such things by organizing them in aluminium foil pans. To secure materials when storing the trays, slip each tray into a large ziplock plastic bag.

TRAIN YOUR DOG

If Rover has a tendency to leap up on the couch or kitchen bench, leave a few aluminium foil pans along the bench edges or the back of the couch when you're not home. The resulting noise will give him a good scare when he jumps and hits them.

KEEP INSECTS OUT OF PET DISHES • Use an aluminium foil pan filled with about 1 inch (2.5 cm) of water to create a metal moat around your pet's food dish. It should help to keep those marauding ants and roaches at bay.

KEEP SQUIRRELS AND BIRDS OFF YOUR FRUIT TREES • Are furry and feathered fiends stealing the fruit off your trees? There's nothing better to scare off those intruders than a few dangling aluminium foil pans. String them up in pairs (to make some noise), and you won't have to worry about finding any half-eaten apples or peaches come harvest time.

MAKE A MINI-DUSTPAN • If you need a spare dustpan for your workplace or bathroom, an aluminium foil pan can fit the bill quite nicely. Simply cut one in half and you're ready to go.

USE AS A DRIP CATCHER UNDER A PAINT CAN • Next time you have something that needs painting, place an aluminium foil pan under the paint can as a ready-made drip catcher. You'll save a lot of time cleaning up, and you can toss the pan in the garbage when you're done. Even better, rinse it off and recycle it for future paint jobs.

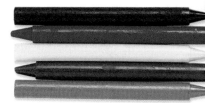

more ALUMINIUM FOIL PANS over →

a 47

STORE SANDING DISKS AND MORE • Since they're highly resistant to corrosion, aluminium foil pans are especially well suited for storing sanding discs, hacksaw blades, and other hardware accessories in your workshop. Cut a circular pan in half and attach it (with staples or duct tape around the edges) open side up to a pegboard. Now get organized!

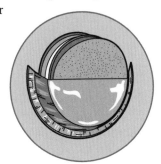

USE AS AN IMPROMPTU ASHTRAY • If you don't have an ashtray on hand when a smoker comes to visit, don't worry. An aluminium foil pan—or even a piece of heavy-duty aluminium foil folded into a square with the sides turned up—should suffice.

PROTECT FINGERS DURING OUTDOOR COOKING • There's nothing like a campfire in the great outdoors. Whether you're planning a day trip or a longer ones, be sure to pack a few aluminium foil pans. Put a small hole in the middle of each pan, and push them up the sticks or barbecue skewers used for toasting bread or marshmallows. The pans deflect the heat of the fire, protecting your and your children's hands.

25 USES!

AMMONIA

in the kitchen

● ● ●

CLEAN YOUR OVEN • Here's a practically effortless way to clean an electric oven. First, turn the oven on, let it warm to 150°F (65°C) and then turn it off. Place a small bowl with ½ cup (125 ml) ammonia on the top shelf and a large dish of boiling water on the bottom shelf. Close the oven door and let it sit overnight. The next morning, remove the bowl and dish, and let the oven air out for a while. Then wipe it clean using the ammonia and a few drops of dishwashing liquid diluted in 4 cups (1 L) warm water—even old burned-on grease should wipe right off.
WARNING: Do not use this cleaning method with a gas oven unless the pilot lights are out and the main gas lines are shut off.

CLEAN OVEN RACKS • Clean baked-on grime from your oven racks by laying them on an old towel in a large laundry tub. You can use your bathtub, though you might need to clean it afterwards. Fill the tub with warm water and add ½ cup (125 ml) ammonia. Let racks soak for at least 15 minutes, remove, rinse, and wipe clean.

MAKE CRYSTAL SPARKLE • Has the twinkle gone out of your good crystal? Bring back its lost luster by mixing several drops of ammonia in 2 cups (500 ml) water and applying with a soft cloth or brush. Rinse it off with clean water and dry with a soft, dry cloth.

REPEL MOTHS • Annoying moths seem to come out of nowhere! Send them back wherever they came from by washing drawers, pantry shelves, or cupboards with 1/2 cup (125 ml) ammonia diluted in 4 cups (1 L) water. Leave drawers and cabinets open to thoroughly air-dry.

CAUTION: Never mix ammonia with bleach or any product containing chlorine. The combination produces toxic fumes that can be deadly. Work in a well-ventilated space and avoid inhaling the vapors. Wear rubber gloves and avoid getting ammonia on your skin or in your eyes. Always store ammonia out of reach of children.

around the house ● ● ●

ELIMINATE PAINT ODORS • A freshly painted home interior looks fantastic, but the lingering paint smell that usually comes with it will drive you up the wall! Absorb the odor by placing small dishes of ammonia in each room that's been painted. If the smell persists after several days, replenish the dishes. Vinegar or onion slices will also do the trick.

CLEAN FIREPLACE DOORS • Think you'll need a blowtorch to remove that blackened-on soot from your glass fireplace doors? Before you get out the goggles, try mixing 1 tablespoon (15 ml) ammonia, 2 tablespoons (30 ml) vinegar and 4 cups (1 L) warm water in a spray bottle. Spray on some of the solution, let it sit for several seconds, then wipe it off with an absorbent cloth. Repeat if necessary— it's worth the extra effort.

CLEAN GOLD AND SILVER JEWELRY • Brighten your gold and silver trinkets by soaking them for 10 minutes in a solution of ½ cup (125 ml) clear ammonia mixed in 1 cup (250 ml) warm water. Gently wipe clean with a soft cloth and allow to dry. **WARNING: Do not do this with jewelry containing pearls, because it could dull or damage the nacre, the delicate, lustrous surface.**

DID YOU KNOW?

During the Middle Ages, ammonia was made in northern Europe by heating the scrapings of deer antlers. Subsequently, it was known as spirits of hartshorn. Before the start of World War I, it was chiefly produced by the dry distillation of nitrogenous vegetable and animal products.

Today, most ammonia is made synthetically using the Haber process, in which hydrogen and nitrogen gases are combined under extreme pressures and medium temperatures. The technique was developed by Fritz Haber and Carl Bosch in 1909, and was first used on a large-scale basis by the Germans during World War I, primarily for the production of munitions.

Testing ammonia

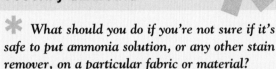

What should you do if you're not sure if it's safe to put ammonia solution, or any other stain remover, on a particular fabric or material?

Always test a drop or two on an inconspicuous part of the garment or object first. Apply, then rub the area with a white washcloth to test the colorfastness. If any color rubs off on the washcloth or if there is any noticeable change in the material's appearance, try another approach.

REMOVE TARNISH FROM BRASS OR SILVER • You can put that sunny shine back in your tarnished silver or lacquered brass by gently scrubbing it with a soft brush dipped in a bit of ammonia. Wipe off any remaining liquid with a soft cloth—or preferably chamois—to protect the metal's surface.

REMOVE GREASE AND SOAP SCUM • To get rid of that ugly grease and soap-scum buildup in your porcelain enamel sink or bathtub, scrub it with a solution of 1 tablespoon (15 ml) ammonia in 1 gallon (4 L) hot water. Rinse thoroughly when done.

RESTORE WHITE SHOES

Brighten up your dingy white sneakers or tennis shoes by rubbing them with a cloth dipped in half-strength ammonia– that is, a solution made of half ammonia and half water.

more AMMONIA over →

AMMONIA

DID YOU KNOW?

Ammonia is a colorless, pungent gas. It is easily soluble in water, however, and the liquid ammonia products sold today contain the gas dissolved in water. Ammonia is one of the oldest cleaning compounds currently in use. It actually dates back to ancient Egypt. In fact, the word ammonia is derived from the Egyptian deity Ammon, whose temple in what is now Libya is credited with producing the earliest form of ammonia, sal ammoniac, by burning camel dung.

REMOVE STAINS FROM CLOTHING • Ammonia is great for cleaning clothes. Here are some ways you can use it to remove a variety of stains. Make sure you dilute ammonia with at least 50 percent water before applying it to silk, wool, or spandex.

■ Rub out perspiration, blood, and urine stains on clothing by dabbing the area with a half-strength solution of ammonia and water before laundering.

■ Remove most non-oily stains with a mixture of equal parts ammonia, water, and dishwashing liquid. Put it in an empty spray bottle, shake well, then apply directly to the stain. Let it set for 2 to 3 minutes before rinsing out.

■ To remove pencil marks from clothing, use a few drops of undiluted ammonia and rinse. If that doesn't work, put a little laundry detergent on the stain and rinse again.

■ You can even remove washed-in paint stains from clothes by saturating them several times with a half-ammonia, half-turpentine solution, then tossing them into the wash.

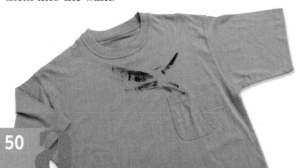

CLEAN CARPETS AND UPHOLSTERY • Lift out stains from carpeting and upholstery by sponging them with 1 cup (250 ml) clear ammonia in 2 quarts (2 L) warm water. Allow to dry thoroughly and repeat if needed.

BRIGHTEN UP WINDOWS • Dirty, grimy windows can make any house look dingy. But it's easy to wipe away the dirt, fingerprints, soot, and dust covering your windows. Just wipe them down with a soft cloth dampened with a solution of 1 cup (250 ml) clear ammonia in 3 cups (750 ml) water. Your windows will not only be crystal-clear, but streak-free to boot.

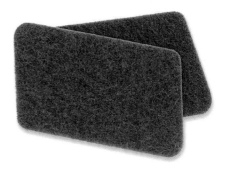

STRIP WAX FROM RESILIENT FLOORING

Wax buildup on resilient flooring causes it to yellow over time. Remove old wax layers and freshen up your floor by washing it with a mixture of 1 cup (250 ml) ammonia in 2 quarts (2 L) water. Let the solution sit for 3 to 5 minutes and scrub with a plastic scouring pad to remove the old wax. Wipe away leftover residue with a clean cloth or sponge, then give the floor a thorough rinse.

CLEAN BATHROOM TILES • Make bathroom tiles sparkle again—and kill mildew—by sponging them with ¼ cup (50 ml) ammonia in 1 gallon (4 L) water.

in the garden ● ● ●

USE AS PLANT FOOD

Give alkaline-loving flowering plants and vegetables in your garden—such as clematis, lilac, hydrangea, and cucumbers—an occasional special treat with a shower of ¼ cup (50 ml) ammonia diluted in 1 gallon (4 L) water. They'll especially appreciate the boost in nitrogen.

STOP MOSQUITO BITES FROM ITCHING • If you forget to put on your insect repellent and mosquitoes start making a meal out of you, stop the itching instantly by applying a drop or two of ammonia directly to the bites. Don't use ammonia on a bite you've already scratched open, though; the itch will be replaced by a nasty sting.

KEEP STRAY ANIMALS OUT OF YOUR GARBAGE • Few things can be quite as startling as a stray cat leaping out of your garbage can just as you're about to make your nightly trash deposit. Keep away those strays and other scavengers by spraying the outside and lids of your garbage bins with half-strength ammonia or by spraying the bags inside.

REMOVE STAINS FROM CONCRETE • If you're tired of those annoying stains on concrete surfaces around the house, get rid of them by scrubbing them with 1 cup (250 ml) ammonia diluted in 1 gallon (4 L) water. Hose them down well when you're done.

FIGHT MILDEW • Ammonia and bleach are equally effective weapons in the battle against mold and mildew. Each has its own distinct applications and under no circumstances should the two ever be combined. Reach for ammonia for the following jobs, but make sure you use it in a well-ventilated area, and don't forget to wear rubber gloves:

■ Clean the mildew off unfinished wooden patio furniture and picnic tables with a mixture of 1 cup (250 ml) ammonia, ½ cup (125 ml) vinegar, ¼ cup (50 g) baking soda and 1 gallon (4 L) water. Rinse off thoroughly and use an old washcloth to absorb excess moisture.

■ To remove mildew from painted outdoor surfaces, use the same combination of ingredients.

■ To remove mildew from wicker furniture, wipe it down with a solution of 2 tablespoons (30 ml) ammonia in 1 gallon (4 L) water. Use an old toothbrush to get into hard-to-reach spots. Rinse well and allow to air-dry.

APPLES

ROAST A JUICY CHICKEN • If your roasted chicken tends to emerge from the oven as dry as shoe leather, don't fret. The next time you roast a chicken, stuff an apple inside the bird before placing it in the roasting dish. When it's finished cooking, toss the used fruit in the garbage and get ready to sit down to a delicious—and juicy—main course.

KEEP CAKES FRESH

Want a simple and effective way to extend the shelf life of homemade or store-bought cakes? Store them with a half an apple. It helps the cake stay moist considerably longer than just popping it in the fridge.

more APPLES over →

51

RIPEN GREEN TOMATOES • If a family member just 'helped' by harvesting a few green tomatoes off the vine for you, don't sweat. You can quickly ripen them up by placing them—along with an already ripe apple—in a paper bag for a couple of days. For the best results, maintain a ratio of about five or six tomatoes per apple.

FLUFF UP HARDENED BROWN SUGAR • Brown sugar has the irritating habit of hardening up when exposed to humidity. Fortunately, it doesn't take much to make this a temporary condition. Simply place an apple wedge in a resealable plastic bag with the chunk of hardened brown sugar. Tightly seal the bag and put it in a dry place for a day or two. Your sugar will once again be soft enough to use.

ABSORB SALT IN SOUPS AND CASSEROLES • Salting to taste is one thing, but it is possible to overdo it. When you find yourself getting heavy-handed with the salt, simply drop a few apple (or potato) wedges into the pot. After cooking for another 10 minutes or so, remove the wedges—along with the excess salt.

DID YOU KNOW?

That old saying 'One bad apple spoils the bunch' just might be true. Apples are among a diverse group of fruits—others include apricots, avocados, bananas, blueberries, cantaloupe, and peaches—that produce ethylene gas, a natural ripening agent. So the increased level of ethylene produced by a single rotten apple in a bag can significantly accelerate the ageing process of the other apples around it.

Ethylene-producing fruits can help speed the ripening of something (like a green tomato; *see 'Ripen green tomatoes', above*). But they can also have unwanted effects. Placing a bowl of ripe apples or bananas too close to freshly cut flowers, for instance, can cause them to wilt. And if your refrigerated potatoes seem to be sprouting buds too soon, they may be too close to the apples. Keep them at least one shelf apart.

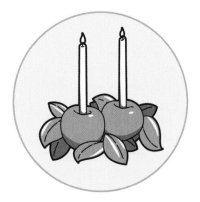

USE AS DECORATIVE CANDLE HOLDERS

Add a cozy, country feel to your table setting by creating a natural candle holder. Use an apple corer to carve a hole three-quarters of the way down into a pair of large apples, insert a tall decorative candle into each hole, surround the apples with a few leaves, branches or flowers and voila! You have a lovely centerpiece.

ASHES

CLEAN FIREPLACE DOORS • You normally wouldn't think of using dirty wood ash to clean glass fireplace doors, but it works. Mix some ash with a bit of water and apply it with a damp cloth, sponge, or paper towel or simply dip a wet sponge into the ash. Rub the mixture over the door's surfaces. Rinse with a wet paper towel or sponge, then dry with a clean cloth. The results will amaze you, but remember that wood ash was a key ingredient in good old-fashioned lye soap.

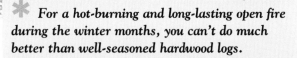

USE AS PLANT FOOD
USE AS PLANT FOOD • Wood ash has a high alkaline content and trace amounts of calcium and potassium, which encourage blooms. If your soil tends to be acidic, sprinkle the ash in spring around alkaline-loving plants such as clematis, hydrangea, lilac, and roses (but avoid acid-lovers like rhododendrons, gardenias, and azaleas). Avoid using ash from preformed logs, which may contain chemicals harmful to plants. And be sparing when adding ash to your compost pile; it can counteract the benefits of manure and other high-nitrogen materials.

REPEL INSECTS • Scatter a border of ash around your garden to deter cutworms, slugs, and snails—it sticks to their bodies and draws moisture out of them. Also sprinkle small amounts of ash over garden plants to manage infestations of soft-bodied insects. Wear eye protection and gloves.

CLEAN PEWTER • Restore the shine to pewter by cleaning it with cigarette ash. Dip a dampened piece of cheesecloth into the ash and rub it over the item. It will turn darker at first, but the shine will come out after a good rinsing.

Selecting firewood
TIP

* *For a hot-burning and long-lasting open fire during the winter months, you can't do much better than well-seasoned hardwood logs.*

Green or wet wood burns poorly and builds up creosote (a leading cause of chimney fires) in your chimney; soft pine is another major producer of creosote. Never burn scraps of pressure-treated wood, as it contains chemicals that can be extremely harmful when burned.

Don't be a fanatic about cleaning ash from your fireplace. Leave a 1 to 2-inch (2.5 to 5-cm) layer of ash under the andiron to reflect heat back up to the burning wood and protect your fireplace floor against hot embers. Just be sure not to let the ash clog up the space under the grate and block the airflow that a good fire needs.

REMOVE WATER SPOTS AND HEAT MARKS FROM WOODEN FURNITURE • Use cigar and/or cigarette ash to remove those white rings left on your wooden furniture by wet glasses or hot cups. Mix the ash with a few drops of water to make a paste and rub lightly over the mark to remove it. Then shine it with your usual furniture polish.

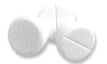

ASPIRIN

REVIVE DEAD CAR BATTERIES • If you get behind the wheel only to discover that your car's battery has given up the ghost—and there's no one around to give you a jump—you may be able to get your vehicle started by dropping two aspirin tablets into the battery. The aspirin's acetylsalicylic acid will combine with the battery's sulphuric acid to produce one last charge. Just make sure that you drive to your nearest service station pronto to find a longer-term solution.

REMOVE PERSPIRATION STAINS

Before you give up all hope of ever getting that perspiration stain out of your good white dress shirt, try this: crush 2 aspirins and mix the powder in 1/2 cup (125 ml) warm water. Soak the stained part of the garment in the solution for around 2 to 3 hours.

more ASPIRIN over →

a 53

DID YOU KNOW?

The bark of the willow tree is rich in salicin—a natural painkiller and fever reducer. In the third century B.C., Hippocrates used it to relieve headaches and pain, and many traditional healers, including Native Americans, used herbs containing salicin to treat cold and flu symptoms. But it wasn't until 1899 that Felix Hoffmann, a chemist at the German company Bayer, developed a modified derivative, acetylsalicylic acid, better known as aspirin.

RESTORE HAIR COLOR • Swimming in a chlorinated pool can have a noticeable, and often unpleasant, effect on your hair coloring if you have light-colored hair. But you can usually return your hair to its former shade by dissolving 6 to 8 aspirins in a glass of warm water. Rub the solution thoroughly into your hair and let it set for 10 to 15 minutes, then rinse.

APPLY TO INSECT BITES AND STINGS

Control the inflammation caused by mosquito bites or bee stings by wetting your skin and rubbing an aspirin over the spot. Of course, if you are allergic to bee stings—or have difficulty breathing, develop abdominal pains, or feel nauseated following a bee sting—seek expert medical attention at once.

TREAT HARD CALLUSES • Soften hard calluses on your feet by grinding 5 or 6 aspirins into a powder. Make a paste by adding ½ teaspoon (2 ml) each lemon juice and water. Apply the mixture to the affected areas, then wrap your foot in a warm towel and cover it with a plastic bag. After staying off your feet for at least 10 minutes, remove the bag and towel and file down the softened callus with a pumice stone.

CONTROL DANDRUFF • If your dandruff problem is getting you down, keep it in check by crushing 2 aspirins into a fine powder and adding it to the normal amount of shampoo you usually use. Leave the mixture on for 1 to 2 minutes, then rinse well and wash again with plain shampoo.

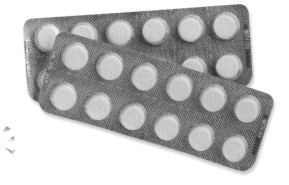

CAUTION: About 10 percent of people with severe asthma are also allergic to aspirin—and, in fact, to all products containing salicylic acid (aspirin's key ingredient), including some cold medications, fruit, and food seasonings and additives. That percentage skyrockets to 30 to 40 percent for older asthmatics who also suffer from sinusitis or nasal polyps. Acute sensitivity to aspirin is also seen in a small percentage of the general population without asthma—particularly people with ulcers and other bleeding conditions.

Always consult your doctor before using any medication, and do not apply aspirin externally if you are allergic to taking it internally.

FOR THOSE WITH GREEN FINGERS ...

HELP CUT FLOWERS LAST LONGER • It's a tried-and-true way to keep roses and other cut flowers fresher longer: Put a crushed aspirin in the water before adding your flowers. Other household items that you can put in the water to extend the life of your flower arrangements include a multivitamin, 1 teaspoon (5 ml) sugar, a pinch of salt, and baking soda. Don't forget to change the vase water every few days.

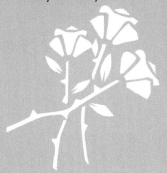

USE AS GARDEN AID • Aspirin is not only a first-aid essential for you, but for your garden as well. Some gardeners grind it up for use as a rooting agent, or mix it with water to treat fungal conditions in the soil. But be careful when using aspirin around plants; too much of it can cause burns or other damage to your greenery. When treating soil, the typical dosage should be a half or a full aspirin tablet in 1 quart (1 L) water.

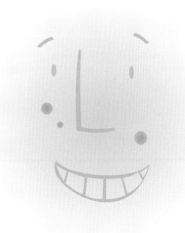

DRY UP PIMPLES • Even those of us who are well past adolescence can get the occasional pimple. Put the kibosh on those annoying blemishes by crushing an aspirin and moistening it with a bit of water. Apply the paste to the pimple and let it sit for a couple of minutes before washing it off with soap and water. The aspirin paste will reduce the redness and soothe the sting. If the pimple persists, repeat the procedure as needed until it's gone.

REMOVE EGG STAINS FROM CLOTHES

Did you drop some raw egg on your clothing while cooking or eating? First of all, scrape off as much of the egg as you can, then try to sponge out the rest with lukewarm water. Don't use hot water—it will set the egg. If that doesn't completely remove the stain, mix water and cream of tartar into a paste and add a crushed aspirin. Spread the paste on the stain and leave it for 30 minutes. Rinse well in warm water and with any luck, the egg will be gone.

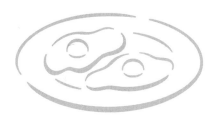

baby oil
baby oil
baby oil
baby oil
baby oil
BABY OIL

BABY OIL

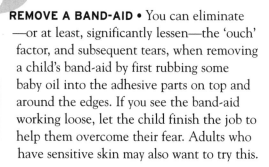

REMOVE A BAND-AID • You can eliminate —or at least, significantly lessen—the 'ouch' factor, and subsequent tears, when removing a child's band-aid by first rubbing some baby oil into the adhesive parts on top and around the edges. If you see the band-aid working loose, let the child finish the job to help them overcome their fear. Adults who have sensitive skin may also want to try this.

BUFF UP YOUR GOLF CLUBS • Don't waste your money on fancy cleaning kits for your chrome-plated, carbon-steel golf club heads. Just keep a small bottle filled with baby oil in your golf bag along with a chamois cloth or towel. Dab a few drops of oil on the cloth and polish the head of your club after each round of golf.

SLIP OFF A STUCK RING • Is that ring jammed on your finger again? First lubricate the ring area with a generous amount of baby oil, then swivel the ring around to spread the oil under it. You should be able to slide the ring off with ease.

POLISH LEATHER BAGS AND SHOES • Just a few drops of baby oil applied with a soft cloth can add new life to an old leather bag or pair of patent leather shoes. Don't forget to wipe away any oil remaining on the leather when you're done.

HIDE SCRATCHES ON DASHBOARD PLASTIC • You can disguise scratches on the plastic lens covering the odometer and other indicators on your car's dash by rubbing over them with a bit of baby oil.

REMOVE ACRYLIC PAINT FROM SKIN • Did you get almost as much paint on your face and hands as you did on the bathroom you just painted? You can quickly get acrylic paint off your skin by first rubbing it with some baby oil, followed by a good washing with soap and hot water.

BATHROOM BLISS

MAKE YOUR OWN BATH OIL • Do you have a favorite perfume or cologne? You can literally bathe in it by making your own scented bath oil. Simply add a few drops of your scent of choice to 1/4 cup (50 ml) baby oil in a small plastic bottle. Shake well and add it to your bath.

CLEAN YOUR BATHTUB OR SHOWER • Remove dirt and built-up soap scum around your bathtub or shower recess by wiping surfaces with 1 teaspoon (2 ml) baby oil on a moist cloth. Use another cloth to wipe away any leftover oil. Finally, spray the area with a disinfectant cleaner to kill any remaining germs. This technique is also great for cleaning soap film and water marks from glass shower doors.

SHINE STAINLESS STEEL SINKS AND CHROME TRIM • Pamper your dull-looking stainless steel sinks by rubbing them down with a few drops of baby oil on a soft, clean cloth. Rub dry with a towel and repeat if necessary. This is also a terrific way to remove stains on the chrome trim of your kitchen appliances and bathroom fixtures.

TREAT CRADLE CAP • Cradle cap may be unsightly, but it is a common, usually harmless, phase in many babies' development. To combat it, gently rub in a bit of baby oil and lightly comb it through your baby's hair. If the baby gets upset, comb it a bit at a time, but do not leave the oil on for more than 24 hours. Thoroughly wash the hair to remove all of the oil. Repeat the process in persistent cases. However, if you notice a lot of yellow crusting, or if the cradle cap has spread behind the ears or on the neck, contact a pediatrician as soon as possible.

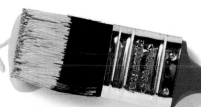

BABY POWDER

GIVE SAND THE BRUSH-OFF • When you return from a day at the beach, do you find that some of the beach has come back with you? Minimize the mess by sprinkling some baby powder over sand-covered, sweaty, kids (and adults) before they enter the house. In addition to soaking up excess moisture, baby powder makes sand incredibly easy to brush off.

COOL SHEETS IN SUMMER • Are those sticky, hot bedsheets giving you the summertime blues when you should be deep in dreamland? Cool things down by sprinkling a bit of baby powder between your sheets before hopping into bed on warm nights.

DRY-SHAMPOO YOUR PET • Give your dog's coat a waterless cleaning by rubbing a few handfuls of baby powder into his fur. Let it settle in for a couple of minutes and follow up with a good brushing. Your dog will look and smell great! You can also dry-shampoo your own hair with the same technique.

ABSORB GREASE STAINS ON CLOTHING • Frying food can be a dangerous business—especially for your clothes. If you get a grease splatter on your clothing, try dabbing the stain with some baby powder on a powder puff. Make sure you rub it in well, then brush off any excess powder. Repeat until the mark is gone.

REMOVE MOLD FROM BOOKS • If your stored books have gotten a bit moldy or mildewed, here's what you can do. First, air-dry them, then sprinkle baby powder between the pages and stand them upright, pages fanned open, for several hours. Afterwards, gently brush out the remaining powder in each book. Now, they'll be in much better shape.

SLIP ON YOUR RUBBER GLOVES • Don't try jamming and squeezing your fingers into your rubber gloves when the powder layer inside the gloves wears out. Instead, give your fingers a light dusting with baby powder. Your rubber gloves should slide on as easily as they did when they were new.

DID YOU KNOW?

When shopping for baby powder, you're faced with three choices: plain, cornstarch, or medicated. Here's the lowdown on each choice:

■ Plain baby powder is primarily talcum powder, not good for infants to breathe and not good for baby girls as studies suggest it could cause ovarian cancer

■ Pediatricians recommend a cornstarch-based powder if needed when changing diapers. It can promote fungal infection so should not be applied in skin folds or to broken skin.

■ Medicated baby powder has zinc oxide added to either talcum powder or cornstarch. It is generally used to soothe diaper rash and to prevent chafing.

DUST OFF FLOWER BULBS • Savvy gardeners use medicated baby powder to dust flower bulbs before planting them. Place 5 to 6 bulbs with 3 tablespoons (45 ml) baby powder in a sealed plastic bag and give it a few gentle shakes. The medicated powder coating helps reduce the chance of rot and keeps away grubs and other bulb-munching garden pests.

CLEAN YOUR PLAYING CARDS

Here's a simple way to keep your playing cards from sticking together. Place the cards in a plastic bag along with a bit of baby powder, seal the bag, and give it a few good shakes. They'll feel fresh and smooth again.

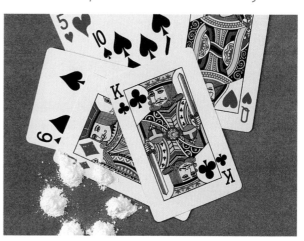

BABY WIPES

USE FOR QUICK, ON-THE-MOVE CLEAN-UPS • Baby wipes can be used for more than just cleaning babies' bottoms. They're great for wiping your hands after pumping gas, mopping up spills in the car, and cooling your sweaty brow after a run. In fact, they make ideal travel companions. Next time you set off on the road, pack a small stack of wipes in a tightly closed ziplock sandwich bag and put it in the glove compartment of your car or in your briefcase, pocketbook, or backpack.

SHINE YOUR SHOES • Most moms know that a baby wipe does a pretty good job of brightening kids' white leather shoes, but you can also use one to put the shine back in your leather pumps—especially with that morning meeting fast approaching!

RECYCLE AS DUST CLOTHS • Believe it or not, some brands of baby wipes—Huggies, for instance—can be laundered and reused as dust cloths and rags for cleaning up around the home. It probably goes without saying, but only 'mildly' soiled wipes should be considered candidates for laundering.

BUFF UP YOUR BATHROOM • Do you have friends coming over and not much time to tidy up the house? Don't break out in a sweat. Try this two-handed trick. Take a baby wipe in one hand and start polishing all the bathroom surfaces. Keep a dry washcloth in your other hand to shine things up as you make your rounds.

REMOVE STAINS FROM CARPET, CLOTHING, AND UPHOLSTERY • Use a baby wipe to blot up coffee spills from your rug or carpet; it absorbs both the liquid and the stain. Wipes can also be effectively deployed when attacking various spills and drips on your clothing and upholstered furniture.

BEAUTY!

SOOTHE YOUR SKIN • Did you get a bit too much sun at the beach? You can temporarily cool a sunburn by gently patting the area with a baby wipe. Baby wipes can also be used to treat cuts and scrapes. Although most wipes don't have any antiseptic properties, there's nothing wrong with using one for an initial cleansing before applying the proper topical treatment to relieve sunburn.

REMOVE MAKE-UP • One of the fashion industry's worst-kept secrets is that many models consider a baby wipe to be their best friend when it comes time to remove that stubborn makeup from their faces, particularly black eyeliner. Try it and see for yourself.

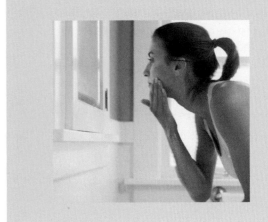

CLEAN YOUR KEYBOARD

Periodically shaking out your computer's keyboard is a good way to get rid of the dust and debris that gather underneath and in between the keys. But that's just half the job. Use a baby wipe to remove the dirt, dried spills, and unspecified gunk that builds up on the keys. Just make sure to turn off the computer or unplug the keyboard before you wipe the keys.

BABY WIPES CONTAINERS

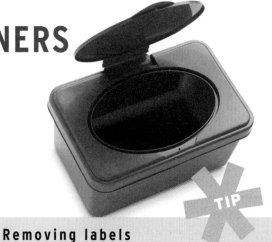

ORGANIZE YOUR STUFF • Don't toss those empty baby wipes containers. Those sturdy plastic boxes are incredibly useful for storing all sorts of items–and the rectangular ones are stackable. Give those containers a good washing, dry thoroughly, and fill them with sewing supplies, recipe cards, coupons, craft and office supplies, loose change, small tools, photos, receipts, and bills. Label the contents with a marker on masking tape and you're all set!

Removing labels

Use a blow-dryer on a high setting to heat up the labels on baby wipes containers to make them easier to pull off. You can get rid of any leftover sticky stuff by applying a little WD-40 oil or orange citrus cleaner.

MAKE A FIRST AID KIT • Every home needs a first aid kit. But you don't have to buy one. Collect your own choice of essentials (such as bandages, sterile gauze rolls and pads, surgical tape, scissors, antibiotic ointment) and use a rectangular baby wipes container to hold it all. Before you add your supplies, give the container a good washing—and after it dries, rub the inside with a cotton ball dipped in alcohol.

USE AS A DECORATIVE WOOL OR STRING DISPENSER • A clean, cylindrical wipes container makes a perfect dispenser for a roll of wool or string. Simply remove the container's cover, insert the roll, thread it through the slot in the lid, and reattach the cover. Paint or paper over the container to give it a more decorative look.

STORE YOUR PLASTIC SHOPPING BAGS • Do you save plastic shopping bags for lining wastebaskets (or perhaps for dog-walking duty)? If so, bring order to the puffed-up chaos they create by storing the bags in cleaned, rectangular wipes containers. Each container can hold 40 to 50 bags—once you squeeze the air out of them. You can also use an empty 250-count tissue box—the kind with a perforated cut-out dispenser—in a similar manner.

HOLD WORKSHOP TOWELS OR RAGS • A used baby wipes container can be a welcome addition in the workshop for storing rags and paper towels—and to keep a steady supply on hand as needed. You can easily keep a full roll of detached paper towels or six or seven decent-sized rags in each container.

MAKE A PIGGY BANK

Well, maybe not a 'piggy' bank, but a bank that gives you a convenient place to dump your extra change. Take a clean rectangular wipes container and use a sharp penknife to cut a slot, wide enough to easily accommodate a quarter on the lid. If you're making the bank for a child, you can either decorate it or let them put their own personal 'stamp' on it.

86 USES!

BAKING SODA
in the kitchen

CLEAN YOUR PRODUCE

You can't be too careful when it comes to food handling and preparation. Wash fruits and vegetables in a pot of cold water with 2 to 3 tablespoons (30-45 ml) baking soda; it will remove some of the impurities tap water leaves behind. Or put a small amount of baking soda on a wet sponge or vegetable brush and scrub your produce. Give everything a thorough rinsing before serving.

SOAK OUT FISH SMELLS • Get rid of that fishy smell from store-bought fish fillets and fish steaks by soaking the raw fish for about an hour (inside your refrigerator) in 4 cups (1 L) water with 2 tablespoons (30 ml) baking soda. Rinse the fish well and pat dry before cooking.

REDUCE ACIDS IN RECIPES • If you or someone in your family is sensitive to the high-acid content of tomato-based sauces or coffee, you can lower the overall acidity by adding a pinch of baking soda while cooking (or, in the case of coffee, before brewing). A bit of baking soda can also counteract the taste of vinegar if you happen to pour in a bit too much. Be careful not to overdo it though—if you add too much, the vinegar–baking soda combo will start foaming.

FLUFF UP YOUR OMELETS

Want to know the secret to making fluffier omelets? For every three eggs used, add 1/2 teaspoon (2 ml) baking soda.

BAKE BETTER BEANS • Do you love baked beans but not their aftereffects? Adding a pinch of baking soda to baked beans as they're cooking will significantly reduce their gas-producing properties.

TENDERIZE MEAT • If you've got a tough cut of meat on your hands, you can soften it by giving it a rubdown with baking soda. Let it sit (in the refrigerator, of course) for 3 to 5 hours, then rinse it off well before cooking.

TIP

Out of baking powder?

* *Instead of baking powder, you can usually substitute 2 parts baking soda mixed with 1 part each cream of tartar and cornstarch.*

To make the equivalent of 1 teaspoon (5 ml) baking powder, mix 1/2 teaspoon (2 ml) baking soda with 1/4 teaspoon (1 ml) cream of tartar and 1/4 teaspoon (1 ml) cornstarch. The cornstarch slows the reaction between the acidic cream of tartar and the alkaline baking soda so it maintains its leavening power longer.

USE AS YEAST SUBSTITUTE • If you need a stand-in for yeast when making dough and you have some powdered vitamin C (or citric acid) and baking soda on hand, you can use a mixture of the two instead. Just mix in equal parts to equal the quantity of yeast required. What's more, the dough you add it to won't have to rise before baking.

RID HANDS OF FOOD ODORS • Chopping garlic or cleaning a fish can leave their 'essence' on your fingers long after the job is done. Get those nasty food smells off your hands by simply wetting them and vigorously rubbing with about 2 teaspoons (10 ml) baking soda instead of soap. The smell should wash off with the baking soda.

CLEAN BABY BOTTLES AND ACCESSORIES • Here's some great advice for new parents. Keep all your baby bottles, nipples, caps, and brushes 'baby fresh' by soaking them overnight in a container filled with hot water and half a box of baking soda. Make sure you give everything a good rinsing afterwards, and dry thoroughly before using. Baby bottles can also be boiled in a full pot of water and 3 tablespoons (45 ml) baking soda for 3 minutes.

CLEAN A CHOPPING BOARD • Keep your wooden or plastic cutting board clean by occasionally scrubbing it with a paste made from 1 tablespoon (15 ml) each baking soda, salt, and water. Rinse thoroughly with hot water and allow to air-dry.

CLEAR A CLOGGED DRAIN • Unclog your kitchen drain by pouring in 1 cup (250 g) baking soda followed by 1 cup (250 ml) hot vinegar (microwave for 1 minute). Give it several minutes to work and add 4 cups (1 L) boiling water. Repeat if necessary. If your drain is clogged with grease, use ½ cup (125 g) each baking soda and salt followed by 1 cup (250 ml) boiling water. Let the mixture work overnight. Rinse with hot tap water in the morning.

DID YOU KNOW?

Baking soda is the main ingredient in many commercial fire extinguishers. You can use it straight out of the box to extinguish small fires throughout your home. For quick access, keep some in buckets placed strategically around the house.

Keep baking soda near your stove and barbecue so you can toss on a few handfuls to quell a flare-up. In the case of a grease fire, first turn off the heat, if possible, and try to cover the fire with a pan lid. Be careful not to let the hot grease splatter on you.

Keep a box or two in your garage and inside your car to quickly extinguish any mechanical or car fires. Baking soda will also snuff out electrical fires and flames on clothing, wood, upholstery, and carpeting.

BOOST POTENCY OF DISHWASHING LIQUID • Looking for a more powerful dishwashing liquid? Try adding 2 tablespoons (30 ml) baking soda to the usual amount of liquid you use, and watch it cut through grease like a hot knife.

MAKE YOUR OWN DISHWASHING DETERGENT • The dishwasher is fully loaded when you discover you're out of your usual powdered dishwashing detergent. What do you do? Make your own by combining 2 tablespoons (30 ml) baking soda with 2 tablespoons (30 ml) borax. You may be so pleased with the results you'll switch for good.

DEODORIZE YOUR DISHWASHER • Eliminate odors inside your automatic dishwasher by sprinkling ½ cup (125 ml) baking soda on the bottom of the dishwasher between loads. Or pour in half a box of baking soda and run the empty machine through its rinse cycle.

more BAKING SODA over →

CLEAN YOUR REFRIGERATOR • To get rid of smells and dried spills inside your refrigerator, remove the contents, then sprinkle some baking soda on a damp sponge and scrub the sides, shelves, and compartments. Rinse with a clean, wet sponge and place a fresh box of baking soda inside afterwards.

CLEAN YOUR MICROWAVE • To clean those splatters inside your microwave, put a solution of 2 tablespoons (30 ml) baking soda in 1 cup (250 ml) water in a microwave-safe container and heat on High for 2 to 3 minutes. Remove the container from the microwave and wipe down the moist interior with a damp paper towel.

REMOVE COFFEE AND TEA STAINS FROM CHINA • Don't let those annoying coffee or tea stains on your good china spoil another special occasion. Remove them by dipping a moist cloth in baking soda to form a stiff paste and gently rubbing your cups and saucers. Rinse clean and then dry.

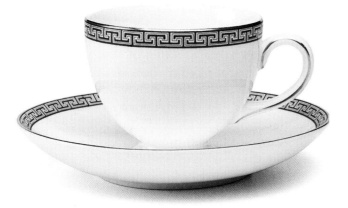

CLEAN A THERMOS • To remove residue on the inside of a thermos, mix ¼ cup (50 g) baking soda in 4 cups (1 L) water. Fill the thermos with the solution—if necessary, give it a going-over with a bottlebrush to loosen things up. Let it soak overnight and rinse clean before using.

FRESHEN A SPONGE OR TOWEL • When a kitchen sponge or dishtowel gets that distinctly sour smell, soak it overnight in 2 tablespoons (30 ml) baking soda and a couple of drops of antibacterial dishwashing liquid dissolved in 2 cups (500 ml) warm water. The following morning, squeeze out the remaining solution and rinse with cold water. It should smell as good as new.

REMOVE OLD STAINS AND SCRATCHES ON COUNTERTOPS • Use a paste of 2 parts baking soda to 1 part water to 'rub out' stains and scratches. For stubborn stains, add a drop of chlorine bleach to the paste. Immediately wash the area with hot, soapy water to prevent the bleach from causing fading.

SHINE UP STAINLESS STEEL AND CHROME TRIM • To put the shine back in your stainless steel sink, sprinkle it with baking soda and give it a rubdown—moving in the direction of the grain—with a moist cloth. To polish dull chrome trim on your appliances, pour a bit of baking soda on a damp sponge and rub over the chrome. Let it dry for an hour or so, then wipe it down with warm water and dry with a clean cloth.

GET RID OF GREASE STAINS ON STOVETOPS • To get rid of grease stains, first wet them with a little water and cover them with a bit of baking soda. Then rub the stains off with a damp sponge.

CLEAN AN AUTOMATIC COFFEEMAKER • Caring for your automatic coffeemaker means never having to worry about bitter or weak coffee. Every two weeks or so, brew a pot of 4 cups (1 L) water mixed with ¼ cup (50 g) baking soda, followed by a pot of clean water. Sweeten your coffee maker's plastic basket by using an old toothbrush to give it an occasional scrubbing with a paste of 2 tablespoons (30 ml) baking soda and 1 tablespoon (15 ml) water. Rinse thoroughly with cold water when you're done.

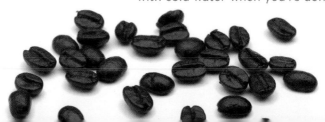

POTS AND PANS

REMOVE STAINS FROM NONSTICK COOKWARE • It may be called nonstick cookware, but a few of those stains seem to be stuck on pretty well. Blast them away by boiling 1 cup (250 ml) water mixed with 2 tablespoons (30 ml) baking soda and ½ cup (125 ml) vinegar for 10 minutes. Wash in hot, soapy water, rinse well and allow to dry. Season with a bit of olive oil.

CLEAN CAST-IRON COOKWARE • It's more prone to stains and rust than nonstick pans, but you can remove even the toughest burned-on food remnants in cast-iron pots. Boil 4 cups (1 L) water with 2 tablespoons (30 ml) baking soda for 5 minutes. Pour off most of the liquid, then lightly scrub it with a plastic scouring pad. Rinse well, dry and season with a few drops of vegetable oil.

CLEAN BURNED OR SCORCHED POTS AND PANS • It usually takes heavy-duty scrubbing to get burned food off the bottom of a pot or pan. But you can make life much easier for yourself by simply boiling a few cups of water (enough to get the pan one-quarter full), adding 5 tablespoons (75 ml) baking soda. Turn off the heat and let the mixture set for a few hours or overnight. When you're ready, that burned-on gunk will practically slip right off.

CARE FOR YOUR COFFEEPOTS AND TEAPOTS • Remove mineral deposits in metal coffeepots and teapots with a solution of 1 cup (250 ml) vinegar and 4 tablespoons (60 ml) baking soda. Bring to a boil and let simmer for 5 minutes. Or try boiling 5 cups (1.25 L) water with 2 tablespoons (30 ml) baking soda and the juice of half a lemon. Rinse with cold water when you're done. To remove annoying exterior stains, wash your pots with a plastic scouring pad in a solution ¼ cup (50 g) baking soda in 4 cups (1 L) warm water. Follow up with a cold-water rinse.

DEODORIZE YOUR GARBAGE CAN • If something smells 'off' in your kitchen, it's probably emanating from your garbage can. Some smells linger even after you dispose of the offending garbage, so make sure you give your kitchen garbage can a cleaning with a wet paper towel dipped in baking soda (wear an old pair of rubber gloves for this job). Rinse the can out with a damp sponge and let it dry before inserting a new bag. You can also ward off bad smells by sprinkling a bit of baking soda into the bottom of the can before inserting the bag.

around the house ● ● ●

REMOVE CRAYON MARKS FROM WALLS

Has a small child redecorated your walls or wallpaper with some original artworks in crayon? Don't lose your cool, just grab a damp rag, dip it in some baking soda and lightly scrub the marks. They should come off with a minimum of effort.

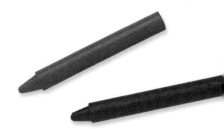

more BAKING SODA over →

WASH WALLPAPER • Wallpaper that's starting to look a bit dingy can be brightened up by wiping it with a rag or sponge moistened in a solution of 2 tablespoons (30 ml) baking soda in (1 L) of water. To remove grease stains from wallpaper, make a paste of 1 tablespoon (15 ml) baking soda and 1 teaspoon (5 ml) water. Rub it on the stain, let it sit for 5 to 10 minutes and rub off with a damp sponge.

CLEAN UP BABY VOMIT • Babies tend to regurgitate —and usually not at opportune moments. Never leave home without a small bottle of baking soda in your diaper bag. If your baby spits up on his or her (or your) shirt after feeding, simply brush off any solid matter, moisten a washcloth, dip it in a bit of baking soda and dab the spot. The odor (and the potential stain) will soon be gone.

DEODORIZE RUGS AND CARPETS • How's this for a simple way to freshen up your carpets or rugs? Lightly sprinkle them with baking soda, let it settle in for about 15 minutes, and vacuum it up.

REMOVE WINE AND GREASE STAINS FROM CARPET • It's bound to happen sometime. Someone drops a slab of butter or a glass of red wine on your beautiful white carpeting. Before you panic, get a paper towel and blot up as much of the stain as possible. Then sprinkle a liberal amount of baking soda over the spot. Give it at least an hour to absorb the stain and vacuum up the remaining powder.

FRESHEN UP MUSTY DRAWERS AND CLOSETS • Put baking soda sachets to work on persistent musty odors in dresser drawers, sideboards, or closets. Just fill the toe of a clean sock or stocking with 3–4 tablespoons (45–60 ml) baking soda, put a knot about 1 inch (2 cm) above the bulge and either hang it up or place it away in an unobtrusive corner. Use a few sachets in large spaces like closets and attic storage areas. Replace them every other month if needed. This treatment can also be used to rid closets of mothball smells.

Kids' Stuff

Make watercolor paints for your kids using ingredients in your kitchen.

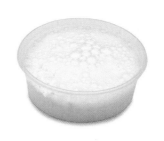

1 In a small bowl, mix 3 tablespoons (45 ml) each baking soda, cornstarch, and vinegar with 1 1/2 teaspoons (7 ml) light corn syrup. Wait for the fizzing to stop.

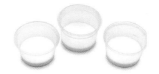

2 Then separate the mixture into several small containers or jar lids (with high edges).

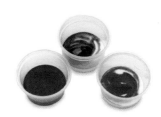

3 Add 8 drops of food coloring to each batch; mix well. Put a different color in each batch or combine colors to make new shades.

Kids can either use the paint right away or wait for them to harden, in which case, they'll need to use a wet brush before painting.

REMOVE MUSTY ODOR FROM BOOKS • If books that have been taken out of storage have a musty smell, place each one in a brown paper bag with 2 tablespoons (30 ml) baking soda. Don't shake the bag, just tie it up and let it sit in a dry place for about one week. When you open the bag, just shake off the remaining powder and the smell should be gone.

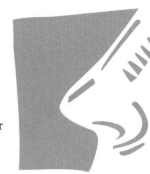

POLISH SILVER AND GOLD JEWELRY • To remove built-up tarnish from your silver, make a thick paste with ¼ cup (50 g) baking soda and 2 tablespoons (30 ml) water. Apply with a damp sponge and gently rub, rinse, and buff dry. To polish gold jewelry, cover with a light coating of baking soda, pour a bit of vinegar over it and rinse clean.

WARNING: Do not use this technique with jewelry containing pearls or gemstones, as it could damage their finish and loosen the glue.

GET YELLOW STAINS OFF PIANO KEYS

That old upright may still sound great, but those yellowed keys definitely hit a sour note. Remove age stains on your ivories by mixing a solution ¼ cup (50 g) baking soda in 4 cups (1 L) of warm water. Apply to each key with a dampened cloth (you can place a thin piece of cardboard between the keys to avoid seepage). Wipe again with a cloth dampened with plain water and buff dry with a clean cloth. (You can also clean piano keys with lemon juice and salt.)

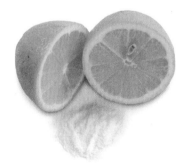

REMOVE STAINS FROM FIREPLACE BRICKS • You may need to use a bit of elbow grease, but you can clean the smoke stains off your fireplace bricks by washing them with a solution of ½ cup (125 g) baking soda in 4 cups (1 L) warm water.

BATHROOM BLITZ

CLEAN BATHTUBS AND SINKS • Get the gunk off old porcelain bathtubs and sinks by applying a paste of 2 parts baking soda and 1 part hydrogen peroxide. Let the paste sit for about half an hour. Then give it a good scrubbing and rinse well. The paste will also sweeten your drain as it washes down.

REMOVE MINERAL DEPOSITS FROM SHOWER HEADS • Get rid of hard water deposits on a showerhead by covering the head with a tough sandwich bag filled with ¼ cup (50 g) baking soda and 1 cup (250 ml) vinegar. Loosely fasten the bag—you need to let some of the gas escape—with adhesive tape or a large twist tie. Let the solution work its magic for about an hour, remove the bag, and turn on your shower to wash off any remaining debris. Not only will the deposits disappear, but your showerhead will be back to its old shining self!

ABSORB BATHROOM ODORS • Keep your bathroom smelling fresh and clean by placing a decorative dish filled with ½ cup (125 g) baking soda either on top of the toilet tank or on the floor behind the bowl. You can also make your own bathroom deodorizers by setting out dishes containing equal parts baking soda and your favorite scented bath salts.

TIDY UP YOUR TOILET BOWL • Instead of using chemicals to clean your toilet bowl, just pour half a box of baking soda into the tank once a month. Let it stand overnight, then give it a few flushes in the morning. This actually cleans both the tank and the bowl. You can also pour 2-3 tablespoons (30-45 ml) baking soda directly into the toilet bowl and scrub any stains. Wait a few minutes, then flush them away.

more BAKING SODA over →

REMOVE WHITE MARKS ON WOOD SURFACES •
Remove those white marks—caused by hot cups
or sweating glasses—on your coffee table or other
wooden furniture by making a paste of 1 tablespoon
(15 ml) baking soda and 1 teaspoon (5 ml) water.
Gently rub the spot in a circular motion until it
disappears. Remember don't use too much water.

SHINE MARBLE-TOPPED FURNITURE • Revitalize
the marble top on a coffee table or counter by
washing it with a soft cloth dipped in a solution of
3 tablespoons (45 ml) baking soda and 4 cups (1 L)
warm water. Let it stand for 15 minutes to a half an
hour, rinse with plain water, and wipe dry.

REMOVE CIGARETTE ODORS FROM FURNITURE •
To eliminate the unpleasant lingering smells
that cigarette or cigar smoke leaves on your
upholstered furniture, lightly sprinkle your chairs
or couches with some baking soda. Let it sit for a
few hours and vacuum it off.

in the medicine cabinet

TREAT MINOR BURNS • If you sustain a minor skin
burn, quickly pour some baking soda into a container
of ice water, soak a cloth or gauze pad in it, and apply
it to the burn. Keep applying the solution until the
burn no longer feels hot. This treatment will also
prevent many burns from blistering.

**COOL OFF SUNBURN AND OTHER SKIN
IRRITATIONS •** For quick relief of sunburn pain,
soak gauze pads or large cotton balls in a solution of
4 tablespoons (60 ml) baking soda mixed in 1 cup
(125 ml) water and apply it to the affected areas. For
a bad sunburn on legs or torso—or for the itching of
chicken pox—take a lukewarm bath with a half to a
full box of baking soda added to the running water.
To ease the sting of razor burns, dab your skin with
a cotton ball soaked in a solution of 1 tablespoon
(15 ml) baking soda in 1 cup (125 ml) water.

SOOTHE POISON IVY RASHES • If you have an
unplanned encounter with poison ivy when
gardening or camping, stop the itch by making a
thick paste from 3 teaspoons (15 ml) baking soda and
1 teaspoon (5 ml) water and apply it to the affected
areas. You can also use baking soda to treat oozing
blisters caused by the rash. Mix 2 teaspoons (10 ml)

baking soda in 4 cups (1 L) water and saturate a few
sterile gauze pads. Cover the blisters with the wet
pads for 10 minutes, four times a day.
WARNING: Do not apply on or near your eyes.

MAKE A SALVE FOR BEE STINGS • Take the
pain out of that bee sting—fast. Make a paste of
1 teaspoon (5 ml) baking soda mixed with drops of
cool water and let it dry on the affected area.

> **CAUTION: Many people have severe
> allergic reactions to bee stings.
> If you have difficulty breathing
> or notice a dramatic swelling,
> seek medical attention at once.**

CONTROL YOUR DANDRUFF • To get dandruff under
control, wet your hair and rub a handful of baking
soda vigorously into your scalp. Rinse thoroughly and
dry. Do this every time you normally wash your hair,
but only use baking soda, not shampoo. Your hair
may dry out at first, but after a few weeks your scalp
will start producing natural oils, leaving your hair
softer and free of flaking skin.

Baking soda and shelf life

How can you tell if the baking soda you've had stashed away in the back of your pantry is still fresh and safe to use?

Just pour out a small amount—a little less than a teaspoon—and add a few drops of vinegar or fresh lemon juice. If it doesn't fizz, it's time to replace it with a new box. By the way, a sealed box of baking soda has an average shelf life of 18 months, while an opened box lasts 6 months.

REMOVE BUILT-UP GEL, HAIR SPRAY, OR CONDITIONER FROM HAIR • When it comes to personal grooming, too much of a good thing can spell bad news for your hair. But a thorough cleansing with baking soda at least once a week will wash all of the gunk out of your hair. Simply add 1 tablespoon (15 ml) baking soda to your hair while shampooing. In addition to removing all the chemicals you put in your hair, it will wash away water impurities and may even lighten your hair.

CLEAN COMBS AND BRUSHES • Freshen up your combs and hairbrushes by soaking them in a solution of 3 cups (750 ml) warm water and 2 teaspoons (10 ml) baking soda. Swirl them around in the water to loosen up all the debris caught between the teeth, and let them soak for about half an hour. Rinse well and let dry thoroughly before using.

USE AS A GARGLE OR MOUTHWASH • The morning after the night you ate too much garlic can be tricky. Try gargling with 1 teaspoon (5 ml) baking soda in a half a glass of water. The baking soda will neutralize the odors on contact. When used as a mouthwash, baking soda will also relieve pain from a mouth ulcer.

BICARB FOR BABIES

FIGHT DIAPER RASH • You can safely and easily soothe your baby's painful diaper rash by adding a couple of tablespoons of baking soda to a lukewarm—not hot—bath. However, if the rash persists, or worsens after several treatments, consult a pediatrician.

COMBAT CRADLE CAP • Cradle cap is a commonplace, and typically harmless, condition in many infants. An old but often effective way to treat it is to make a paste of about 3 teaspoons (15 ml) baking soda and 1 teaspoon (5 ml) water. Apply it to a baby's scalp about an hour before bedtime and rinse it off the next morning, but do not use it with shampoo. You may need to apply it consecutive nights before the cradle cap recedes. *(See page 67 for ways to treat cradle cap with baby oil.)*

SCRUB TEETH AND CLEAN DENTURES • If you run out of your usual toothpaste, or if you're looking for an all-natural alternative to commercial toothpaste, just dip your wet toothbrush in some baking soda, brush and rinse as usual. You can also use baking soda to clean mouthpieces and dentures. Use a solution of 1 tablespoon (15 ml) baking soda dissolved in 1 cup (250 ml) warm water. Let the object soak for half an hour and rinse well before using.

CLEAN AND SWEETEN TOOTHBRUSHES • Keep your family's toothbrushes squeaky clean by immersing them in a solution of ¼ cup (50 g) baking soda and ¼ cup (50 ml) water. Let brushes soak overnight about once every week or two. Make sure you give them a good rinsing before using.

more BAKING SODA over →

USE AS AN ANTIPERSPIRANT • Looking for an effective, all-natural deodorant? Try applying a small amount—about 1 teaspoon (5 ml)—baking soda under each arm with a powder puff. You won't smell like a flower or some exotic spice, but then you won't smell like the locker room after the big game either.

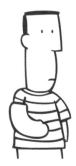

RELIEVE ITCHING INSIDE A CAST • Having a plaster cast on your arm or leg is a misery any time of year, but wearing one during summer can be torture. The sweating and itchiness you feel underneath that 'shell' can drive a person insane. Find temporary relief by using a hair dryer–on the coolest setting–to blow a bit of baking soda down the edges of the cast. It's a good idea, though, to have someone help you, to avoid getting the powder in your eyes.

ALLEVIATE ATHLETE'S FOOT • You can deploy wet or dry baking soda to combat a case of athlete's foot. First, try dusting your feet (along with your socks and shoes) with dry baking soda to dry out the infection. If that doesn't work, make a paste of 1 teaspoon (5 ml) baking soda and ½ teaspoon (2 ml) water and rub it between your toes. Let it dry and wash it off after 15 minutes. Dry your feet thoroughly afterwards.

SOOTHE TIRED, STINKY FEET • When your feet are hot, tired and aching, treat them to a soothing bath of 4 tablespoons (60 ml) baking soda in 4 cups (1 L) warm water. Besides relaxing your aching feet, baking soda will remove the sweat and lint between the toes. Regular footbaths can also be an effective treatment for persistent foot odor.

DEODORIZE SHOES AND SNEAKERS

A smelly shoe or sneaker is no match for the power of baking soda. Liberally sprinkle some into the offending shoe and let it sit overnight. Shake out the powder in the morning. (Be careful when using baking soda with leather shoes, as repeated applications can dry them out.) You can also make reusable 'odor eaters' by filling the toes of old socks with 2 tablespoons (30 ml) baking soda and tying them up in a knot. Stuff the socks into each shoe at night before retiring. Remove the socks in the morning and you'll breathe easier.

SCIENCE **WORKS!**

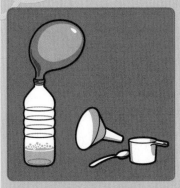

Use the gas produced by mixing baking soda and vinegar to blow up a balloon.

First, pour ½ cup (125 ml) vinegar into the bottom of a narrow-necked bottle (such as an empty water bottle) or jar. Insert a funnel into the mouth of an average-size balloon and fill it with ⅓ cup (75 g) baking soda. Carefully stretch the mouth of the balloon over the opening of the bottle, then gently lift it up so that the baking soda empties into the vinegar at the bottom of the bottle. The fizzing and foaming you see is actually a chemical reaction between the two ingredients. This reaction results in the release of carbon dioxide gas–which will soon inflate the balloon!

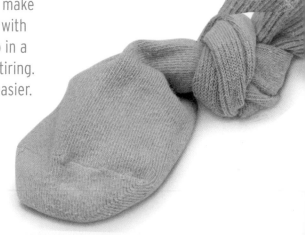

in the laundry

BOOST STRENGTH OF LIQUID DETERGENT AND BLEACH • It may sound like a cliché, but adding ½ cup (125 g) baking soda to your usual amount of liquid laundry detergent really will give you 'whiter whites' and brighter colors. The baking soda also softens the water, so you can actually use less detergent. Adding ½ cup (125 g) of baking soda in top-loading machines (¼ cup/50 g) for front-loaders) also increases the potency of bleach, so you need only half the usual amount of bleach.

REMOVE MOTHBALL SMELL FROM CLOTHES

If your clothes come out of storage reeking of mothballs, take heed: Adding ½ cup (125 g) baking soda during your washing machine's rinse cycle will get rid of the smell.

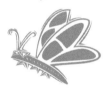

WASH NEW BABY CLOTHES • Get all of the chemicals out of newborn baby's clothing—without using any harsh detergents. Wash new baby clothes with some mild soap and ½ cup (125 g) baking soda.

RUB OUT PERSPIRATION AND OTHER STAINS • Pre-treat clothes with a paste made from 4 tablespoons (60 ml) baking soda and ¼ cup (50 ml) warm water can help vanquish a variety of stains. For example, rub it into shirts to remove perspiration stains. For really bad stains, let the paste dry for about 2 hours before washing. Rub out tar stains by applying the paste and washing in plain baking soda. For collar stains, rub in the paste and add a bit of vinegar when you put the shirt in the wash.

WASH MILDEWED SHOWER CURTAINS • If your plastic shower curtain or liner gets dirty or mildewed you don't have have to throw it away. Try cleaning it in your washing machine with two bath towels on gentle setting. Add ½ cup (125 g) cup baking soda to your detergent during the wash cycle and ½ cup (125 ml) cup vinegar during the rinse cycle. Allow it to drip-dry; don't put it in the dryer.

for the do-it-yourselfer

CLEAN BATTERY TERMINALS • Eliminate the corrosive buildup on your car's battery terminals by scrubbing them clean using an old toothbrush and a mixture of 3 tablespoons (45 ml) baking soda along 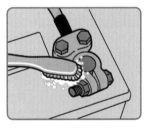 with 1 tablespoon (15 ml) warm water. Wipe them off with a wet towel and dry with another towel. Once the terminals have completely dried, apply a bit of petroleum jelly around each terminal, to deter future corrosive buildup.

USE AS DEICER IN WINTER

Salt can stain–or actually eat away–the concrete around your house. For an equally effective, but completely innocuous, way to melt the ice on your steps and paths during cold winter months, try sprinkling them with generous amounts of baking soda. You can also add some sand for improved traction.

more BAKING SODA over →

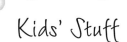

Kids' Stuff

Spies use it and so can you. Send a message or draw a picture with invisible ink. Here's how to do it. Mix 1 tablespoon (15 ml) each baking soda and water. Dip a toothpick or paintbrush in the mixture and write your message or draw a picture or design on a piece of plain white paper. Let the paper and the 'ink' dry completely. To reveal your message or see your picture, mix 6 drops food coloring with 1 tablespoon (15 ml) water. Dip a clean paintbrush in the solution and lightly paint over the paper. Use different food coloring combinations for a really cool effect.

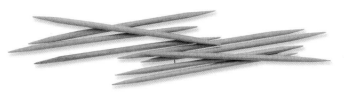

GIVE YOUR DECK THE WEATHERED LOOK • You can instantly give your wooden deck a weathered look by washing it in a solution of 2 cups (500 g) baking soda in 1 gallon (4 L) water. Use a stiff straw brush to work the solution into the wood and rinse with cool water.

TIGHTEN CANE CHAIR SEATS • The bottoms of cane chairs can start to sag with age, but it's possible to tighten them up again easily enough. Just soak two cloths in a solution of ½ cup (125 g) baking soda in 4 cups (1 L) hot water. Saturate the top surface of the caning with one cloth, while pushing the second up against the bottom of the caning to saturate the underside. Use a clean, dry cloth to soak up the excess moisture and put the chair in the sun to dry.

REMOVE TAR FROM YOUR CAR • It may look pretty bad, but it's not that hard to get road tar off your car without damaging the paint. Make a soft paste of 3 parts baking soda to 1 part water and apply to the tar spots with a damp cloth. Let it dry for 5 minutes, then rinse clean.

CLEAN AIR CONDITIONER FILTERS • Clean washable air conditioner filters each month they're in use. First vacuum off as much dust and dirt as possible, then wash in a solution of 1 tablespoon (15 ml) baking soda in 4 cups (1 L) water. Let the filters dry thoroughly before replacing.

KEEP YOUR HUMIDIFIER ODOR-FREE • Kill musty smells in a humidifier by adding 2 tablespoons (30 ml) baking soda to the water each time it's changed. **WARNING: Check your owner's manual or consult the unit's manufacturer before trying this.**

in the great outdoors

KEEP WEEDS OUT OF CEMENT CRACKS • Looking for a safe way to keep weeds and grasses from growing in the cracks of your paved patios, driveways, and paths? Sprinkle a few handfuls of baking soda on the concrete and simply sweep it into the cracks. The added sodium will make it much less hospitable to dandelions and their friends.

CLEAN RESIN GARDEN FURNITURE • Most commercial cleaners are too abrasive to be used on resin garden furniture. But you won't have to worry about scratching or dulling the surface if you clean your resin furniture with a wet sponge dipped in baking soda. Wipe using circular motions and rinse well.

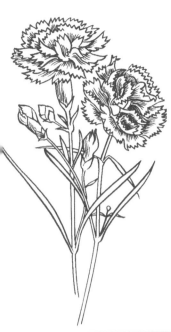

USE AS PLANT FOOD • Give your flowering, alkaline-loving plants, such as clematis, delphiniums, and dianthus an occasional shower in a mild solution of 1 tablespoon (15 ml) baking soda in 8 cups (2 L) water. They'll give a show with fuller, healthier blooms.

MAINTAIN PROPER POOL ALKALINITY • Add 2¾ cups (680 g) baking soda for every 10,000 gallons (38,000 L) water in your swimming pool to raise the total alkalinity by 10 ppm (parts per million). Most pools require alkalinity in the 80–150 ppm range. Maintaining the right pool alkalinity level is vital for minimizing changes in pH if acidic or basic pool chemicals or contaminants are introduced into the water.

SCOUR BARBECUE GRATES • Keep your barbecue grate in top condition by making a soft paste of ¼ cup (50 g) baking soda and ¼ cup (50 ml) water. Apply the paste with a wire brush and let dry for 15 minutes. Then wipe it down with a dry cloth and place the grate over the hot coals for at least 15 minutes to burn off remaining residue before placing any food on it.

for your pet

MAKE DEODORIZING DOG SHAMPOO • The next time your dog rolls around in the compost heap, pull out the baking soda to freshen him up. Just rub a few handfuls of the powder into his coat and give it a thorough brushing. In addition to removing the smell, it will leave his coat shiny and clean.

WASH INSIDE PETS' EARS • If your pet constantly scratches her ears, it could indicate the presence of an irritation or ear mites. Ease the itch (and wipe out any mites) by using a cotton ball dipped in a solution of 1 teaspoon (5 ml) baking soda in 1 cup (250 ml) warm water to gently wash the insides of her ears.

DEODORIZE THE LITTER BOX • Don't waste money on expensive deodorized cat litter, just put a thin layer of baking soda under the bargain-brand litter to absorb the odor. Or mix baking soda with the litter as you're changing it.

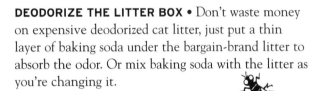

KEEP INSECTS AWAY FROM PETS' DISHES

Placing a border of baking soda around your pet's food bowls will keep away six-legged intruders. And it won't harm your pet if he happens to lap up a little (though most pets aren't likely to savor baking soda's bitter taste).

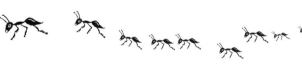

BALLOONS

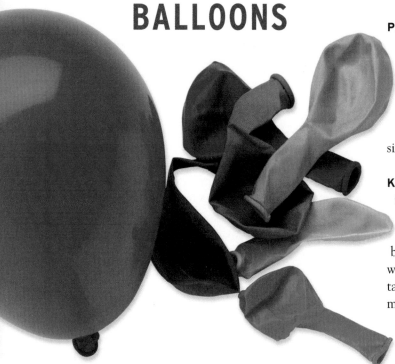

PROTECT A BANDAGED FINGER • Bandaging a minor injury on your finger is easy, but keeping the bandage dry as you go about you business can be a different story. Here's the secret to skipping those wet-bandage changes: Just slip a small balloon over your finger when doing dishes, bathing or even simply washing your hands.

KEEP TRACK OF YOUR CHILD • Those inexpensive, floating, helium-filled balloons sold in most shopping centers can be more than just a treat for a small child; they could be invaluable in locating a child who tends to wander off into a crowd. Even if you keep close tabs on your kids, you can buy a little peace of mind by simply tying (though not too tightly) a balloon to a young child's wrist on those weekend shopping trips.

MAKE A PARTY INVITATION • Here's an imaginative invitation! Inflate a balloon (for the purpose of cleanliness, use an electric pump, if possible). Pinch off the end, but don't tie a knot in it. Write your invitation details on the balloon with a bright permanent marker, making sure the ink is dry before you deflate it. Place the balloon in an envelope and mail one out to each guest. When your guests receive it, they'll have to blow it up to see what it says.

TRANSPORT CUT FLOWERS • Don't bother with awkward, water-filled plastic bags and that sort of thing when you're traveling with freshly cut flowers. Simply fill up a balloon with about ½ cup (125 ml) water and slip it over the cut stem ends of your flowers. Wrap a rubber band several times around the mouth of the balloon to keep it from slipping off.

USE AS A HAT MOLD • To keep the shape in your freshly washed knitted beanie or cloth hat, fit it over an inflated balloon while it dries. You can use a piece of masking tape to stop the balloon from tilting over or falling onto the ground.

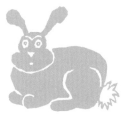

REPEL UNWANTED GARDEN VISITORS

Put those old, deflated, shiny metallic balloons—the ones lying around your house from past birthday parties—to work in your garden. Cut them into vertical strips and hang them from bamboo garden stakes placed around your vegetables and attach them to your fruit trees to scare off invading birds, rabbits, and deer.

SCIENCE **WORKS!**

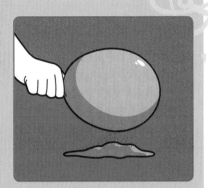

You experience a discharge of static electricity when you touch a doorknob after shuffling across a carpet. However, you rarely see this phenomenon, which is static electricity on a grand scale, with the exception of lightning. Here's an experiment that offers a dazzling display of static electricity in action.

Empty the contents of a packet of unflavored gelatine powder onto a piece of paper. Blow up a balloon, rub it on a woolen sweater and then hold it about 3/4 inch (2 cm) above the powder. The gelatine particles will arch up towards the balloon. The slightly negatively charged electrons—the builtup static electricity on the balloon—are attracting the positively charged protons in the gelatine powder.

MARK YOUR CAMPSITE • On your next camping trip, bring along a few helium-filled balloonsto attach to your tent or a post. They'll make it easier for the members of your party to locate your campsite when hiking or foraging in the woods.

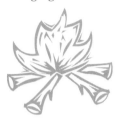

PROTECT A RIFLE • If you are a licensed gun owner, you already know that a dirty rifle can jam up and be dangerous to use. You can keep dust and debris from accumulating in your rifle barrel by putting a sturdy latex balloon over the barrel's front end.

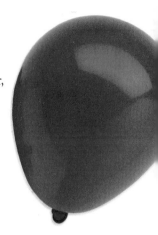

COLD-AIR BALLOONS!

MAKE AN ICE PACK • Looking for a flexible ice pack you can use for everything from soothing a sore back to keeping food cold in a cooler? Just fill a large, extra-strong balloon with as much water as you need and put it in your freezer. You can even mold it to a certain extent into specific shapes—for example, put it under something flat like a box of frozen spinach if you want a flat ice pack for your back. Use smaller latex balloons for making smaller ice packs for lunch boxes.

FREEZE FOR PARTY PUNCH • To keep your party punch bowl cold and well filled, pour juice in several balloons (using a funnel) and place them in your freezer. When it's party time, peel the latex off the ice and periodically drop a couple into the punch bowl.

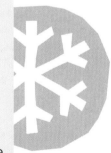

more BALLOONS over →

BANANAS

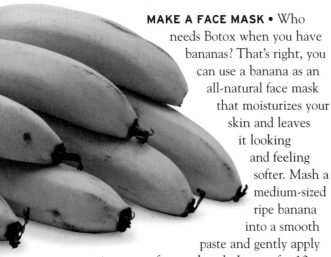

MAKE A FACE MASK • Who needs Botox when you have bananas? That's right, you can use a banana as an all-natural face mask that moisturizes your skin and leaves it looking and feeling softer. Mash a medium-sized ripe banana into a smooth paste and gently apply it to your face and neck. Let set for 10 to 20 minutes and rinse off with cold water. Another popular mask recipe uses ¼ cup (50 ml) plain yogurt, 2 tablespoons (30 ml) honey and 1 medium banana, mixed together.

EAT A FROZEN BANANA • As a summer treat for friends and family, peel and cut four ripe bananas in half (across the middle). Stick a wooden popsicle stick into the flat end of each piece. Place them all on a piece of waxed paper and put in the freezer. A few hours later, serve them up as yummy frozen treats. If you want to go all out, quickly dip your frozen bananas in ¾ cup (170 g) melted white chocolate or milk chocolate (chopped nuts or shredded coconut are optional) and refreeze.

TENDERIZE A ROAST • Banana leaves are used in many Asian countries to wrap meat while it's cooking to make it more tender. And some people claim that the banana itself also has the same ability. So the next time you're cooking a roast, add a ripe, peeled banana to the baking dish.

POLISH SILVERWARE AND LEATHER SHOES • Using a banana peel is actually a great way to put the shine back on your silverware and leather shoes. First, remove any of the leftover stringy material from the inside of the peel, then just start rubbing the inside of the peel on your shoes or silver. When you're done, buff with a paper towel or soft cloth. You might even want to use this technique to restore your leather furniture. Test it on a small section first before you take on the whole piece.

ATTRACT BUTTERFLIES AND BIRDS • Bring more butterflies and various bird species to your backyard by putting out overripe bananas (as well as other fruit such as mangos and oranges) on a raised platform. Punch a few holes in the bananas to make the fruit more accessible to the butterflies. Some enthusiasts swear by adding a drop of Gatorade to further mush things up. The fruit is also likely to attract more bees and wasps as well, so make sure that the platform is well above head level and not centrally located. Moreover, you'll probably want to clear it off before sunset, to discourage visits from raccoons and other nocturnal creatures.

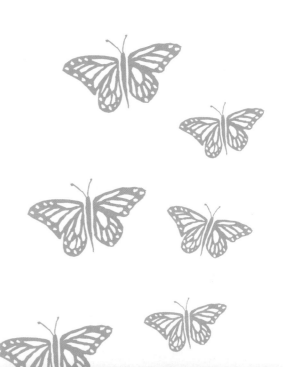

FOR THOSE WITH GREEN FINGERS ...

BRIGHTEN UP HOUSE PLANTS • Are the leaves on your houseplants looking dingy or dusty? Don't bother misting them with water—that just spreads the dirt around. Instead, wipe down each leaf with the inside of a banana peel. It'll remove all the gunk on the surface and replace it with a clean, lustrous shine.

DETER APHIDS • If aphids are attacking your rosebushes or other plants, bury dried or cut-up banana peels a few inches deep around the base of the plants, and the aphids soon will leave. Don't use whole peels or bananas themselves, though; they tend to be viewed as tasty treats by possums, racoons, rabbits, and other animals, who will just dig them up.

USE AS FERTILIZER OR MULCH • Banana peels, like the fruit itself, are rich in potassium—an important nutrient for both you and your garden. Dry out banana peels on screens during the winter months. In early spring, grind them up in a food processor or blender and use the mixture as a mulch to give new plants and seedlings a healthy start. Many cultivars of roses and other plants, like staghorn ferns, also benefit from the nutrients found in banana peels. Simply cut up some peels and use them as plant food around established plants.

ADD TO COMPOST PILE • With their high content of potassium and phosphorus, whole bananas and peels are welcome additions to any compost pile—particularly in so-called compost tea recipes (made by brewing compost in water for a couple of days to produce energy-rich liquid). The fruit breaks down especially fast in hot temperatures. But don't forget to remove any stickers from the peels, and make sure you bury bananas deep within your compost pile—otherwise they could turn out to be a meal for a four-legged visitor.

BASTERS

POUR PERFECT BATTER • To make picture-perfect pancakes, cookies, and muffins, simply fill your baster with batter so that you can pour just the right amount in a frying pan, on a cookie sheet, or in a muffin tin.

REMOVE EXCESS WATER FROM A COFFEEMAKER • The perfect cup of coffee is determined by using the proper balance of water and ground coffee in your automatic coffeemaker. If you pour in too much water, you'll have to add more coffee or suffer through a weak pot. But there's another, often overlooked option, which is to simply use your kitchen baster to remove the excess water and bring it down to just the right level.

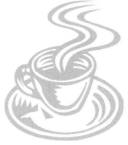

WATER HARD-TO-REACH PLANTS • Do you get drips all over yourself, the floor, or furniture when trying to water hanging plants or other difficult-to-reach houseplants? Instead, fill a baster with water and squeeze it directly into the pot. You can also use a baster to water a Christmas tree and to add small, precise amounts of water to cups containing seedlings or germinating seeds.

REFRESH WATER IN FLOWER ARRANGEMENTS • It's a well-known fact that cut flowers last longer with periodic water changes. But pouring out the old water and adding the new is not a particularly easy or pleasant task—unless, that is, you use a baster to suck out the old water and squirt in the fresh water.

more BASTERS over →

TRANSFER PAINTS AND SOLVENTS • The toughest part of any touch-up paint job is pouring the paint from a large can into a small cup or container. To avoid the inevitable spills, and just to make life easier in general, use a baster to take the paint out of the paint can. In fact, it's a good idea to make a baster a permanent addition to your workshop for transferring any solvents, varnishes, and other liquid chemicals.

CURE A MUSTY-SMELLING AIR CONDITIONER • If you detect a musty odor blowing out of the vents of your room air conditioner, chances are it's caused by a clogged drain hole. First, unscrew the front of the unit and find the drain hole. It's usually located under the barrier between the evaporator and compressor, or under the evaporator. Use a bent wire hanger to clear away any obstacles in the hole or use a baster to flush it clean. You may also need

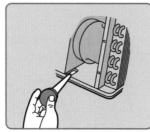

to use the baster to remove any water that may be pooling up at the bottom of the unit to gain access to the drain.

FIX A LEAKY REFRIGERATOR • Is water leaking inside your refrigerator? The most likely cause is a blocked drain tube. This plastic tube runs from a drain hole in the back of the freezer compartment along the back of your fridge and drains into an evaporation pan underneath. Try forcing hot water through the drain hole in the freezer with a baster. If you can't access the drain hole, try disconnecting the tube on the back to blow water through it. After clearing the tube, pour 1 teaspoon (5 ml) ammonia or bleach into the drain hole to prevent a recurrence of algae spores, which are the probable culprit.

CREATURE COMFORTS

PLACE WATER IN YOUR PET'S BOWL • Are you getting tired of chasing the bunny, guinea pig, or other caged pet around the house whenever you change its water? Use a baster to fill the water dish. You can usually fit the baster between the slats without having to open the cage.

CLEAN YOUR FISH TANK • A baster makes it incredibly easy to change the water in your fish tank or to freshen it up a bit. Simply use the baster to suck up the greenish gunk that tends to collect in the corners and in the gravel at the bottom of your fish tank.

BLOW AWAY ROACHES AND ANTS • If you've had it with sharing your living quarters with roaches or ants, give them the heave-ho by sprinkling boric acid (borax) along any cracks or crevices where you've spotted the intruders. Use a baster to blow small amounts of the powder into hard-to-reach corners and any deep voids you come across. However, keep in mind that boric acid can be toxic if ingested by young children or pets, so keep it out of their reach.

CAUTION: Never use your kitchen baster for tasks such as cleaning out a fish tank or spreading or transferring chemicals. Basters are staples at discount stores so it's worth a visit to pick up a few to keep around the house specifically for noncooking jobs. Label them with a piece of masking tape to make sure you always use the same baster for the same task.

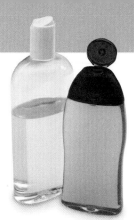

BATH OIL

REMOVE GLUE FROM LABELS OR BANDAGES

Get rid of those sticky leftover adhesive marks from bandages, price tags, and labels. Rub them away with a bit of bath oil applied to a cotton ball. It works well on glass, metal, and most plastics.

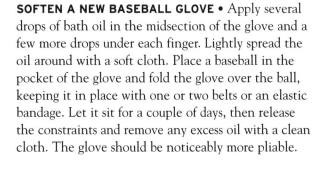

PRY APART STUCK DRINKING GLASSES • When moisture seeps in between stacked glasses, separating them can get mighty tough—not to mention being dangerous. But you can break the seal by applying a few drops of bath oil along the sides of the glasses. Give the oil a few minutes to work its way down and simply slide your glasses apart.

LOOSEN CHEWING GUM FROM HAIR AND CARPETING • If your child comes home with chewing gum in his or her hair—or tracks a wad on your rug or carpet—hold off on reaching for the scissors. Instead, rub a liberal amount of bath oil into the gum. It should loosen it up enough to comb it out. On a carpet, test the oil on an inconspicuous area before applying to the spot with gum on it.

REMOVE SCUFF MARKS • You can get those annoying scuff marks off your patent leather shoes or handbags just by applying a bit of bath oil to a clean, soft cloth or towel. Gently rub in the oil and polish with another dry towel.

USE AS A HOT-OIL TREATMENT • Heat ½ cup (125 ml) bath oil mixed with ½ cup (125 ml) water on High in your microwave for 30 seconds. Place the solution in a deep bowl and soak your fingers or toes in it for 10 to 15 minutes to soften cuticles or calluses. After drying, use a pumice stone to smooth over calluses or a file to push down cuticles. Follow up by rubbing in hand cream until it is fully absorbed.

SOFTEN A NEW BASEBALL GLOVE • Apply several drops of bath oil in the midsection of the glove and a few more drops under each finger. Lightly spread the oil around with a soft cloth. Place a baseball in the pocket of the glove and fold the glove over the ball, keeping it in place with one or two belts or an elastic bandage. Let it sit for a couple of days, then release the constraints and remove any excess oil with a clean cloth. The glove should be noticeably more pliable.

CLEAN GREASE OR OIL FROM SKIN • It doesn't take much tinkering around the inside of a car or mower engine to get your hands coated in grease or oil. But before you reach for any heavy-duty grease removers, rub a few squirts of bath oil onto your hands and wash them in warm, soapy water. It works, and it's a lot easier on the skin than harsh chemicals.

DID YOU KNOW?

It appears we *Homo sapiens* have had a penchant for perfumed body oils since the beginning of history. The first use of such oils is believed to have occurred in the Neolithic period (7000-4000 B.C.), when Stone Age people began combining olive and sesame seed oils with fragrant plants. The ancient Egyptians also used scented oils, primarily in religious rituals. And the use of body oils, such as myrrh and frankincense, for both religious and secular uses is documented in the Bible. Indeed, fragrant oils have been an integral part of most cultures—including those of Native Americans and many Asian peoples.

more BATH OIL over →

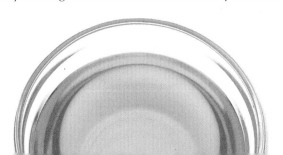

REVITALIZE VINYL UPHOLSTERY • Give your car's dreary-looking vinyl upholstery a makeover by using a small amount of bath oil on a soft cloth to wipe down the seats, dashboard, armrests, and other surfaces. Polish with a clean cloth to remove any excess oil. As an added bonus, a scented bath oil will make the interior smell better, too.

SLIDE TOGETHER PIPE JOINTS • If you can't find the all-purpose lubricating oil or the WD-40 when you're trying to join pipes together, a few drops of bath oil should provide sufficient lubrication to fit the pipe joints together with ease.

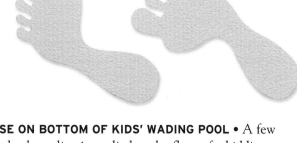

BATHTUB APPLIQUÉS

PLACE ON THE BOTTOM OF PC CASES • Has your desktop computer's case lost its 'legs'—those small rubber feet that invariably fall off over time from moving your computer around? To steady the casing, and to minimize vibrations, cut small squares from a nonslip bathtub appliqué and apply them to the four bottom corners of the computer's case.

APPLY TO DANCE SLIPPERS, SHOES, AND PAJAMAS • Avoid nasty falls caused by slippery plastic dance slippers—and even new shoes. Cut small pieces of bathtub appliqués and apply them to the sole of each slipper or shoe. You can also sew cutout pieces of an appliqué to the soles of a small child's 'onesie' pajamas to prevent slips.

USE ON BOTTOM OF KIDS' WADING POOL • A few bathtub appliqués applied to the floor of a kiddie pool will make it a lot less slippery for little feet and help prevent falls—especially when the water games turn rowdy. Also put a couple of appliqués along the edges of the pool to give kids places to hold onto.

AFFIX TO TRAINING CUPS AND HIGH CHAIR SEATS • Cut pieces of a bathtub appliqué to put on the base of toddlers' sippy cups to minimize spills. You can also attach appliqués to high chair seats to keep small children from sliding down—or out.

BEANS (DRIED)

USE FOR PLAYING PIECES

We know you had your heart set on being the racing car in the next game of Monopoly, but if the car has taken a trip to parts unknown, would you settle for a bean? Beans work fine as replacement pieces for everything from checkers to Snakes and Ladders to bingo.

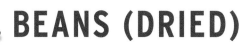
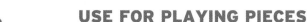
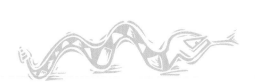

TREAT SORE MUSCLES • Is your bad back or tennis elbow acting up again? A hot beanbag may be just the cure you need. Place a couple of handfuls of dried beans in a cloth shoe bag, an old sock, or a folded dishtowel (tie the ends tightly) and microwave it on High for 30 seconds to 1 minute. Let it cool for a minute or two and apply it to your aching muscles.

PRACTICE YOUR PERCUSSION • Make yourself a homemade percussion shaker or maraca or one for your children. Add ½ cup (125 g) dried beans to a small plastic jar or a soft-drink or juice can—even an empty coconut shell. Cover any openings with electrical or duct tape. You can use this noisemaker at sporting events or as a dog-training tool by giving it a couple of shakes when the dog misbehaves.

MAKE A BEANBAG • Pour ¾ to 1½ cups (175–375 g) dried beans in an old sock, shaking them down to the toe section. Tie a loose knot and tighten it up as you work it down against the beans. Then cut off the remaining material about 1 inch (2.5 cm) above the knot. You now have a beanbag for tossing around or juggling. Or you can use it as a squeeze bag for exercising your hand muscles.

RECYCLE A STUFFED ANIMAL • Make your own beanie toy by removing the stuffing from one of your child's old, unused stuffed animals. Replace the fluff with dried beans and sew it closed. It's bound to rekindle some interest in the old toy.

DECORATE A JACK-O'-LANTERN

Embellish the fright potential of your Halloween jack-o'-lantern by gluing on various dried beans for the eyes and teeth.

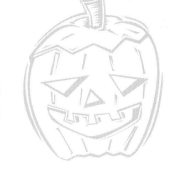

BEER

USE AS SETTING LOTION • Put some life back into flat hair with some flat beer. Before you get into the shower, mix 3 tablespoons (45 ml) beer in ½ cup (125 ml) warm water. After you shampoo your hair, rub in the solution, let it set for a couple of minutes, and rinse it off. When you see the result, you'll want to keep a six-pack in the bathroom!

SOFTEN UP TOUGH MEAT • Who would have guessed that beer makes a great tenderizer for tough, inexpensive cuts of meat? Pour a can over the meat and let it to soak in for about an hour before cooking. Even better, marinate it overnight in the fridge or put the beer in your slow cooker with the meat.

POLISH GOLD JEWELRY • Get the shine back in your solid gold rings (without gemstones) and other jewelry by pouring a bit of beer (not dark ale!) on a soft cloth and rubbing it gently over the piece. Use a clean second cloth or dish towel to dry it thoroughly.

CLEAN WOODEN FURNITURE • Have you got some beer that's old or gone flat? Use it to clean wooden furniture. Just wipe it on with a soft cloth and off with another dry cloth.

more BEER over →

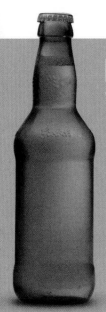

DID YOU KNOW?

The art of beer brewing is almost as old as civilization itself and, along with breadmaking, is probably the most ancient form of manufacturing known to man. The Chinese were known to have brewed beer some 5,000 years ago and the ancient Babylonians perfected the art—a tablet in New York's Metropolitan Museum records their production of several types of beer. Native Americans brewed beer from corn before the arrival of Europeans and the earliest record of nonnatives brewing beer was 1587.

MAKE A TRAP FOR SLUGS AND SNAILS • Like some people, some garden pests find beer irresistible—especially slugs and snails. If you're having problems with these slimy invaders, bury a container, such as a clean, empty juice container cut lengthwise in half, in the area where you've seen the pests, pour in about half a can of warm, leftover beer, and leave it overnight. You'll probably find a horde of them, drunk and drowned, the next morning.

REMOVE COFFEE OR TEA STAINS FROM RUGS • Getting that coffee or tea stain out of your rug may seem impossible, but you can literally lift it out by pouring a bit of beer right on top. Lightly rub the beer into the material and the stain should disappear. You may have to do this a couple of times to remove all traces of the stain.

BERRY BASKETS

KEEP PEELINGS OUT OF THE DRAIN • Don't clog up your kitchen drain with peelings from potatoes or carrots. Use a berry basket as a sink strainer to catch those vegetable shavings as they fall.

STORE SOAP PADS AND SPONGES • Are you tired of throwing away prematurely rusted steel wool soap pads or smelly sponges? Place a berry basket near the corner of your kitchen sink, cut off one corner and line the bottom with a layer of heavy-duty aluminium foil. Fashion a spout on a corner of the foil closest to the sink that can act as a drain, to keep water from pooling up at the bottom of the basket. Now sit back and enjoy the added longevity of your soap pads and sponges.

USE AS A COLANDER • When you need a small colander to wash individual servings of fruits and vegetables, or to drain off a child's portion of hot pasta shells, use an empty berry basket. They make a very effective colander for these sorts of jobs.

HOLD RECYCLED PAPER TOWELS • Don't toss out those barely used paper towels in your kitchen. You can reuse them to wipe down countertops or to soak up serious spills. Keep a berry basket in a convenient location in your kitchen to have your recycled towels at the ready when needed.

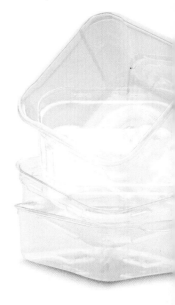

USE AS A DISHWASHER BASKET • If the smaller items you place in your dishwasher, such as baby bottle caps, jar lids, and food-processor accessories, won't stay in the same spot, try putting them in a berry basket. Place the items inside one basket and cover over with a second basket. Fasten them together with a thick rubber band and place on your dishwasher's upper rack.

Kids' Stuff

Berry baskets can be particularly useful for all sorts of children's crafts. For example, you can cut apart the panels and carve out geometric shapes for kids to use as stencils. You can also turn one into an Easter basket by adding a bit of cellophane grass and a colored pipe cleaner for a handle. Or use one as a multiple bubble maker; simply dip it in some water mixed with dishwashing liquid and wave it through the air to create swarms of bubbles. Lastly, let kids decorate the baskets with ribbons or construction paper and use them to store their own little trinkets and toys.

ORGANIZE YOUR PILLS • A clean berry basket could be just what the doctor ordered for organizing your vitamins and medicine bottles. If you're taking several medications regularly, a berry basket offers a simple and convenient way to place them all—or prepackaged individual doses—in one, easy-to-remember location. You can also use baskets to organize medications in a cupboard or medicine cabinet according to their expiration dates or uses.

MAKE A BULB CAGE • Squirrels and other rodents view freshly planted flower bulbs as nothing more than tasty morsels and easy pickings. But you can put a damper on their meal by planting bulbs in berry baskets. Be sure to place the basket at the correct depth, insert the bulb and cover with soil.

FLOWER POWER

ARRANGE FLOWERS • Droopy or lopsided flower arrangements just don't cut it. That's why the professionals use something known as a frog to keep cut flowers in place when they're arranged. To make your own frog, insert an inverted berry basket into a vase (cut the basket to fit, if necessary). It will keep your stalks standing tall.

PROTECT SEEDLINGS • Help young plants thrive in your garden by placing inverted berry baskets over them. The baskets will let water, sunlight and air in, but keep birds and squirrels out. Make sure the basket is buried below ground level and tightly secured (placing a few decent-sized stones around it may do the trick).

BUILD A HANGING ORCHID PLANTER • Orchids are said to be addictive. Once you start collecting them, you can't stop. If you've got the bug, you can at least save yourself a bit of money by making your own hanging baskets for them. Fill up a berry basket with sphagnum moss mixed with a bit of potting mix, then suspend it with a length of monofilament fishing line.

FASHION A STRING DISPENSER OR SCREWDRIVER HOLDER

If you don't want to bother untangling knots every time you need a piece of string, ribbon, or wool, build your own string dispenser with two berry baskets. Place the ball inside one berry basket. Feed the cord through the top of a second, inverted basket, then tie the two baskets together with twist ties. Mount an inverted berry basket on your workshop's pegboard and use it to hold and organize different-size screwdrivers. They'll fit neatly through the holes.

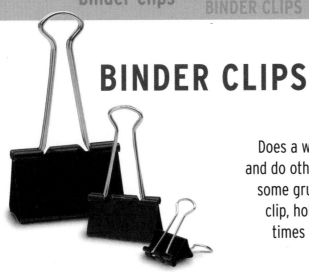

BINDER CLIPS

STRENGTHEN YOUR GRIP

Does a weak grip or arthritis make it hard for you to open jars and do other tasks with your hands? Use a large binder clip to add some grunt to your grip. Squeeze the folded-back wings of the clip, hold for a count of five and relax. Do this a dozen or so times with each hand a few times a day. It will strengthen your grip and release tension, too.

MOUNT A PICTURE • Here's a great way to mount and hang a picture so that it has a clean, frameless look. Sandwich the picture between a sheet of glass or clear plastic and piece of hardboard or stiff cardboard. Use tiny binder clips along the edges to clamp the pieces together and two or three clips on each side. After the clips are in place, remove the clip handles at front, then tie picture wire to the rear handles for hanging the picture.

KEEP YOUR PLACE • A medium-sized binder clip makes an ideal bookmark. If you don't want it to leave impression marks on the pages, just tape a soft material, such as felt or even just some adhesive tape, to the inside jaws of the clip before using.

MAKE A MONEY CLIP • To keep paper money in a neat bundle in your pocket or purse, stack the bills, fold them in half, and put a small binder clip over the fold.

KEEP ID HANDY • You're at the airport and you know you'll be asked to show your ID a few times. Instead of fishing in your wallet or trying to figure out in which pocket you stuck your driver's license, use a binder clip to firmly and conveniently attach your ID and other documents to your belt or the inside of a bag. You can also use a small binder clip to secure your office ID to your belt or a breast pocket.

BLEACH

CLEAN OFF MOLD AND MILDEW • Bleach and ammonia are useful for removing mold and mildew both inside and outside your home. However, the two should never be used together. Bleach is especially suited for the following jobs:

■ Wash mildew out of washable fabrics. Wet the mildewed area and rub in some powdered detergent. Then wash the garment in the hottest water setting permitted by the clothing manufacturer using ½ cup (125 ml) chlorine bleach. If the garment can't be washed in hot

water and bleach, soak it in a solution of ¼ cup (50 g) oxygen bleach in 1 gallon (4 L) warm water for 30 minutes before washing.

■ Remove mold and mildew from grout. Just mix equal parts of chlorine bleach and water in a spray bottle and spray it over the grout. Let it sit for 15 minutes, then scrub with a stiff brush and rinse off.

■ Get mold and mildew off shower curtains. Wash them—along with a couple of bath towels (to prevent the plastic curtains from crinkling)—in warm water with ½ cup (125 ml) chlorine bleach and ¼ cup (50 g) laundry detergent Run the washing machine for a couple of minutes before loading. Put the shower curtain and towels in the dryer on the lowest temperature setting for 10 minutes, then immediately hang out to dry.

■ Rid your rubber shower mat of mildew. Soak in a solution of 2 tablespoons (30 ml) chlorine bleach in 1 gallon (4 L) water for 3 to 4 hours. Rinse well.

■ Get mildew and other stains off unpainted cement, patio stones or stucco. Mix a solution of 1 cup (250 ml) chlorine bleach in 7 quarts (7 L) water. Scrub vigorously with a stiff or wire brush and rinse. If stains remain, scrub again using ½ cup (125 g) cup washing soda (sodium carbonate, not baking soda) dissolved in 7 quarts (7 L) warm water.

■ Remove mildew from painted surfaces and siding. Make a solution of ¼ cup (50 ml) chlorine bleach in 2 cups (500 ml) water and apply with a brush to mildewed areas. Let the solution set for 15 minutes, then rinse. Repeat as necessary.

CLEAN BUTCHER BLOCK, CUTTING BOARDS, AND COUNTERTOPS • Don't even think about using furniture polish or any other household cleaner to clean butcher block, cutting boards, or countertops. Instead, scrub the surface with a brush dipped in a solution of 1 teaspoon (5 ml) bleach diluted in 8 cups (2 L) water. Scrub in small circles and don't saturate the wood. Wipe with a slightly damp paper towel and immediately buff dry with a clean cloth.

> **CAUTION:** Never mix bleach with ammonia, caustic soda, rust removers, oven or toilet bowl cleaners, or vinegar. Any combination can produce toxic chlorine gas fumes, which are potentially deadly. Some people are even sensitive to the fumes of undiluted bleach itself. Always make sure you have adequate ventilation in your work area before you start pouring bleach.

STERILIZE SECONDHAND ITEMS

Remember being told: 'Put that down. You don't know where it's been'? It's not a bad point—especially when it comes to toys or kitchen utensils picked up at secondhand shops and garage sales. Just to be on the safe side, take your used, waterproof items and soak them for 5 to 10 minutes in a solution containing ¾ cup (175 ml) bleach, a few drops of antibacterial dishwashing liquid and 1 gallon (4 L) warm water. Rinse well, then air-dry, preferably in sunlight.

BRIGHTEN UP GLASSES AND GLASSWARE • Put the sparkle back in your drinking glasses and glass dishes by adding 1 teaspoon (5 ml) bleach to your soapy dishwater water as you're washing your glassware. Make sure you rinse well and dry with a soft towel.

SHINE WHITE PORCELAIN • It's easy to get a white porcelain sink, a candlestick, or pottery looking as good as new. In a well-ventilated area on a work surface protected by heavy plastic, place several paper towels over the item (or across the bottom of the sink) and carefully saturate them with undiluted bleach. Let it soak for 15 minutes to half an hour, then rinse and wipe dry with a clean towel.
WARNING: Do not try this with antiques; it can cause damage. And never use bleach on colored porcelain because the color will fade.

MAKE A HOUSEHOLD DISINFECTANT SPRAY • Want a good, all-purpose disinfectant? Mix 1 tablespoon (15 ml) bleach in 1 gallon (4 L) hot water, fill a clean, empty spray bottle and wet a paper towel to clean countertops, garden furniture, tablecloths—wherever it's needed. Just don't use it with ammonia or other household cleaners.

more BLEACH over →

INCREASE CUT FLOWERS' LONGEVITY • Freshly cut flowers will stay fresh longer if you add 1/4 teaspoon (1 ml) bleach per 4 cups (1 L) vase water. Another popular recipe calls for 3 drops of bleach and 1 teaspoon (5 ml) sugar in 4 cups (1 L) water. This will also keep the water from becoming cloudy and inhibit the growth of bacteria.

CLEAN PLASTIC GARDEN FURNITURE • Is your plastic garden furniture looking dingy? Before you toss it, try washing it with some mild detergent mixed with 1/2 cup (125 ml) bleach in 1 gallon (4 L) water. Rinse it clean and air-dry.

KILL WEEDS IN PATHS • Do weeds seem to thrive in the cracks and crevices of your paths? Try pouring a bit of undiluted bleach over them. After a day or two, you can simply pull them out, and the bleach will keep them from coming back. Just be careful not to get bleach on the grass or plantings bordering the path.

GET RID OF MOSS AND ALGAE • To remove slippery and unsightly moss and algae on your brick, concrete, or stone paths, scrub them with a solution of 3/4 cup (175 ml) bleach in 1 gallon (4 L) water. Be careful not to get bleach on your grass or ornamental plants.

SANITIZE GARDEN TOOLS • If you cut a diseased stalk from a plant with a pair of clippers, you'll need to clean the blades to prevent spreading the disease the next time you use them. Sterilize garden tools by washing them in 1/2 cup (125 ml) bleach in 4 cups (1 L) water. Allow them to air-dry in the sun, then rub on some oil to prevent rust.

DISINFECT GARBAGE CANS • Even the cleanest housekeeper confronts a revolting kitchen garbage can every now and then. On such occasions, take the can outside and flush out any loose debris with a garden hose. Then add 1/2 to 1 cup (125–250 ml) bleach and several drops of dishwashing liquid to 1 gallon (4 L) warm water. Use a clean (unused) toilet brush or long-handled scrubbing brush to splash and scour the solution on the bottom and sides of the container. Empty, rinse well, empty, and air-dry.

CAUTION: Some people skip the bleach when cleaning their toilets, fearing that lingering ammonia from urine—especially in households with young children—could result in toxic fumes. Unless you are sure there is no such problem, you may be better off sticking with ammonia for this particular job.

BLOW-DRYER

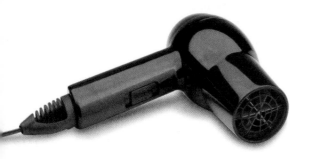

GET WAX OFF WOODEN FURNITURE • It may have been a romantic evening, but that hardened candle wax on your wooden table or chest of drawers is not what lingering memories are made of. Melt the wax with a blow-dryer on its slowest, hottest setting. Remove the softened wax with a paper towel, then wipe the area with a cloth dipped in equal parts vinegar and water. Repeat if necessary. To remove wax from silver candlestick holders with a blow-dryer, use the blow-dryer to soften the wax, then just peel it off.

CLEAN OFF RADIATORS • Cast-iron radiators around the home have a tendency to become unsightly dust catchers. To clean them, hang a large, damp cloth behind each radiator and use a blow-dryer on its highest, coolest setting to blow dust and hidden dirt onto the cloth.

REMOVE BUMPER STICKERS • To remove those cutesy stickers your kids used to decorate your car bumper, use a blow-dryer on its hottest setting to soften the adhesive. Move the dryer slowly back and forth for several minutes. Next, use your fingernail or a credit card to lift up a corner and slowly peel the sticker off.

DUST OFF SILK FLOWERS AND ARTIFICIAL HOUSE PLANTS

They may require less care than their living counterparts, but silk flowers and artificial house plants are apt to collect dust and dirt. Use a blow-dryer on its highest, coolest setting for a quick, efficient way to clean them off. Since this will blow the dust onto the furniture surfaces and floor around the plant, do this just before you vacuum those areas.

BORAX

CLEAR A CLOGGED DRAIN • Before you reach for a caustic drain cleaner to unclog the kitchen or bathroom drain, try this much gentler approach. Use a funnel to insert ½ cup (125 g) borax into the drain and slowly pour in 2 cups (500 ml) boiling water. Let the mixture sit for 15 minutes, then flush with hot water. Repeat for stubborn clogs.

RUB OUT HEAVY SINK STAINS • Get rid of those stubborn stains—even rust—in your stainless steel or porcelain sink. Make a paste of 1 cup (250 g) borax and ¼ cup (50 ml) lemon juice. Put some of the paste on a cloth or sponge and rub it into the stain and rinse with running warm water. The stain should wash away with the paste.

CLEAN WINDOWS AND MIRRORS • To get windows and mirrors spotless and streakless, just wash them with a clean sponge dipped in 2 tablespoons (30 ml) borax dissolved in 3 cups (750 ml) water.

REMOVE MILDEW FROM FABRIC • To remove mildew from upholstery and other fabrics, soak a sponge in ½ cup (125 g) borax dissolved in 2 cups (500 ml) hot water and rub it into the affected areas. Let it soak in for several hours until the stain disappears and rinse well. To remove mildew from clothing, soak it in a solution of 2 cups (500 g) borax in 8 cups (2 L) water.

GET OUT RUG STAINS • Remove stubborn stains from rugs and carpets by thoroughly dampening the area, then rubbing in some borax. Let the area dry, vacuum or blot it with a solution of equal parts vinegar and soapy water and allow to dry. Repeat if necessary. Don't forget to first test the procedure on an inconspicuous corner of the rug or on a carpet scrap before applying it to the stain.

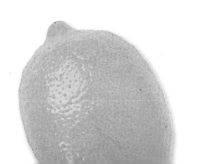

more BORAX over →

Kids' Stuff

Help your children make some slime—that gooey, stretchy stuff kids love to play with. Mix 1 cup (250 ml) water, 1 cup (250 ml) white school glue, and 10 drops food coloring in a medium bowl. In a second, larger bowl, stir 4 teaspoons (20 ml) borax into 1 1/3 cups (325 ml) water until fully dissolved. Slowly pour the contents of the first bowl into the second. Use a wooden spoon to roll (don't mix) the glue solution around in the borax solution several times. Lift out the globs of glue mixture and knead it into a larger glob for 2 to 3 minutes. Store your homemade slime in an airtight container or a large ziplock plastic bag. (Do not eat this mixture!)

CLEAN YOUR TOILET • Disinfect the toilet bowl without having to worry about dangerous fumes, by using a stiff brush to scrub it in a solution of ½ cup (125 g) borax in 1 gallon (4 L) water.

ELIMINATE URINE ODOR ON MATTRESSES • Toilet training can be a rough experience for all parties involved. If your child has an 'accident' in bed, here's how to get rid of any lingering smell. Dampen the area and rub in some borax. Let it dry, then vacuum up the powder.

MAKE YOUR OWN DRIED FLOWERS • To give your homemade dried flowers a professional look, start by mixing 1 cup (250 g) borax with 2 cups (500 ml) polenta. Put a 1-inch (2.5 cm) layer of the mixture in the bottom of an airtight container, such as a large, flat, plastic food-storage container. Cut the stems off the flowers for drying, lay them on top of the powder and lightly sprinkle more of the mixture on top of them (be careful not to bend or crush the petals or other flower parts). Cover the container and let it sit for 7 to 10 days. Remove the flowers and brush off any excess powder with a soft brush.

> **CAUTION:** Borax, like its close relative boric acid, has relatively low toxicity levels, and is considered safe for general household use, but the powder can be harmful if ingested in sufficient quantities by young children or pets. Store it safely out of their reach.
>
> However, borax is toxic to plants. When you're in the garden, take care when applying borax on or near soil. It doesn't take much to leach into the ground to kill off nearby plants and prevent future growth.

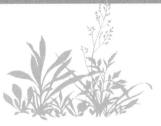

KEEP WEEDS AND ANTS AWAY

Get the jump on those weeds that grow in the cracks of the concrete outside your house by sprinkling borax into all the crevices where you've seen weeds grow in the past. It will kill them off before they have a chance to take root. When applied around the foundation of your home, it will also keep ants and other insect intruders from entering your house. But be very careful when applying borax—it is toxic to plants (see the CAUTION box, above).

CONTROL WANDERING JEW • If your garden is being overrun by Wandering Jew, you may be able to conquer it with borax. Dissolve 1 cup (250 g) borax in ½ cup (125 ml) warm water. Pour the solution into 9 quarts (9 L) warm water. This is enough to cover 1,000 ft² (93 m²). Apply the treatment only once in each of two years. If you still have problems, switch to a standard herbicide. (*See the CAUTION box, above, for using borax in the garden.*)

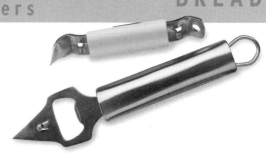

BOTTLE OPENERS

REMOVE CHESTNUT SHELLS • An easy way to remove the shells from chestnuts is to use the pointed end of a bottle opener to pierce the tops and bottoms of the shells and boil the chestnuts for 10 minutes.

CUT PACKING TAPE ON CARTONS • It's hard to resist opening that long-awaited package on your doorstep, so if you don't have a knife handy just run the sharp end of a bottle opener along the tape. It should do the job quite nicely.

DEPLOY AS A SHRIMP DEVEINER

If you don't have a small paring knife on hand when you're getting ready to devein a batch of shrimp, don't worry. Just use the sharp end of a bottle opener. It just happens to be the perfect shape to make this messy job a breeze.

SCRAPE A BARBECUE GRATE • An easy way to clean off the burned remnants of last weekend's meal from your barbecue grate is to use a bottle opener and a metal file. All you have to do is file a notch about ⅛-inch (3 mm) wide into the flat end of the opener and you're ready to go.

DID YOU KNOW?

The old-fashioned bottle opener with one flat end and one pointed end is often referred to as a 'church key'. Although no one is exactly sure how or when this association came into being, it originated years ago in the brewery industry and was used to describe a flat opener with a hooked cutout used to pry off beer bottle caps. It is widely believed that the term derived from the early openers' resemblance to the heavy, ornate keys used to unlock big, old doors, such as those found on churches. Ironically, the term is now applied only to openers with both flat and pointed ends.

LOOSEN PLASTER OR REMOVE GROUT • It may not be the carpenter's best friend, but the sharp end of a bottle opener can be handy for removing loose plaster from a wall before patching it. It's great for running along cracks, and you can use it to undercut a hole—that is, make it wider at the bottom than at the surface—so that the new plaster will 'key' into the old. The sharp end of the opener is equally useful for removing old grout between your bathroom tiles before regrouting.

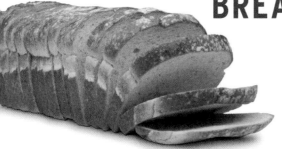

BREAD

REMOVE SCORCHED TASTE FROM RICE • Did you leave the rice cooking too long and let it burn? To get rid of the scorched taste, place a slice of white bread on top of the rice while it's still hot. Replace the pot lid and wait several minutes. When you remove the bread, the burned taste should be gone.

more BREAD over →

BUBBLE WRAP

SOFTEN UP HARD MARSHMALLOWS • If you reach for your bag of marshmallows, only to discover that they've gone stale, just put a couple of slices of fresh bread in the bag (or first transfer them to a ziplock plastic bag) and seal it shut. Let it sit for a couple of days. When you reopen the bag, your marshmallows should be as fresh as new.

ABSORB VEGETABLE ODORS • Love cabbage or broccoli, but hate the smell while it's cooking? Try putting a piece of white bread on top of the pot when cooking up a batch of 'smelly' vegetables. It will absorb most of the unpleasant odors.

CLEAN WALLS AND WALLPAPER • Most kids have a hard time understanding how easily the dirt on their hands can be transferred to walls. But you can remove most dirty or greasy fingerprints from painted walls by rubbing the area with a slice of white bread. Bread also does a good job cleaning nonwashable wallpaper. Just cut off the crusts first to minimize the chance of scratching the paper.

PICK UP GLASS FRAGMENTS

Picking up the large pieces of a broken glass or dish is usually easy enough, but picking up those tiny slivers can be a real pain (figuratively if not literally). The easiest way to make sure you don't miss any is to press a slice of bread over the area. Just be careful not to cut yourself when you toss the bread in the garbage.

SOAK UP GREASE AND STOP FLARE-UPS • One of the best ways to prevent a grease flare-up when grilling meat is to place a couple of slices of white bread in your drip pan to absorb the grease. It will also cut down on the amount of smoke produced.

DUST OIL PAINTINGS • You wouldn't want to try this with a valuable oil painting, or with any museum-quality painting for that matter, but you can clean off everyday dust and grime that collects on an oil painting by very gently rubbing the surface with a piece of white bread.

BUBBLE WRAP

PREVENT TOILET-TANK CONDENSATION • If your toilet tank sweats in warm, humid weather, bubble wrap could be just the right antiperspirant. Lining the inside of the tank with bubble wrap will keep the outside of the tank from getting cold and causing condensation when it comes in contact with warm, moist air. To line the tank, shut off the supply valve under the tank and flush to drain the tank, then wipe the inside walls clean and dry. Use silicone sealant to glue appropriate-sized pieces of bubble wrap to the major flat surfaces.

PROTECT PATIO PLANTS • You can keep your outdoor container plants warm and protected from winter frost damage, just by wrapping each container with bubble wrap. And use duct tape or string to hold the wrap in place. Make sure the wrap extends 1 to 2 inches (3 to 5 cm) above the lip of the container. The added insulation will also help keep the soil warm all winter long.

KEEP SODA COLD • Wrap soft-drink cans with bubble wrap to keep beverages refreshingly cold on hot summer days. Do the same for packages of frozen or chilled picnic foods. Wrap ice cream just before you leave for the picnic to help keep it firm en route.

PROTECT PRODUCE IN THE FRIDGE • Line your refrigerator's crisper drawer with bubble wrap to keep fruit and produce from bruising. Cleanup will be easier, too. When the lining gets dirty, just throw it out and replace with fresh bubble wrap.

ADD INSULATION • In cold areas, cut window-sized pieces of wide bubble wrap and duct tape them to inside windows for added warmth and savings on fuel bills in winter. Lower the blinds to make it less noticeable.

MAKE A BEDTIME BUFFER • Keep cold air from creeping into your bed on a chilly night by placing a large sheet of bubble wrap between your bedspread or quilt and your top sheet. You'll be surprised at how effective it is in keeping warm air in and cold air out.

CUSHION YOUR WORK SURFACE • When repairing delicate glass or china, cover the work surface with bubble wrap to help prevent breakage.

PROTECT TOOLS • You can reduce wear and tear on your good-quality household tools and extend their lives by lining your toolbox with bubble wrap. Use duct tape to hold it in place.

CUSHION SEATS AND BENCHES • Take some bubble wrap with you to sports events to soften those hard stadium seats or benches. Or stretch a length along a picnic bench for more comfy dining.

DID YOU KNOW?

Bubble wrap wallpaper? Yep, that's what inventors Alfred Fielding and Marc Chavannes had in mind when they began developing the product in Saddle Brook, New Jersey in the late 1950s. Perhaps they were looking to capture the padded-cell market. In any case, they soon realized their invention had greater potential as packaging material. In 1960, they raised $85,000 and started the Sealed Air Corporation.

Today, Sealed Air is a top U.S. company with $4.5 billion annual revenues. The company produces bubble wrap cushioning in a multitude of sizes, colors, and properties, along with other protective packaging materials such as Jiffy padded mailbags.

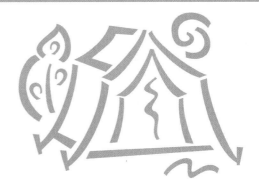

SLEEP ON AIR WHILE CAMPING

Get a better night's sleep on your next camping trip, by simply carrying a 6-foot (2 m) roll of wide bubble wrap to use as a mat under your sleeping bag. If you don't have a sleeping bag, fold a 12-foot (4 m) long piece of wide bubble wrap in half—bubble side out—and duct tape the edges. Then slip in and enjoy a restful night in your makeshift padded slumber bag.

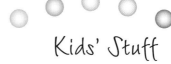

BUCKETS

MAKE YOUR OWN LOBSTER POT

If you don't have a large stockpot, boil lobsters in an old metal bucket. Make sure to use pot holders and tongs when cooking and removing the lobster, and let the bucket cool before handling it again.

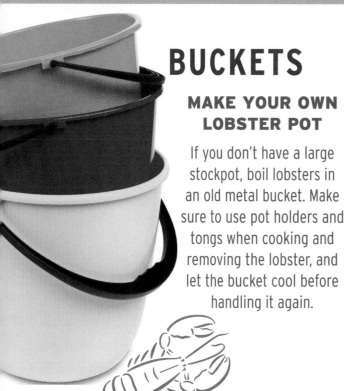

IN THE WILD

CREATE A FOOD STORAGE BIN • A tightly-sealed 5 gallon (20 L) bucket is an ideal waterproof (and animal-proof) food storage bin to take with you on trips that involve rafting or canoeing.

BUILD A CAMP WASHING MACHINE • Here's a great way to wash clothes while camping. Make a hole in the lid of a 5 gallon (20 L) plastic bucket and insert a new toilet plunger. Add clothes and detergent, snap on the lid, and move the plunger up and down as an agitator. You can even safely clean delicate garments.

CAMP SHOWER • A bucket perforated with holes on the bottom makes an excellent campsite shower. Hang it securely from a sturdy branch, and fill it using another bucket or jug, and take a quick shower as the water comes out. Want to shower in warm water? Paint the outside of another bucket matte black. Fill it with water and leave it out in the sun all day to absorb heat.

Kids' Stuff

Add the beat of bucket tom-toms to create an exciting, fun atmosphere around the firepit on your next family camping trip. Cut plastic buckets to different lengths to create a distinct tone for each drum or use a mix of various-sized plastic and galvanized buckets. For more musical accompaniment, make a broom-handle string bass using a bucket as the sound box.

PAINT HIGH • Avoid messy paint spills on a scaffold or ladder when painting by putting your paint can and brush in a large bucket and use paint can hooks to hang the bucket and the brush. If the bucket is large enough, you'll even have room for your paint scraper, putty knife, rags, or other painting tools you may need. A 5 gallon (20 L) plastic bucket is ideal.

PAINT LOW • Use the lids from 5 gallon (20 L) plastic buckets as trays for 1 gallon (4 L) cans of paint. The lids act as platforms for the paint cans and are also large enough to hold a paintbrush.

KEEP EXTENSION CORDS TANGLE-FREE • A 5 gallon (20 L) bucket can help you keep a long extension cord free of tangles. Just cut or drill a hole near the bottom of the bucket, making sure it is large enough for the cord's plug end to pass through, then coil the rest of the cord into the bucket. The cord will come out when pulled and is easy to coil back in. Plug the ends of the cord together when it's not in use. Use the center space to carry tools to a worksite.

SOAK YOUR SAW • The best way to clean saw blades is to soak them in acetone or turpentine in a shallow tray with a lid on it to contain the fumes. Make your own shallow tray by cutting 2 inches (5 cm) from the bottom of a plastic 5 gallon (20 L) bucket with a craft knife. The bucket's lid can serve as the cover. Remember to wear rubber gloves and use a stick to remove the sharp blades.

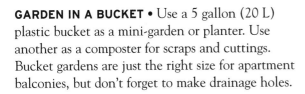

GARDEN IN A BUCKET • Use a 5 gallon (20 L) plastic bucket as a mini-garden or planter. Use another as a composter for scraps and cuttings. Bucket gardens are just the right size for apartment balconies, but don't forget to make drainage holes.

MAKE A CHRISTMAS TREE STAND • Partially fill a bucket with sand or gravel and insert the base of the tree in it. Then fill it the rest of the way and pour water on the sand or gravel to help keep the tree from drying out.

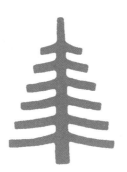

Finding five-gallon (20 L) buckets

Five-gallon (20 L) plastic buckets are versatile, virtually indestructible, with many handy uses. You can even get them for free!

Ask nicely and your local fast food outlet or supermarket deli section may be happy to give you the buckets that various deli items came in. Or check with neighborhood plasterers, who use 5 gallon (20 L) buckets of cement. Keep an eye open for neighbors doing home improvements. And don't forget to take the lids. Wash out a bucket with water and household bleach and let it dry in the sun for a day or two. Put some scented kitty litter, charcoal, or a couple of drops of vanilla inside to help remove any lingering odors.

BUTTER

GET RID OF A FISHY SMELL

Your fishing trip may have been a big success, but now your hands reek of fish. What to do? Just rub some butter on your hands, wash with warm water and soap, and your hands will smell clean and fresh again.

KEEP MOLD OFF CHEESE • Why waste good cheese by letting the cut edges get hard or moldy? Give semi-hard cheeses a light coat of butter when you get them home from the supermarket to keep them fresh and free of mold. Each time you use the cheese, coat the cut edge with a smear of butter before you rewrap it and put it back in the fridge.

MAKE THE CAT FEEL AT HOME • Is the family feline freaked out by your move to a new home? Moving is often traumatic for pets as well as family members. Here's a good way to help an adult cat adjust to the new house or apartment. Spread a bit of butter on the top of one of its front paws. Cats love the taste of butter so much they'll keep coming back for more.

SWALLOW TABLETS WITH EASE • If you have difficulty getting tablets to go down, try rolling them in a small amount of butter or margarine first. The pills will slide down your throat more easily.

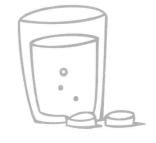

more BUTTER over →

Kids' Stuff

Making butter is fun and easy. You'll need a jar, a marble and 1 to 2 cups (250-500 ml) heavy whipping cream or double cream (preferably without gum or other stabilizers added). Use the freshest cream possible and leave it out of the refrigerator until it reaches a temperature of 60°F (15°C). Pour the cream into the jar, add the marble, close the lid, and let the kids take turns shaking (churning), about one shake per second. It may take anywhere from 5 to 30 minutes, but the kids will see the cream go through various stages from sloshy to coarse whipped cream. When the whipped cream suddenly seizes and collapses, fine-grained bits of butter will be visible in the liquid buttermilk. Before long, a glob of yellowish butter will appear. Drain off the buttermilk and enjoy the delightful taste of freshly made butter.

SOOTHE ACHING FEET • To soothe tired feet, massage them with butter, wrap in a damp, hot towel, sit back, and relax for 10 minutes. Your feet will feel revitalized—and they'll smell like popcorn, too.

REMOVE SAP FROM SKIN • You've just got home from a pleasant walk in the woods, but your hand is still covered with sticky tree sap that feels like it will never come off. Don't worry, just rub butter on your hand and the gunky black sap will wash right off with soap and water.

EMERGENCY SHAVING CREAM • If you run out of shaving cream, try slathering some butter on your wet skin for a smooth, close shave.

KEEP LEFTOVER ONION FRESH • If a recipe calls for half an onion and you want to keep the remaining half fresh as long as possible, rub butter on the cut surface and wrap it in aluminium foil before putting it in the fridge. The butter will help keep it fresh.

FIX INK MARKS ON A DOLL'S FACE • Many favorite dolls have been given an ink-pen makeover by an overzealous, underage beautician. You can undo the handy work by rubbing butter on the pen stains and leaving the doll face-up in the sun for a few days. Then wash it off with soap and water.

CUT STICKY FOODS WITH EASE • Rub butter on your knife or scissor blades before cutting sticky foods like dates, figs, or marshmallows. The butter will act as a lubricant and help to prevent the food from sticking to the blades as you cut.

PREVENT POTS FROM BOILING OVER • You take your eye off the pasta for 2 seconds and the next thing you know, the pot is boiling over onto the stovetop. Keep the boiling water in the pot next time by adding a tablespoon or two of butter.

TREAT DRY HAIR • Is your hair dry and brittle? Try buttering it up for a luxuriant shine. Massage a small chunk of butter into your dry hair, cover it with a shower cap for about 30 minutes, then shampoo and rinse thoroughly.

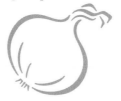

BUTTONS

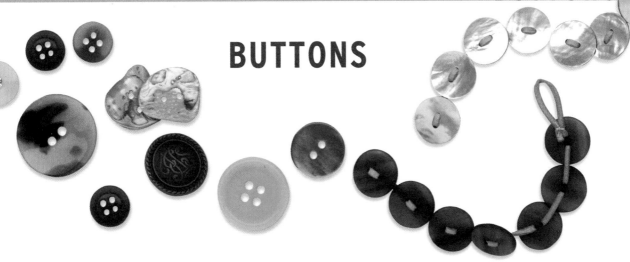

DECORATE A DOLLHOUSE • Use buttons as wall lights, plates, and wall hangings in a child's dollhouse. The more variety, the better.

BEANBAG FILLER • The next time you need to make beanbags, use up all the leftover buttons that are in your sewing box and save the dried beans for soup.

KEEP TAPE UNSTUCK • You're trying to wrap a present and you can't find the start of the tape roll. Instead of scratching in frustration, the next time you use the tape, stick a button on the end when you're done. As you use the tape, keep moving the button.

USE AS GAME PIECES OR POKER CHIPS • Don't let lost pieces stop you from playing backgammon, bingo, or checkers. You can substitute buttons for the lost pieces and keep playing to your heart's content. For an impromptu game of poker, use buttons as chips, with each color representing a different value.

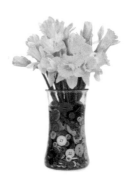

MAKE A COLORFUL FLOWER ARRANGEMENT • Buttons can create a unique and beautiful look. Select a large glass vase, another narrower one that fits inside it, and enough buttons to fill the space between them. Choose colors that will complement your flowers. Fill the bottom of the large vase with buttons and place the second one on top. Add enough buttons to fill the space between them, and add water. Finally, fill the smaller vessel with water and arrange your flowers inside.

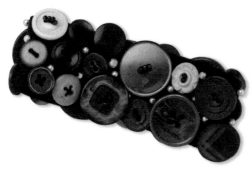

MAKE A BRACELET

String attractive buttons on 1/8-inch (3-mm) wide leather thonging, available from craft stores, or make a 'cuff' bracelet simply by sewing buttons on wide elastic. Make an attractive design by alternating large and small buttons of various colors.

DECORATE A CHRISTMAS TREE • Give your Christmas tree an old-fashioned look by making a garland by knotting large buttons on a sturdy length of string or dental floss.

C CANDLES

UNSTICK A DRAWER • If you have a desk drawer or a chest drawer that always sticks, remove it and rub a white candle on the runners. The drawer will open more smoothly when you slip it back in place.

MAKE A PINCUSHION • A wide candle makes an ideal pincushion. The wax will help pins and needles glide more easily through fabric, too. Just make sure the wax is soft enough for the pins to go in easily.

DID YOU KNOW?

Beeswax–the substance secreted by honeybees to make honeycombs–didn't make its debut in candles until the Middle Ages. Until then, candles were made of the rendered animal fat called tallow, which produced a smoky flame and gave off acrid odors. Beeswax candles, by contrast, burned pure and clean. But they were not widely used at the time, being far too expensive for ordinary serfs and peasants.

The growth of whaling in the late 1700s brought a major change to candlemaking as spermaceti– a waxlike substance derived from sperm whale oil– became available in bulk. The nineteenth century witnessed the advent of mass-produced candles and low-cost paraffin wax. Made from oil and coal shale, paraffin burned cleanly with no unpleasant odor.

MAKE A SECRET DRAWING

Let your kids make an 'invisible' drawing with a white candle, and then cover it with a wash of watercolor paint to reveal the picture. The image will show up because the wax laid down by the candle will keep the paper in the areas it covers from absorbing the paint. If you have a few kids around, they can all make secret drawings and messages to swap and reveal.

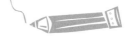

USE A TRICK CANDLE TO IGNITE FIRES • Don't let a draft blow out the flame when you're trying to light your fireplace or fire up the barbecue grill. Start your fire with one of those trick, blow-proof birthday candles, designed as a practical joke to prevent birthday celebrants from blowing out the candles on their cakes. Once your fire is roaring, smother the candle's flame and save your trick candle for future use.

WEATHERPROOF YOUR LABELS • After you address a package with a felt-tip pen, weatherproof the label by rubbing a white candle over the writing. Neither rain, nor sleet, nor snow will smear the label.

MEND SHOELACE ENDS • When those plastic or metal tips come off the ends of your shoelaces, don't wait for the laces to fray. Do something to prevent the hassle that comes from having to force a scraggly shoelace end through a tiny eyelet. Dip the end into melted candle wax and the lace will hold until you can buy a new one.

MAKE A SQUEAKY DOOR QUIET • If a squeaky door is driving you crazy, take it off its hinges and rub a candle over the hinge surfaces that touch each other. The offending door will squeak no more.

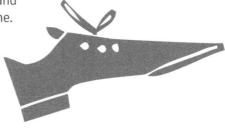

CANDY TINS

MAKE A BIRTHDAY KEEPSAKE •
Decorate the outside of a small candy tin, line it with felt or silk, and include a penny or silver dollar from the birth year of a friend or loved one.

STORE WORKSHOP ACCESSORIES • Candy tins are great for storing brads, glazing points, setscrews, lock washers, and other small items that might otherwise clutter up your workshop.

CAR FUSES • You'll always know where to find your spare car fuses if you store them in a little candy tin in the glove compartment of your car.

JEWELRY BOXES

STORE BROKEN JEWELRY • Don't lose little pieces of broken jewelry you plan to repair someday. Keep them together in a candy tin.

PREVENT TANGLES • Keep necklaces and chains tangle-free in their own individual tins.

KEEP EARRINGS TOGETHER • To prevent pairs of small earrings from going their separate ways, store them together in a little candy tin and you'll never have to search for them.

EMERGENCY SEWING KIT • A small candy tin is just the size to hold a handy selection of needles, thread, and buttons to put in your purse or briefcase for speedy on-the-spot repairs.

CANS

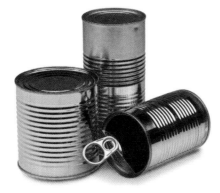

MAKE LIGHT REFLECTORS • It's simple to make reflectors for your campsite or backyard lights. Just remove the bottom of a large empty can with a can opener and take off the label that's wrapped around the can. Using strong kitchen scissors, cut the can in half lengthwise, and you'll have two reflectors.

TUNA CAN EGG POACHER

An empty 5-ounce (150 g) tuna can is the perfect size to use as an egg poacher. Remove the bottom of the can as well as the top and remove any paper label. Then place the metal ring in a frying pan of simmering water and crack an egg into it.

MAKE A QUICK FLOOR PATCH • Nail can lids to a wooden floor to plug knotholes and keep rodents out. If you can get access to the hole from the basement or under the house, nail the lid in place from below and the patch won't be obvious.

STORE SCISSORS SAFELY • Use a punch-type can opener to pierce evenly spaced holes around the bottom of a large, clean can. Place the inverted can on your countertop or worktable and slip the points of your scissors into the holes. This is also a good way to store screwdrivers.

FEED THE BIRDS • A bird doesn't care if the feeder is plain or fancy as long as it is filled with suet or seed. For a feeder that's about as basic as you can get, wedge a small can filled with suet or seed between tree branches or posts.

MAKE A MINIATURE GOLF COURSE •
Arrange cans with both ends removed so the ball must go through them, go up a ramp into them, or ricochet off a board through them.

more CANS over →

95

MAKE A PEDESTAL • Fill several wide, same-sized cans with rocks or sand and glue them together, one on top of another. Screw a piece of wood into the bottom of the topmost can before attaching it, upside down, to the others. Paint your pedestal and place a potted plant, lamp, or statue on top. (*See the TIP box at right, for suggestions on the type of glue to use.*)

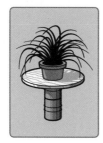

CREATE DECORATIVE LUMINARIAS • Fill clean, empty cans of different sizes with water and freeze. Use a hammer and a large nail or an electric drill to pierce a pattern of holes in the sides of the cans, defrost the ice and insert small candles or tealights.

MAKE PIGEONHOLES • Assemble half a dozen or more empty cans and paint them with bright enamel. After they dry, glue the cans together and place them on their sides on a shelf. Store silverware, nails, office supplies, or other odds and ends in them.

ORGANIZE YOUR DESK • If your office desk is a mess, a few empty cans can be the start of a nifty solution. Just attach several empty cans of assorted sizes together in a group to make an office-supplies holder for your desk. Start by cleaning and drying the cans and removing any labels and spray paint them (or wrap them in felt or jute string). When the paint is dry, glue them together using a hot glue gun. Your desk organizer is now ready to hold pens, pencils, paperclips, scissors, and whatever else you need.

MAKE A PAIR OF CHILD'S STILTS

Pierce a hole in opposite sides of the bottom of two identical, large, sturdy cans. Knot thin rope or nylon cord through the holes to form handles. The length of the handles will depend on the height of the child, but they need to reach up as far as their hands. Step up onto the cans, pull the handles taut, and off you go!

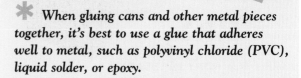

Glue for cans

When gluing cans and other metal pieces together, it's best to use a glue that adheres well to metal, such as polyvinyl chloride (PVC), liquid solder, or epoxy.

If the joint won't be subject to stress, you can use a hot glue gun. Make sure to wash and dry the cans and to remove any labels first. Also, let any paint dry thoroughly before gluing.

MAKE A TOOL TOTE • Tired of fumbling around in your tool pouch to find the tool you need? Use empty fruit juice cans to transform the deep, wide pockets of a nail pouch into a convenient tote for wrenches, pliers, and screwdrivers. Make sure to remove the bottom of the can as well as the top. Glue or tape the cylinders together to keep them from shifting around and slip them in the pouches to create dividers.

KEEP TABLES TOGETHER

When you're having a large dinner party, lock card tables together by setting adjacent pairs of legs into empty cans. You won't have to clean up any spills from tables moving this way and that.

DID YOU KNOW?

Tin cans are often described as 'hermetically sealed', but do you know the origin of the term? The word hermetic comes from Hermes Trismegistus, the Egyptian god Thoth, who is reputed to have lived sometime in the first three centuries AD and to have invented a magic seal that keeps a vessel airtight.

The hermetically sealed can was invented in 1810 by British merchant Peter Durand. His cans were so thick they had to be hammered open! An Englishman called Thomas Kensett patented the process in 1825 in America, and more than a century later, in 1957, the first all-aluminium can appeared.

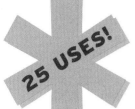

25 USES!

CARDBOARD BOXES
around the house

MAKE A BED TRAY • Have breakfast in bed on a tray made from a cardboard box. Just remove the top flaps and cut arches from the two long sides to fit over your lap. Decorate the bottom of the box—which is now the top of your tray—with colored or decorative contact paper and serve up the bacon and eggs.

SHIELD DOORS AND FURNITURE •
Use cardboard shields to protect doors and furniture from stains when you polish doorknobs and furniture pulls. Cut an appropriate-sized shield and slide it over the item you are going to polish. This works best when you make shields that slip over the neck of knobs or knobby pulls. You can also make shields for hinges and U-shaped pulls.

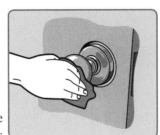

CREATE GIFT-WRAP SUSPENSE

Take a cue from the Russians and their nesting matryoshka dolls. Next time you are giving a small but sure-to-be-appreciated gift to a friend, place the gift-wrapped little box inside a series of increasingly bigger, festively decorated or wrapped boxes.

MAKE DUSTCOVERS • Keep dust and dirt out of a small appliance, power tool, or keyboard by cutting the flaps off a cardboard box that will fit over the item, decorate it or cover it with self-adhesive contact paper, and use it as a dustcover.

MAKE AN OFFICE IN-BOX • Making an in-box (or out-box) for your office desk is easy. Simply cut the top and one large panel off a cereal box and slice the narrow sides at an angle. Wrap what remains of the box in colored contact paper.

A good box source

TIP

Even if you don't drink alcohol, the proprietors of your local liquor store will often be happy to provide you with empty wine and liquor boxes. And don't forget to ask that the handy divider sections be left intact.

DID YOU KNOW?

The Chinese invented cardboard in the early 1500s, thus anticipating the demand for containers for Chinese takeaway food by several hundred years.

In 1871, New Yorker Albert Jones patented the idea of gluing a piece of corrugated paper between two pieces of flat cardboard to create a material rigid enough to use for shipping. But it wasn't until 1890 that another American, Robert Gair, invented the corrugated cardboard box. His boxes were pre-cut flat pieces manufactured in bulk that folded into boxes, just like the cardboard boxes that surround us today.

more CARDBOARD BOXES over →

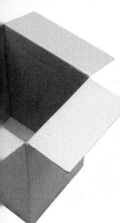

MAKE PLACE MATS • Cut out several 12 x 18-inch (30 x 45 cm) pieces of cardboard and cover them with decorative adhesive paper or use other paper with clear contact on top.

PLAY LIQUOR-BOX SKEE BALL • Transform your playroom or backyard into a carnival alley. Leave the dividers in place in an empty wine or liquor box. Place the box at an angle and erect a small ramp in front (a rubber mat over a pile of books will do the trick). Assign numbered values to each section of the carton, grab a few tennis or golf balls, and you're ready to roll.

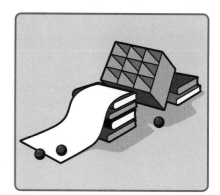

for storing things

PROTECT GLASSWARE OR LIGHTBULBS • A good way to safely store fine crystal glassware is to put it in an empty wine or liquor box with partitions. You can also use these boxes for storing lightbulbs, but make sure you sort the bulbs by wattage so that it's easy to find the right one when you need a replacement.

MAKE A MAGAZINE HOLDER • You can store your growing collection of magazines in holders made from empty detergent boxes. Remove the top of the box, then cut it at an angle, from the top of one side to the bottom third of the other. Cover your new holders with decorative self-adhesive paper.

POSTER AND ARTWORK HOLDER

A clean liquor box with its dividers intact is a great place to store rolled-up posters, drawings on paper, and canvases. Just insert the items upright between the partitions.

STORE CHRISTMAS DECORATIONS • When you take down your Christmas tree, wrap each ornament in newspaper or tissue paper and store it in an empty wine box with partitions. You can keep a few wrapped ornaments, stacked vertically, in each partition.

for the kids

CREATE AN IMPROMPTU SLED • Use a large cardboard box to pull a small child (or a load of firewood) over the snow or to slide down snowy hills.

GARAGE FOR TOY VEHICLES • Turn a large empty appliance box on its side and let the kids use it as a 'garage' for their wheeled vehicles. They can also use a smaller box as a garage for miniature cars, trucks, and buses.

MAKE A PUPPET THEATER • Stand a large cardboard box on end. Cut a big hole in the back for puppeteers to crouch in and a smaller one high up in the front for the stage. Decorate it with felt pens or glue on pieces of fabric for curtains.

ORGANIZE KIDS' SPORTING GOODS • Keep a decorated empty wine or liquor box with partitions, with the top cut off, in your child's room and use it for easy storage of tennis racquets, baseball bats, fishing rods, and such.

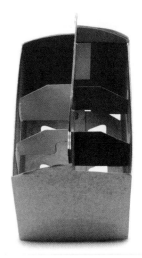

C

SCIENCE **WORKS!**

Making a simple cardboard sundial is a great way for kids to observe how the sun's path changes every day.

Just take a 10 x 10-inch (25 x 25 cm) piece of cardboard and poke a stick through the middle. If necessary, screw or nail a small board to the bottom of the stick to hold it upright. Place the sundial in a sunny spot. At each hour, have the kids mark where the stick's shadow falls on the cardboard. Check again the next day, and sure enough, the sundial seems pretty accurate. Check a week later, though, and the shadows won't align to the marks at the right times. Encourage the kids to start searching the Internet for an explanation for this, which is that the earth is tilted on its axis.

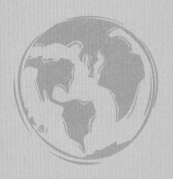

MAKE A PLAY CASTLE

Turn a large-appliance cardboard box into a medieval castle. Cut off the top flaps and make battlements by cutting notches along the top. To make a notch, use a craft knife and make a cut on either side of the section you want to remove, then fold the cut section forward and cut along the fold. To make a drawbridge, cut a large fold-down opening on one side that is attached at the bottom. Connect the top of the drawbridge to the side walls with ropes on either side, punching holes for the rope and knotting the rope on the other side. Use duct tape to reinforce the holes. Also cut out narrow window slits in the walls. Let the kids draw stones and bricks on the walls.

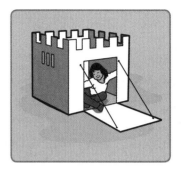

for the do-it-yourselfer

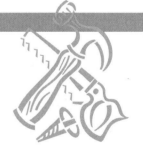

REPAIR A ROOF • For temporary repair on your roof, put a piece of cardboard into a plastic bag and slide it under the shingles.

ORGANIZE YOUR WORKSHOP • Use a partitioned wine or liquor box as a place to store dowels, moldings, battens, brackets, weather stripping, and metal rods.

STORE TALL GARDEN TOOLS • Turn three empty liquor boxes into a partitioned storage bin for your long-handled garden tools. Put a topless box on the floor with the box dividers left in. Then cut the tops and bottoms off two similar boxes and stack them so dividers match up. Use duct tape to

attach the boxes together. Use the divided bin to store hoes, rakes, and other long-handled garden tools.

PROTECT WORK SURFACES • To keep work surfaces from being damaged, flatten a large box or cut a large, flat piece from a box and use it to protect your countertop, workbench, table, or desk from ink, paint, glue, or nicks from knives and scissors. Just replace it when it becomes messed up.

more CARDBOARD BOXES over →

PROTECT YOUR FINGERS

Ouch! You just hammered your finger instead of the tiny nail you were trying to drive into a piece of wood. To keep this from happening again, stick the little nail through a small piece of thin cardboard before you start hammering. Hold the cardboard by an edge, position the nail, and pound it home. When you're finished, use your bruise-free fingers to tear away the piece of protective cardboard.

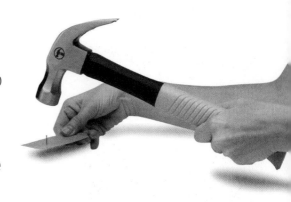

KEEP UPHOLSTERY TACKS STRAIGHT • Reupholstering a chair or sofa? Here's a great way to get a row of upholstery tacks perfectly straight and evenly spaced. Mark the spacing along the edge of a lightweight cardboard strip and press the tacks into it. After driving all of the tacks most of the way in, tug on the strip to pull the edge free before driving the tacks in the rest of the way.

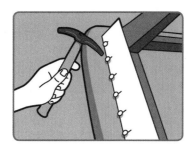

MAKE A DRIP PAN • Prevent an oil leak from soiling your garage floor or driveway by making a drip pan. All you need to do is place a few sheets of corrugated cardboard on a cookie sheet or a shallow baking dish and place the pan under your car's drip. For better absorption, just sprinkle some cat litter, sawdust, or oatmeal into the pan on top of the cardboard. Replace with fresh cardboard as needed.

HELP YOUR MECHANIC • Something is dripping from your car's engine, but you don't know what. Instead of blubbering helplessly to your mechanic about it, place a large piece of cardboard under the engine overnight and bring it with you when you take the car in for service. The color and location of the leaked fluid will help the mechanic identify the nature of the problem.

CARDBOARD TUBES

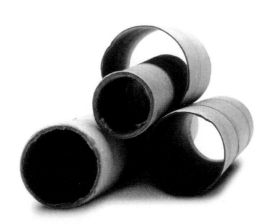

EXTEND VACUUM CLEANER REACH

Can't reach that cobweb on the ceiling with your regular vacuum cleaner attachment? Try using a long, empty cardboard tube to extend the reach. You can even crush the end of the cardboard tube to create a crevice tool. Use duct tape to make the connection airtight.

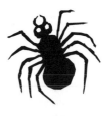

MAKE A SHEATH • Flatten a cardboard paper towel tube, duct tape one end shut, and you have a perfect sheath for a picnic or camp knife. You can use toilet paper rolls for smaller cutlery.

KEEP ELECTRICAL CORDS TANGLE-FREE • To keep computer and appliance cords tangle-free, fanfold the cord and pass it through a toilet-paper tube before plugging in. You can also use the tubes 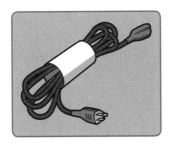 to store extension cords when they're not in use. Paper towel tubes will also work well. Just cut them in half before using them to hold the cords.

FOR THOSE WITH GREEN FINGERS ...

MAKE A PLANT GUARD • It's easy to accidentally scar the trunk of a young tree when you are whacking weeds around it. To avoid doing this, cut a cardboard poster tube in half lengthwise and tie the two halves around the trunk while you work around the tree. Then slip it off and use it on another tree.

START SEEDLINGS • Don't go to the garden supply store to buy biodegradable starting pots for seedlings, just use the cardboard tubes from paper towels and toilet paper. Use scissors to cut each toilet paper tube into two pots, or each paper towel tube into four. Fill a tray with the cut cylinders packed against each other so they won't tip when you water the seedlings. This will also prevent them from drying out too quickly. Now fill each pot with seed-starting mix, gently pack it down, and sow your seeds. When you plant the seedlings, make sure to break down the side of the roll and be sure that all the cardboard is completely buried in the soil.

DID YOU KNOW?

It took nearly 500 years for toilet paper to make the transition from sheets to rolls. Toilet paper was first produced in China in 1391 for the exclusive use of the emperor in sheets that measured 24 x 36 inches (60 x 90 cm) each! Toilet paper in rolls was first made in the US in 1890 by Scott Paper Company. Scott began making paper towels in 1907, thanks to a failed attempt to develop a new crepe toilet tissue. This paper was so thick it couldn't be cut and rolled into toilet paper, so Scott made larger rolls, perforated into 13 x 18-inch (33 x 45 cm) sheets and sold them as Sani-Towels.

MAKE A FLY AND PEST STRIP • It's easy to get rid of annoying flies and mosquitoes with a homemade pest strip. Just cover an empty paper towel or toilet paper tube with transparent double-stick transparent tape, and hang where needed.

USE AS KINDLING AND LOGS • Turn toilet paper and paper towel tubes into kindling and logs for your fireplace. For fire starters, use scissors to cut the cardboard into 1/8-inch (3 mm) strips. Keep the strips in a bin near the fireplace so they'll be handy to use next time you make a fire. To make logs, tape over one end of the tube and pack shredded newspaper inside, then tape the other end closed. The tighter you pack the newspaper, the longer your log will burn.

MAKE BOOT TREES • To keep the tops of long, flexible boots from flopping over and developing ugly creases, insert cardboard poster tubes into them to help them hold their shape.

PROTECT IMPORTANT DOCUMENTS • Before storing diplomas, marriage certificates, and other important documents in a chest of drawers, roll them tightly and insert them into cardboard tubes. This prevents creases and keeps the documents clean and dry.

more CARDBOARD TUBES over →

STORE KNITTING NEEDLES

To keep your knitting needles from bending and breaking, try this: Use a long cardboard tube from aluminium foil or plastic wrap. Cover one end with sticky tape. Pinch the other end closed and secure it tightly with tape. Slide the needles in through the tape on the taped end. The tape will hold them in place for secure, organized storage.

STORE FABRIC SCRAPS • Roll up leftover fabric scraps tightly and insert them inside a cardboard tube from your bathroom or kitchen, depending on the volume. For easy identification, tape or staple a sample of the fabric to the outside of the tube.

STORE STRING • Nothing is more useless and frustrating than tangled string. To keep your string ready to use, cut a notch into each end of a toilet paper tube. Secure one end of the string in one notch, wrap the string tightly around the tube, and secure the remaining end in the other notch.

KEEP LINENS CREASE-FREE • Wrap tablecloths and napkins around cardboard tubes after laundering to avoid the creases they would get if they were folded. Use long tubes for tablecloths and paper towel or toilet paper tubes for napkins. Cover the tubes with plastic wrap first.

KEEP PANTS CREASE-FREE • Go to your closet for that good pair of pants you haven't worn in a while, and you find an ugly crease where they've been folded on a wire coat hanger. It won't happen again if you cut a paper towel tube lengthwise, fold it in half horizontally, and place it over the hanger before you hang up your pants. Before hanging pants, tape the sides of the cardboard together at the bottom to keep it from slipping.

MAKE SOME NOISE!

MAKE A KAZOO • Got a bunch of bored kids driving you crazy on a rainy day? Cut three small holes in the middle of a paper towel tube. Cover one end of the tube with waxed paper, secured with a strong rubber band. Now hum into the other end, while using your fingers to plug one, two or all three holes to vary the pitch. Make one for each kid. They may still drive you crazy, but they'll have a ball doing it!

INSTANT MEGAPHONE • Don't shout yourself hoarse when you're calling outside for a child or pet to come home *right now*. Give your vocal cords a rest by using a wide cardboard tube as a megaphone to amplify your voice.

KEEP CHRISTMAS LIGHTS TIDY

Spending more time untangling your Christmas lights than it takes to put them up? Make life easier by wrapping your lights around a cardboard tube and securing them with masking tape. Put small strands of lights or garlands inside cardboard tubes and seal the ends of the tubes with masking tape.

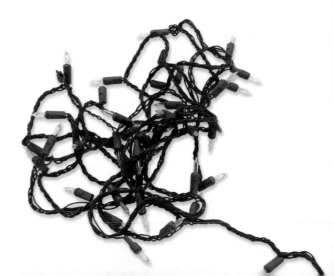

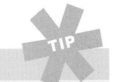

Carpet tubes

✳ *Carpet retailers regularly discard long, thick cardboard tubes that they will probably be happy to give you free for the asking.*

Because the tubes can be up to 12 feet (3.6 m) long, you might want to ask for them to cut one to the size you would like before you take it away.

PROTECT FLUORESCENT LIGHTS • Prevent fragile fluorescent light tubes from breaking before you use them. They will fit neatly into long cardboard tubes sealed with tape at one end.

MAKE A HAMSTER TOY

Place a couple of paper towel or toilet paper tubes in the hamster (or guinea pig) cage. Your little critters will love running and walking through them, and they'll like chewing on the cardboard, too. When the tubes start looking ragged, just replace them with fresh ones.

PRESERVE KIDS' ARTWORK • If you want to save some of your kids' precious artwork for posterity (or you don't want it to clutter up the house), simply roll up the artwork and place it inside a paper towel tube. Label the outside with the child's name and date. The tubes are easy to store, and you can safely preserve the work of your budding young artists. Use this method to hold and store common documents, such as certificates and licenses, too.

BUILD A TOY LOG CABIN • Notch the ends of several long tubes with a craft knife and help your children build log cabins, fences, or huts with them. Use different-sized tubes for added versatility. For a bit of realism, have the kids paint or color the tubes before construction begins.

MAKE CHRISTMAS CRACKERS • Use toilet paper tubes to make Christmas crackers, which 'explode', revealing tiny gifts. For each cracker, tie a string about 8 inches (20 cm) long around a small gift such as candy, a balloon, a pencil eraser, or a small toy. After tying, the string should have about 6 inches (15 cm) to spare. Place the gift into the tube so the string dangles out one end. Cover the tube with brightly colored crepe paper or tissue and twist the ends. When you pull the string, out pops the gift.

CARPET SCRAPS

CATCH A FALLING SOCK • You may never be able to stop socks and other pieces of clothing from falling to the floor en route from your washing machine to dryer, but you can make retrieval a lot easier by placing a narrow piece of carpet on the floor between the two appliances. When something falls, pull out the strip and the article will come back on it.

MUFFLE CLUNKY APPLIANCE NOISE

Does your washing machine or dryer shake, rattle, and roll when you're doing a load? Put a piece of scrap carpet underneath it, and with any luck that'll be all you'll need to calm things down.

more CARPET SCRAPS over →

EXERCISE IN COMFORT • To make an instant exercise mat, cut a length of old carpet around 3 feet (1 m) wide and as long as your height. When you're not using it for yoga or sit-ups, roll it up and store it underneath your bed.

MAKE YOUR OWN CAR MATS • Why buy expensive floor mats for your car when you can make your own? Cut carpet remnants to fit the floor space of your car and drive off in comfort.

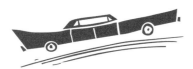

PROTECT YOUR KNEES • To protect your knees when you're washing the floor, weeding, or doing other work on all fours, make your own kneepads. Cut two pieces of carpeting 10 inches (25 cm) square and cut two parallel slits or holes in each. Run old neckties or scarves through the slits and use them to tie the pads to your knees.

KEEP FLOORS DRY • Don't let the floor get soaked when you water your indoor plants. Place 12-inch (30 cm) round carpet scraps under the drip trays of your house plants to absorb any accidental overwatering excess.

PREVENT SCRATCHED FLOORS • Stop screeching chairs from scratching or making black marks on wood or vinyl floors. Glue small circles of carpet remnants to the bottom of chair and table legs.

MAKE A SHOE BUFFER • Use epoxy resin to glue an old piece of carpet to a block of wood for buffing shoes. Make several and use another one to wipe blackboards, and one to clean window screens.

CUSHION KITCHEN SHELVES • To reduce the noisy clattering when putting away pots and pans, cushion kitchen shelves and cupboards with pieces of carpet.

ADD TRACTION • When driving in cold areas, keep good-sized carpet scraps in the trunk of your car to add traction when you're stuck in snow or ice. And keep one piece with your spare tire. When you have a flat, you won't have to kneel or lie on the dirty ground when you have to work under the car.

PROTECT WORKSHOP TOOLS • Is your workshop floor made of concrete or another hard material? If so, put down a few carpet remnants in the area closest to your workbench. Now when tools or containers accidentally fall to the floor, they will be far less likely to break.

KEEP GARDEN PATHS WEED-FREE • Place a series of carpet scraps upside down and cover them with bark mulch or straw for a weed-free garden path. Use smaller scraps as mulch around your vegetable garden.

PET PROTECTION

KEEP DOGGY'S HOME DRY • Don't let raindrops keep falling on your dog's head. Weatherproof the doghouse: Make a rain flap by nailing a carpet remnant over the entrance to your dog's domicile. In colder climates, you can also use small pieces of carpet to line interior walls and the floor to add insulation.

MAKE A SCRATCHING POST • If your cat is clawing up the living room couch, this might do the trick. Make a scratching post by stapling carpet scraps to a post or board and place it near the cat's favorite target. If you want it to be freestanding, nail a board to the bottom of the post to serve as a base.

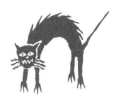

CAR WAX

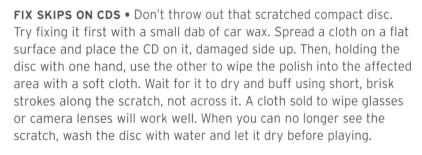

FIX SKIPS ON CDS • Don't throw out that scratched compact disc. Try fixing it first with a small dab of car wax. Spread a cloth on a flat surface and place the CD on it, damaged side up. Then, holding the disc with one hand, use the other to wipe the polish into the affected area with a soft cloth. Wait for it to dry and buff using short, brisk strokes along the scratch, not across it. A cloth sold to wipe glasses or camera lenses will work well. When you can no longer see the scratch, wash the disc with water and let it dry before playing.

KEEP BATHROOM MIRRORS FOG-FREE • To prevent your bathroom mirror from steaming up after your next hot shower, apply a small amount of car paste wax to the mirror, let it dry, and buff it off with a soft cloth. Next time you step out of the shower, you'll be able to see your face in the mirror immediately. You can rub the wax on bathroom fixtures to prevent water spots, too.

ERADICATE FURNITURE STAINS • If there's an ugly white ring on the dining room table, and your regular furniture polish doesn't work, try using a dab of car wax. Trace the ring with your finger to apply the wax and allow it to dry, then buff with a soft cloth.

ELIMINATE BATHROOM MILDEW • To chase grime and mildew from your shower, follow these two simple steps. First, clean the soap and water residue off the tiles or shower wall. Then rub on a layer of car paste wax and buff with a clean, dry cloth. You'll only need to reapply the wax about once a year. But don't wax the bathtub—it will become very slippery.

KEEP SNOW FROM STICKING • When it's time to clear the driveway after a snowstorm, you don't want snow sticking to your shovel. Apply two thick coats of car paste wax to the work surface of the shovel before you begin shoveling. The snow won't stick and there will be less wear and tear on your cardiovascular system. If you use a snow blower, wax the chute.

CASTOR OIL

SOFTEN CUTICLES • If you were ever forced to swallow castor oil as a child, this may come as a pleasant surprise: The high vitamin-E content of that awful-tasting thick oil can work wonders on brittle nails and ragged cuticles. And you don't have to swallow the stuff to get the benefits, just massage a small amount into your cuticles and nails each day and within about three months you will have supple cuticles and healthy nails.

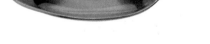

SOOTHE TIRED EYES

Before going to bed, rub odorless castor oil all around your eyes. Rub some on your eyelashes, too, to keep them shiny. However, be very careful not to get the oil in your eyes.

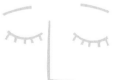

more CASTOR OIL over →

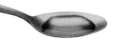

LUBRICATE KITCHEN SCISSORS • Use castor oil instead of toxic petroleum oil to lubricate kitchen scissors and other utensils that touch food.

REPEL MOLES • If moles are destroying your garden and lawn, try using castor oil to get rid of them. Mix ½ cup (125 ml) castor oil and 7½ quarts (7 L) water together and drench the lawn with the mixture. It won't kill them, but it will certainly get them looking for another place to dig up.

ENJOY A MASSAGE • Castor oil is just the right consistency to use as a soothing massage oil. For a real treat, warm the oil on the stovetop or on half-power in the microwave. Relax and enjoy.

PERK UP AILING FERNS • Give your sickly ferns a tonic made by mixing 1 tablespoon (15 ml) castor oil and 1 tablespoon (15 ml) baby shampoo with 4 cups (1 L) lukewarm water. Give the fern about 3 tablespoons (45 ml) of the tonic and follow up with plain water. Your plants will be perky by the time you use up your supply of tonic.

DID YOU KNOW?

Native to India, castor oil is extracted from the seeds of the castor oil plant. It is more than an old-fashioned medicine cabinet staple, as it has hundreds of industrial uses. Large amounts are used in paints, varnishes, lipsticks, hair tonics, and shampoos. Castor oil is also converted into plastics, soaps, waxes, hydraulic fluids, and inks. It is also made into lubricants for jet engines and racing cars because it does not become stiff with cold or overly thin with heat.

CONDITION YOUR HAIR • For healthy, shiny hair, mix 2 teaspoons (10 ml) castor oil with 1 teaspoon (5 ml) glycerine and 1 egg white. Massage it into wet hair, wait for a few minutes, then wash it out.

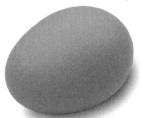

CAT LITTER

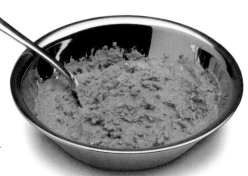

MAKE A MUD MASK

Make a deep-cleansing mud mask. Mix two handfuls of fresh, clumping, clay-based cat litter with enough warm water to make a thick paste. Smear the paste over your face, let it set for 20 minutes, and rinse clean with water. The clay from cat litter detoxifies your skin by absorbing dirt and oil from the pores. When your friends compliment you on your complexion and ask how you did it, just tell them it's your little secret.

SNEAKER DEODORIZER • If your running shoes and sneakers reek, fill a couple of old socks with scented clay-based cat litter, tie them shut, and place them in the sneakers overnight. Repeat if necessary until the sneakers are stink-free.

ADD TRACTION ON ICE • In cold areas, keep a bag of clay-based cat litter in the trunk of your car. Use it to add traction when you're stuck in ice or snow.

PREVENT GREASE FIRES • Don't let a grease fire spoil your next barbecue. Pour a layer of clay-based cat litter into the bottom of the barbecue's drip tray for trouble-free outdoor cooking.

STOP MUSTY ODORS • You can get rid of that musty smell when you open the closet door just by placing a shallow box filled with clay-based cat litter in each musty closet or room. Because it absorbs odors, cat litter works great as a deodorant.

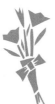

PRESERVE FLOWERS • The fragrance and beauty of freshly cut flowers is such a fleeting thing. You can't save the smell, but you can preserve their beauty by drying your flowers on a bed of clay-based cat litter in an airtight container for 7 to 10 days.

REMOVE A FOUL STENCH • Just because garbage cans hold garbage doesn't mean they have to smell disgusting. Sprinkle some clay-based cat litter into the bottom of garbage cans to keep them smelling fresh. Change the litter after a week or so or when it becomes damp. If you have a baby in the house, use cat litter the same way to freshen diaper pails.

KEEP TENTS FREE OF MUSTY ODORS • Keep tents and sleeping bags fresh smelling and free of musty odors when not in use. Pour cat litter into an old sock, tie the end and store it inside the bag or tent.

MAKE GREASE SPOTS DISAPPEAR • Get rid of ugly grease and oil spots on your driveway or garage floor by simply covering them with clay-based cat litter. If the spots are fresh, the litter will soak up most of the oil right away. To remove old stains, pour some paint thinner on the stain before tossing on the cat litter. Wait about 12 hours and sweep it clean.

FRESHEN OLD BOOKS

You can rejuvenate old books that smell musty by sealing them overnight in a container with clean, clay-based cat litter.

CREATE INSTANT PAPIER-MÂCHÉ • Simply add water to clean recycled paper-based cat litter in a bucket and allow it to soften overnight. You'll have instant paper pulp for your next craft project.

DID YOU KNOW?

American salesman Ed Lowe might not have had the idea for cat litter if a neighbor hadn't asked him for some sand for her cat litter tray one day in 1947. Ed, who worked for his father's company selling industrial absorbents, suggested clay instead because it was more absorbent and would not leave tracks around the house. When she returned for more, he knew he had a winner. Soon he was crisscrossing the country, selling bags of his Kitty Litter from the back of his Chevy Coupe. By 1990, Edward Lowe Industries, Inc. was America's largest producer of litter tray filler with sales of more than $210 million annually.

CHALK

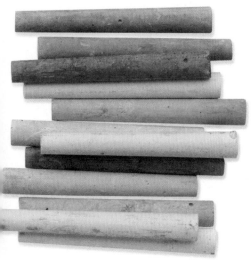

REPEL ANTS • The easiest way to keep ants at bay is by drawing a chalk line around home entry points. The ants will be repelled by the calcium carbonate in the chalk, which is actually made up of ground-up and compressed shells of marine animals. And you can scatter powdered chalk around garden plants to repel ants and slugs.

POLISH METAL AND MARBLE • To make metal shine like new, put some chalk dust on a damp cloth and wipe. (You can make chalk dust by pulverizing pieces of chalk.) Buff with a soft cloth for an even shinier finish. Wipe marble with a damp, soft cloth dipped in powdered chalk. Rinse with clear water and dry thoroughly.

KEEP SILVER FROM TARNISHING • You love serving friends with your fine silver, but polishing it before each use is another story. Put one or two pieces of chalk in the drawer with your good silver; it will absorb moisture and slow tarnishing. Put some in your jewelry box to delay tarnishing there, too.

REMOVE GREASE SPOTS • Rub chalk on a grease spot on clothing or table linen and let it absorb the oil before you brush it off. If the stain lingers, rub chalk into it again before laundering. To get rid of ring-around-the-collar stains, mark the stains heavily with chalk before laundering. The chalk will absorb the oils that hold dirt in.

STOP SCREWDRIVER SLIPS

Does your screwdriver slip when you try to tighten a screw? It won't slip nearly as much if you rub some chalk on the tip of the blade.

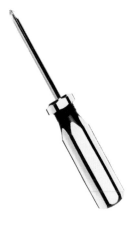

DID YOU KNOW?

The first 'street painting' took place in sixteenth-century Italy, when artists began using chalk to make drawings on the pavement. The artists, who became known as *madonnari*, often made paintings of the Virgin Mary. These *madonnari* of old were itinerant artists known for a life of freedom and travel. But they always managed to attend the many regional holidays and festivals that took place in each Italian province. Today, *madonnari* and their quaint street paintings continue to be a colorful part of the celebrations that take place every day in modern Italy.

REDUCE CLOSET DAMPNESS • Tie a dozen pieces of chalk together and hang them up in a damp closet. The chalk will absorb moisture and help prevent mildew. Replace the chalk bundle with a new one every few months.

HIDE CEILING MARKS • Temporarily cover up water or scuff marks on the ceiling until you have time to paint or make a permanent repair. Rub a stick of white chalk over the mark until it lightens or disappears.

KEEP TOOLS RUST-FREE • You can eliminate moisture and prevent rust from invading your toolbox by simply putting a few pieces of chalk in the box. Your tools will be rust-free and so will the toolbox.

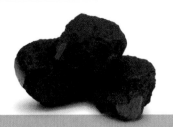

CHARCOAL BRIQUETTES

MAKE A DEHUMIDIFIER • A humid closet, attic, or cellar can wreak havoc on your health as well as your clothes. Get rid of all that humidity with several homemade dehumidifiers. To make one, just put some charcoal briquettes in a large, clean, lidded can, punch a few holes in the lid and place in the humid areas. Replace the charcoal every few months.

KEEP ROOT WATER FRESH • Put a piece of charcoal in the water when you're rooting plant cuttings. The charcoal will keep the water fresh.

BANISH BATHROOM MOISTURE AND ODORS • Hiding a few pieces of charcoal in the nooks and crannies of your bathroom is a great way to soak up moisture and cut down on unpleasant odors. Replace them every couple of months.

KEEP BOOKS MOLD-FREE • Professional librarians use charcoal to get rid of musty odors on old books, and you can do the same. If your bookcase has glass doors, it may provide a damp environment that can lead to mustiness and mold. A piece or two of charcoal placed inside will help keep the books dry and mold-free.

DID YOU KNOW?

Henry Ford was the originator of charcoal briquettes? The first mass-produced charcoal briquettes were, surprisingly enough, manufactured by the Ford Motor Company. They were made from waste wood from a Ford-owned sawmill in Kingsford, Michigan, built to provide wood for the bodies of Ford's popular 'Woody' station wagons. The remaining charcoal was manufactured into briquettes and sold as Ford Charcoal Briquettes. Henry Ford II closed the sawmill in 1951 and sold the plant to some local businessmen, who formed the Kingsford Chemical Company.

CHEESECLOTH

MAKE A HOMEMADE BUTTERFLY NET • Just sew cheesecloth into a bag and glue or staple it to a hoop formed from a wire coat hanger—and send the kids on a hunt. Or make a smaller cheesecloth net for when you take the kids fishing and let them use it as a bait net to catch minnows. For an inexpensive Halloween costume, wrap a child in cheesecloth from head to toe and send your mini-mummy out to collect treats.

REMOVE TURKEY STUFFING WITH EASE • To keep turkey stuffing from sticking to the bird's insides, pack the stuffing in cheesecloth before you stuff it into the turkey's cavity. When the turkey is ready to serve, pull out the cheesecloth and the stuffing will slide out with it.

more CHEESECLOTH over →

CONVERT A COLANDER INTO A STRAINER • If you can't find a strainer when you need one, a colander lined with cheesecloth will do the trick just as well.

CUT VACUUMING TIME • Here is a fabulous, time-saving way to vacuum the contents of a drawer filled with small objects without having to remove the contents. Simply cover the nozzle of your vacuum cleaner with cheesecloth, secured with a rubber band, and the vacuum will pick up only the dust.

REDUCE WASTE DRYING HERBS • When you're drying fresh herbs, first wrap them in cheesecloth to prevent seeds and the smaller crumbled pieces from falling through.

PICNIC FOOD TENT • Keep insects and dirt away from your picnic-food serving plates. Wrap a piece of cheesecloth around an old wire umbrella form and place it over the plates. Remove the umbrella handle and tack the cheesecloth to the umbrella ribs with a needle and thread.

MAKE INSTANT FESTIVE CURTAINS • Brighten any room with inexpensive, colorful, and festive cheesecloth curtains. Dye inexpensive cheesecloth (available in bulk from fabric stores) in bright colors and cut it to the lengths and widths you need. Attach clip-on café-curtain hooks and your new curtains are ready to hang.

CHEST RUB

REPEL TICKS AND OTHER INSECTS • Going for a walk in the woods? Smear some chest rub on your legs and pants before you leave the house. It will keep ticks from biting and spare you from getting Lyme disease, which is spread by ticks. Annoying insects like gnats and mosquitoes will go elsewhere for victims if you apply chest rub to your skin before venturing outdoors. They hate the smell.

STOP INSECT-BITE ITCH FAST • Apply a generous coat of chest rub for immediate relief from itchy insect bites. The eucalyptus and menthol in the ointment are what do the trick.

MAKE CALLUSES DISAPPEAR • Coat calluses with chest rub and cover them with a suitable-sized band-aid overnight. Repeat as needed. Most calluses will disappear after several days.

SOOTHE ACHING FEET • Are your feet aching after that long walk in the woods? Try applying a thick coat of chest rub and cover them with a pair of socks before going to bed at night. When you wake up, your feet will be moisturized and rejuvenated.

TREAT TOENAIL FUNGUS • If you have a toenail fungus, try applying a thick coat of chest rub to the affected nail several times a day. Many users and even some medical pros swear that it works (just check the Internet). But if you don't see results after a few weeks, consult a dermatologist or podiatrist.

DID YOU KNOW?

Lunsford Richardson, the pharmacist who created Vick's VapoRub in 1905, also originated America's first 'junk mail'. Richardson was working in his brother-in-law's pharmacy when he blended menthol and other ingredients into an ointment to clear sinuses and ease congestion. He called it Richardson's Croup and Pneumonia Cure Salve, but soon realized he needed something catchier for the product to sell successfully. He changed the name to Vick's after his brother-in-law, Joshua Vick, and convinced the U.S. Post Office to institute a new policy allowing him to send the advertisements addressed only to 'Boxholder'. Sales of Vick's first surpassed a million dollars during the Spanish flu epidemic of 1918.

CHEWING GUM

RETRIEVE VALUABLES • Oops, you just lost an earring or other small valuable down the drain. Try retrieving it with a freshly chewed piece of chewing gum stuck to the bottom of a fishing weight. Dangle it from a string tied to the weight, let it take hold, and reel the earring back up the drain.

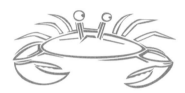

LURE A CRAB

You'll be eating plenty of crab cakes if you try this trick. Briefly chew a piece of gum so that it is soft but still hasn't lost its flavor, then attach it to a crab line. Lower the line and wait for the crabs to go for the gum.

FILL CRACKS • Fill a crack in a clay flowerpot or a dog bowl with a piece of well-chewed chewing gum.

DID YOU KNOW?

Humans have been chewing gum a long time. Ancient Greeks chewed *mastiche*, a chewing gum made from the resin of the mastic tree. And ancient Mayans chewed *chicle*, the sap from the sapodilla tree. Native Americans chewed the sap from spruce trees, then passed the habit on to the Pilgrims. And other early American settlers made chewing gum from spruce sap and beeswax. John B. Curtis produced the first commercial chewing gum in the U.S. in 1848 and called it State of Maine Pure Spruce Gum.

USE AS MAKESHIFT WINDOW PUTTY • Worried that a loose pane of glass may tumble and break before you get around to fixing it? Hold it in place temporarily with a wad or two of freshly chewed gum.

REPAIR GLASSES • When your glasses suddenly have a lens loose, put a small piece of chewed gum in the corner of the lens to hold it in place until you can get the glasses properly repaired.

TREAT FLATULENCE AND HEARTBURN • Settle stomach gases and relieve heartburn by chewing a stick of spearmint gum. The oils in the spearmint act as an antiflatulent. Chewing stimulates the production of saliva, which neutralizes stomach acid and corrects the flow of digestive juices. Spearmint also acts as a digestive aid.

CHICKEN WIRE

REPEL DEER • Are the deer tearing up your garden again? Here's a simple method to keep them away. Stake chicken wire *flat* around the perimeter of your garden. Deer don't like to walk on it and it looks better than the usual chicken-wire fencing.

FIRMER FENCE POSTS • Before setting a fence post in concrete, wrap the base with chicken wire. This will make the anchoring firmer and the post more secure.

more CHICKEN WIRE over →

MAKE A CHILDPROOF CORRAL

Garages and sheds are often full of dangerous tools and toxic substances. Keep kids away from these hazardous items by enclosing them in a childproof corral. Make it by first attaching standard-width chicken wire to the walls in a corner. Then staple 1 x 2s to the cut ends of the wire and install screw eyes in the wood to accommodate two padlocks.

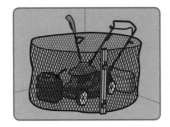

SECURE INSULATION • After you place fiberglass batting between roof rafters or floor joists, staple chicken wire across the joists to secure it and, in the case of the rafters, to keep it from sagging.

FOR THOSE WITH GREEN FINGERS ...

CROWN CATNIP PLANTS • If you are growing catnip for your cat, put a crown of chicken wire over the plant, close to the ground. As the catnip grows through the wire and gets eaten, the roots will remain intact, growing new catnip. Make sure the edges of the wire are tucked in securely. Catnip is a hardy plant, even in very low temperatures, so if the roots remain it will grow back year after year.

PROTECT BULBS FROM RODENTS • You can keep annoying burrowing rodents from damaging your flower bulbs by lining the bottom of a prepared bed with chicken wire, planting the bulbs, and covering them with soil.

FLOWER HOLDER • To keep cut flowers aligned in a vase, squish some chicken wire together and place it in the bottom of the vase before inserting the flower stems.

CLIPBOARDS

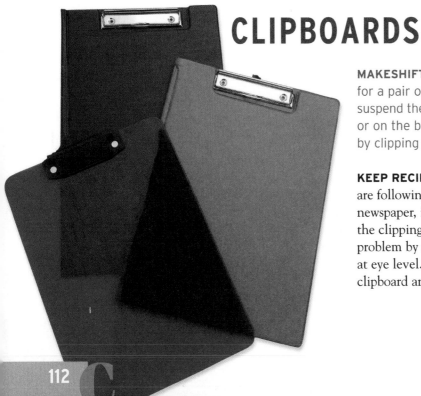

MAKESHIFT PANTS HANGER • Can't find a hanger for a pair of pants? Use a clipboard instead. Just suspend the clipboard from a hook inside the closet or on the bedroom door. Hang the pants overnight by clipping the cuffs to the board.

KEEP RECIPES AT EYE LEVEL • When you are following a recipe taken from a magazine or newspaper, it's hard to read and keep clean when the clipping is lying on the countertop. Solve the problem by attaching a clipboard to a wall cupboard at eye level. Just snap the recipe of the day on the clipboard and you're ready to start cooking.

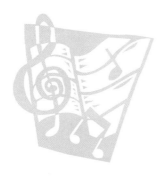

KEEP SHEET MUSIC IN PLACE

Flimsy pages of sheet music are susceptible to drafts and sometimes seem to spend more time on the floor than on the music stand. To eliminate this problem, attach the music sheets to a clipboard before placing it in the stand. The pages will remain upright and in place.

HOLD PLACEMATS • Hang a clipboard inside a kitchen cupboard or pantry door and use the clamp as a convenient, space-saving way to store placemats.

AID ROAD-TRIP NAVIGATION • Before starting out on a long drive, fold the map to the area where you will be traveling. Attach it to a clipboard and keep it nearby to check your progress during rest stops.

ORGANIZE YOUR SANDPAPER • Most of the time, sandpaper is still good after the first or second time it's been used. The trick is to find the used sandpaper again. Hang a clipboard on a hook on your workshop pegboard. Just clip still-usable sandpaper to the board when you are done and it will be on hand the next time you need it.

CLOTHESPINS

KEEP SNACKS FRESH • Tired of biting into stale potato chips from a previously opened bag? Use clothespins to reseal bags of chips and other snacks, cereal, crackers, and seeds. The foods will stay fresh longer and you won't have as many spills in the pantry, either. Use a clothespin for added freshness insurance when you store food in a freezer bag, too.

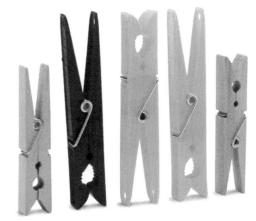

FASTEN CHRISTMAS LIGHTS • The trick to keeping your outdoor Christmas lights in place and ready to withstand the elements isn't as tricky as you might think. As you fix the lights to gutters, trees, or bushes, fasten them securely with clip-on clothespins.

MAKE A CLOTHESPIN CLIPBOARD • Organize your workshop, kitchen, or bathroom with a homemade rack made with straight clothespins. Space several pins evenly apart on a piece of wood and screw them on with screws coming through from the back of the board (pre-drill the holes so you don't split the peg). Now your rack is ready to hang.

ORGANIZE YOUR WARDROBE • Sometimes it's not just finding children's shoes that's the problem; it's finding *both* shoes. Try using clothespins to hold together pairs of shoes, boots, or sneakers, and put an end to those unscheduled hunting expeditions in the closet. It's a good idea for gloves, too.

KEEP GLOVES IN SHAPE

After washing wool gloves, insert a straight wooden clothespin into each finger. The pins will keep the gloves in their proper shape.

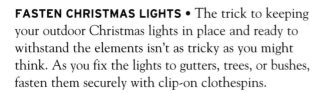

more CLOTHESPINS over →

C **113**

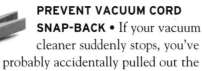

PREVENT VACUUM CORD SNAP-BACK • If your vacuum cleaner suddenly stops, you've probably accidentally pulled out the plug, which means the cord will automatically retract and snap back into the machine. To avoid similar annoyance in the future, simply clip a clothespin to the cord at the length you want.

MAKE AN INSTANT BIB • Make bibs for your child by using a clip-on clothespin to hold a dish towel around the child's neck. Use bigger towels to make lobster bibs for adults. It's much faster than tying on a bib.

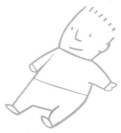

MAKE CLOTHESPIN PUPPETS • Traditional straight clothespins are ideal for making little puppets. Using the knob as a head, have kids paste on bits of wool for hair and scraps of cloth or colored paper for clothes to give each one its own personality.

HOLD A LEAF BAG OPEN • If you've ever tried to fill a large leaf bag all on your own, only to see half the leaves fall to the ground because the bag won't stay open, we have a solution for you. Next time use a couple of clip-on clothespins as helpers. After you shake open the bag and spread it wide, use the clothespins to clip one side of the bag to a chain-link fence or other convenient site. The bag will stay open for easy filling.

DID YOU KNOW?

Between 1852 and 1857 the U.S. Patent Office granted patents for 146 different clothespins. Today wooden pin makers have all but disappeared, as plastic pins take the place of the wooden ones. The small family-owned, secondary wood-processing companies have died off, to be replaced by imported wooden pins made overseas. Ironically, these days wooden pins are more likely to be found in craft and discount stores than in supermarkets.

MARK A BULB SPOT • What to do when a flower that is supposed to bloom in the spring doesn't? Just push a straight clothespin into the soil at the spot where it didn't grow. In the autumn you will know exactly where to plant new bulbs to avoid gaps.

GRIP A NAIL

Hammer the nail and not your fingers. Just remember to use a clip-on clothespin to hold nails when hammering in hard-to-reach places.

CLAMP THIN OBJECTS • You can use clip-on clothespins as clamps when you're gluing two thin objects together. Just let the clothespin hold them in place until the glue sets.

KEEP A PAINTBRUSH AFLOAT • To keep your paintbrush from sinking into the solvent residue when you soak it, just clamp the brush to the container with a clothespin.

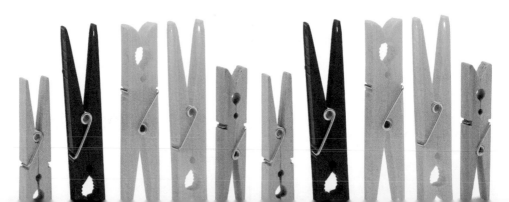

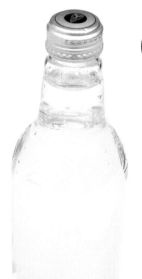

CLUB SODA

MAKE PANCAKES AND WAFFLES FLUFFIER • If you like your pancakes and waffles on the fluffy side, substitute club soda for the liquid called for in the recipes. You'll be amazed at how light and fluffy your breakfast treats turn out. The bubbles really give the batter a lift.

REMOVE FABRIC STAINS • Clean grease stains from double-knit fabrics by pouring club soda on the stains and scrubbing gently. Scrub stains on carpets, or less delicate articles of clothing, more vigorously.

HELP SHUCKING OYSTERS • If you love oysters but find shucking them to be a near-impossible job, try soaking them in club soda before you shuck. The oysters won't exactly jump out of their shells, but they will be much easier to open.

ELIMINATE URINE STAINS • Did someone have an accident? After blotting up as much urine as possible, pour club soda over the stained area and immediately blot again. The club soda will get rid of the stain and help reduce the foul smell.

TAME YOUR TUMMY

Cold club soda with a dash of bitters will work wonders on an upset stomach caused by indigestion or a hangover.

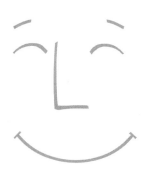

CLEAN CAST IRON EASILY • Food tastes delicious when it's cooked in cast iron, but cleaning those heavy pots and pans isn't much fun. You can make the cleanup a lot easier by pouring some club soda into the cookware while it's still warm. The bubbly soda will prevent the mess from sticking.

CLEAN YOUR CAR WINDSHIELD • Keep a spray bottle filled with club soda in the trunk of your car and use it to help remove bird droppings, and greasy stains from your windshield. The fizzywater speeds the cleaning process.

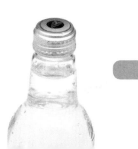

more CLUB SODA over →

CLEAN PRECIOUS GEMS • Soak your diamonds, rubies, sapphires, and emeralds in club soda to give them a bright sheen. Simply place them in a glass full of club soda and let them soak overnight.

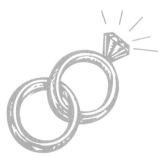

CLEAN COUNTERTOPS AND FIXTURES • Pour club soda directly on stainless steel countertops, ranges, and sinks, wipe with a soft cloth, rinse with warm water, and wipe dry. To clean porcelain fixtures, simply pour club soda over them and wipe with a soft cloth. There's no need for soap or rinsing, and the soda will not mar the finish. Give the inside of your fridge a good cleaning with a weak solution of club soda and a little bit of salt.

REMOVE RUST • To loosen rusty nuts and bolts, pour some club soda over them. The carbonation helps to bubble the rust away.

GIVE YOUR PLANTS A MINERAL BATH • Don't throw out that leftover club soda—use it to water your indoor and outdoor plants. The minerals in the club soda help green plants grow. For maximum benefit, try to water your plants with club soda at least once a week.

DID YOU KNOW?

Bubbling water has been associated with good health since the time of the ancient Romans, who enjoyed drinking mineral water almost as much as they liked bathing in it. The first club soda was sold in North America at the end of the 1700s. That's when pharmacists figured out how to infuse plain water with carbon dioxide, which they believed was responsible for giving natural bubbling water health-inducing qualities. Club soda and sparkling mineral water are essentially the same. However, true mineral water (originally called seltzer, after the region in Germany where it is plentiful) is a natural effervescent water whereas club soda is manufactured.

RESTORE HAIR COLOR

If your blonde hair turns green when you swim in a pool with too much chlorine, don't panic. Rinse your hair with club soda and it will return to its original color.

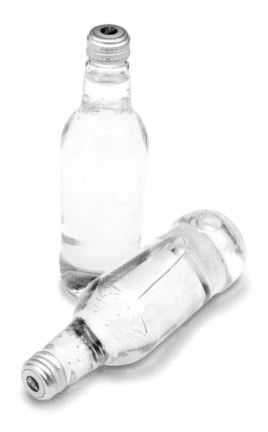

COAT HANGERS

STOP CAULK-TUBE OOZE

To prevent caulk from oozing out of the tube once the job is done, cut a 3-inch (7.5 cm) piece of coat hanger wire and shape one end into a hook and insert the other, straight end into the tube. Now you can easily pull out the stopper as needed.

SECURE A SOLDERING IRON • Keeping a hot soldering iron from rolling away and burning something on your workbench can be a real problem. To solve this, just twist a wire coat hanger into a holder 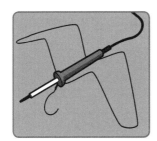 for the iron to rest in. To make the holder, simply bend an ordinary coat hanger in half to form a large V. Then bend each half in half so that the entire piece is shaped like a W.

CREATE ARTS AND CRAFTS • Make mobiles for the kids' room using wire coat hangers, and paint them in bright colors. Or use hangers to make wings and other accessories for costumes.

UNCLOG TOILETS AND VACUUM CLEANERS • If your toilet is clogged by a foreign object, fish out the culprit with a straightened wire coat hanger. Use a straightened hanger to unclog a jammed vacuum cleaner hose.

LIGHT A HARD-TO-REACH PILOT LIGHT • The pilot light has gone out way inside your stove or furnace and you'd rather not risk a burn by lighting a match and sticking your hand all the way in there. Instead, open up a wire hanger and tape the match to one end. Strike the match, then use the hanger to reach the pilot to light it.

FOR THOSE WITH GREEN FINGERS ...

MAKE A MINI-GREENHOUSE • To convert a window box into a mini-greenhouse, bend three or four lengths of coat hanger wire into U shapes and place the ends into the soil. Punch small holes in a dry-cleaning bag and wrap it around the box before putting it back in the window.

HANG A PLANT • Wrap a straightened wire coat hanger around a 6 to 8-inch (15–20 cm) flowerpot just below the lip, twist it back on itself to secure it, and hang.

MAKE PLANT MARKERS • Need some waterproof plant signs for your outdoor plants? Just cut up little rectangles from an empty plastic milk carton or similar rigid but easy-to-cut plastic. Write the name of the plant with an indelible marker. Cut short stakes from wire hangers. Make two small slits in each marker and pass the wire stakes through the slits. Neither rain nor sprinkler will obscure your signs.

more COAT HANGERS over →

SCIENCE **WORKS!**

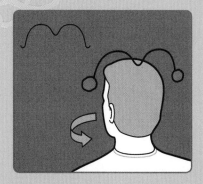

Here's a fun and easy way to demonstrate Newton's first law of motion.

Bend a wire coathanger into a large loopy M shape, as shown. Holding the wire in the middle, attach a same-sized modeling-clay ball to each of the hooks. Then place the low center point of the M on top of your head. If you turn your head to the left or right, the inertia of the balls will be enough to keep them in place, demonstrating Newton's law that 'Objects at rest tend to stay at rest'. With practice, you'll be able to turn right around and the balls will remain still.

DID YOU KNOW?

All Albert J. Parkhouse wanted to do when he arrived at work was to hang up his coat and get busy doing his job. It was 1903, and Albert worked at Timberlake Wire and Novelty Company in Jackson, Michigan. But when he went to hang his clothes on the hooks the company provided for workers, all were in use. Frustrated, Albert picked up a piece of wire, bent it into two large, oblong hoops opposite each other and twisted both ends at the center into a hook. He hung his coat on it and went to work. The company thought so much of the idea they patented it and made a fortune. Poor old Albert never got a penny for inventing the wire coat hanger.

EXTEND YOUR REACH

Can't reach that object that has fallen behind the refrigerator or stove? Try using a straightened wire coat hanger (except for the hook at the end), and use it to fish for the object.

MAKE A GIANT BUBBLE WAND • Kids will love to make giant bubbles with a homemade bubble wand fashioned from a wire coat hanger. Shape the hanger into a hoop with a handle and dip it into a bucket filled with 1 part dishwashing liquid in 2 parts water. You can add a few drops of food coloring to make the bubbles more visible. One or two teaspoons (5-10 ml) glycerine will also keep the bubbles shiny and stable.

MAKE A HANDY DISPOSABLE STRAINER • If you need a strainer for paint or any other messy liquid, use a wire coat hanger to make a disposable one. Pull the hanger wire into a roughly round shape, leaving the hook as a handle. Cover it by stretching the leg from a pair of pantyhose over the frame. Strain whatever you need to, toss the nylon hose, and keep the frame. If you cover it with an onion-bag mesh, it makes a handy lightweight net to catch fish or other little critters.

MAKE A PAINT CAN HOLDER • When you are up on a ladder painting your house, one hand is holding on while the other is painting, so how do you hold onto the paint can? Grab a pair of wire-cutting scissors and cut the hook plus 1 inch (2.5 cm) of wire from a wire coat hanger. Use a pair of pliers to twist the 1-inch (2.5 cm) section firmly around the handle of your paint can. Now you have a handy hanger.

COFFEE BEANS

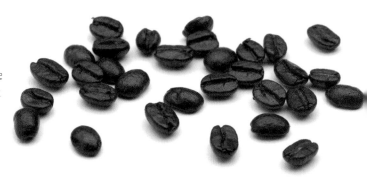

FRESHEN YOUR BREATH • What to do when you're all out of peppermints or breath fresheners? Just suck on a coffee bean for a while and your mouth will smell clean and fresh again.

REMOVE FOUL ODORS FROM HANDS • If your hands smell of garlic, fish, or other strong foods you've been handling, a few coffee beans may be all you need to get rid of the odor. Put the beans in your hands and rub them together. The oil released from the coffee beans will absorb the foul smell. When the odor is gone, wash your hands thoroughly in warm, soapy water.

FILL A BEANBAG • They don't call them beanbags for nothing. Coffee beans are ideal for using as beanbag filler, but with the price of coffee these days it's a good idea to wait for a sale and then buy the cheapest beans available.

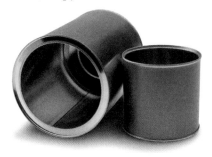

COFFEE CANS

SEPARATE HAMBURGERS • Before you put those hamburger patties in the freezer, stack them with a plastic coffee-can lid between each and put them in a plastic bag. Now, when the patties are frozen you'll be able to easily peel off as many as you need.

BAKE PERFECTLY ROUND BREAD • Use small coffee cans to bake perfectly cylindrical loaves of bread. Use your favorite recipe but put the dough in a well-greased coffee can instead of a loaf pan. For yeast breads use two cans and fill each only half full. Grease the inside of the lids and place them on the cans. For yeast breads, you will know when it is time to bake when the rising dough pushes the lids off. Place the cans—without the lids—upright in the oven to bake.

HOLD KITCHEN SCRAPS • Line a coffee can with a small plastic bag and keep it near the sink to hold kitchen scraps and peelings. Instead of walking back and forth to the garbage can, you'll make one trip to dump all the scraps at the same time.

MAKE A BANK • To make a bank for the kids or a collection can for a favorite charity, use a craft knife to cut a 1/8-inch (3 mm) slit in the centrer of the plastic lid of a coffee can. Tape decorative paper or adhesive plastic to the sides of the kids' bank; for a collection can, use the sides of the can to highlight the charity you are helping.

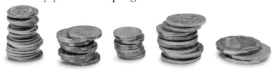

KEEP THE LAUNDRY NEAT • Have an empty coffee can nearby as you're going through the kids' pockets before putting up a load of laundry. Use it to deposit chewing gum and candy wrappers, paper scraps, and other assorted items that kids like to stuff into their pockets. Keep another can handy for coins and bills.

more COFFEE CANS over →

CREATE A TOY HOLDER • Coffee cans are perfect decorative containers for kids' miniature books and small toys. Wash and dry a coffee can and file off any sharp edges. Sponge on two coats of white acrylic paint, letting it dry between coats. Cut out a design from an old sheet or pillowcase to wrap around the can. Mix 4 tablespoons (60 ml) white school glue with enough water to make the consistency of paint. Paint on the glue mixture and gently press the fabric onto the can. Trim the bottom and tuck top edges inside the can. Apply two coats of glue mixture over the fabric overlay, letting it dry between coats.

KEEP CARPETS DRY • Place plastic coffee-can lids under house plants as saucers. They will protect carpets and wooden floors and catch excess water.

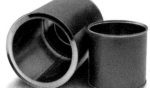

STORE BELTS • If you have more belts than places to hang them up, just roll them up and store them in a cleaned-out coffee can with a clear lid. Coffee cans are just the right size to keep belts from creasing, and clear lids will let you find each belt easily.

MAKE A DEHUMIDIFIER • If you have below-ground rooms that are excessively damp, try this easy-to-make dehumidifier. Fill an empty coffee can with salt and leave it in a corner where it will sit undisturbed. Replace the salt at monthly intervals or as needed.

KEEP TOILET PAPER DRY WHEN CAMPING • Take a few empty coffee cans with you on your next camping trip and use them to keep toilet paper dry in rainy weather, or when you're transporting camping supplies in a canoe or boat.

FOR THE DO-IT-YOURSELFERS

ELIMINATE WORKSHOP CLUTTER • If you want small items like screws, nuts, and nails to be handy, but don't want them to take up workbench space, here's a way to get the small stuff up out of the way. Drill a hole near the top of empty coffee cans so you can hang them on nails on your workshop wall. Label the cans with masking tape so you will know what's inside.

SOAK A PAINTBRUSH • An empty coffee can is perfect for briefly soaking a paintbrush in thinner before continuing a job the next day. Cut an X into the lid and insert the brush handles so the bristles clear the bottom of the can by about an 1/2 inch (1 cm). If the can has no lid, attach a stick to the brush handle with a rubber band to keep the bristles off the bottom of the can.

CATCH PAINT DRIPS • Turn the plastic lids from old coffee cans into drip catchers under paint cans and under furniture legs when you're painting. Protect cupboard shelves by putting them under jars of cooking oil and honey, too.

GAUGE RAINFALL OR SPRINKLER COVERAGE • Next time it starts to rain, place empty coffee cans in several places around the garden. When the rain stops, measure the depth of the water in the cans. If they measure at least 1 inch (2.5 cm), there's no need for additional watering. This is also a good way to test if your irrigation system is getting sufficient water to the areas it is supposed to cover.

DID YOU KNOW?

Once it has been ground, coffee loses its flavor immediately unless it is specially packaged or brewed. While freshly roasted and ground coffee is often sealed in special combination plastic-and-paper bags, vacuum-sealed cans can keep coffee fresh for up to three years. The U.S. is the world's largest consumer of coffee. In 2016-2017, American coffee drinkers consumed 3 billion pounds (1.5 million kg) of coffee. The typical U.S. coffee drinker has more than 3 cups of coffee per day.

MAKE A COFFEE-CAN BIRD FEEDER

To transform a coffee can into a sturdy bird feeder, begin with a full can and open the top only halfway. (Pour the coffee into an airtight container.) Open the bottom of the can the same way. Carefully bend the cut ends down inside

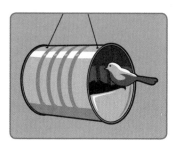

the can so the edges are not exposed to cut you. Punch a hole in the side of the can at both ends, where it will be the 'top' of the feeder, and put a length of wire through each end to make a hanger for it.

MAKE A SPOT LAWN SEEDER • When it's time to re-seed bare spots on your lawn, don't use a regular spreader. It wastes seed by throwing it everywhere. For precision seeding, fashion a spot seeder from an empty coffee can and a pair of plastic lids. Drill small holes in the bottom of the can, just big enough to let grass seeds pass through. Put one lid over the bottom of the can, fill the can with seeds and cap it with the other lid. When you're ready to spread the seeds, take off the bottom lid. When you're finished, replace it to seal in any unused seed for safe storage.

COFFEE FILTERS

COVER FOOD IN THE MICROWAVE • Coffee filters are microwave-safe. Use them to cover bowls or dishes to prevent splattering when cooking or baking in your microwave oven.

FILTER CORK CRUMBS FROM WINE • Don't let cork crumbs ruin your enjoyment of a good glass of wine. If your attempt at opening the bottle results in floating cork crumbs, just decant the wine through a coffee filter.

LINE A SIEVE • If you save your cooking oil for reuse after deep-frying, line your sieve with a basket-style coffee filter to remove smaller food remnants and impurities.

HOLD A TACO • Serve tacos, hot dogs, popcorn, and other messy foods in cone or basket-style coffee filters. The filter is a perfect sleeve, will help keep fingers clean, and make the cleanup a snap.

CATCH ICE-CREAM DRIPS • Next time the kids scream for ice cream cones or popsicles, serve them with a drip catcher made from basket-style coffee filters. Just poke the stick or cone through the center of two filters and the drips will fall into the paper, not on the child or your carpet.

MAKE AN INSTANT FUNNEL • Cut the end off a cone-style coffee filter to make an instant funnel. Keep a few in your car and use them to avoid spillage when you add a quart or two of oil.

CLEAN YOUR SPECS • Next time you clean your glasses, try using a coffee filter instead of a tissue. Good-quality coffee filters are made from 100 percent virgin paper, so you can use them to clean your glasses without leaving lint. You can also use them to safely polish mirrors and TV and computer-monitor screens.

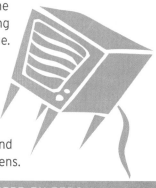

more COFFEE FILTERS over →

KEEP SKILLETS RUST-FREE • To prolong the life of your good cast-iron cookware, put a coffee filter in the frying pan or casserole dish when it's not in use. The filter will absorb moisture and prevent rusting.

PREVENT SOIL LEAKAGE • When you're repotting a plant, line the pot with a coffee filter to keep the soil from leaking out through the drain hole.

MAKE AN AIR FRESHENER

Fill a coffee filter with baking soda, twist-tie it shut, and you have just made an air freshener. Make several and tuck them into shoes, closets, fridge, or wherever else they may be needed.

COFFEE GROUNDS

DEODORIZE THE FREEZER • You can easily get rid of the smell of spoiled food after a freezer failure. Simply fill a couple of bowls with used or fresh coffee grounds and place them in the freezer overnight. For a flavored-coffee scent, add a couple of drops of vanilla to the grounds.

DID YOU KNOW?

The coffee filter was invented in 1908 by a housewife from Dresden, Germany. Melitta Bentz was looking for a way to brew a perfect cup of coffee without the bitterness often caused by overbrewing. She decided to try making a filtered coffee, pouring boiling water over ground coffee and filtering out the grounds. Melitta experimented with different materials, until she found that the blotter paper her son used for school worked best. She cut a round piece of blotting paper, put it in a metal cup, and the first Melitta coffee filter was born. Shortly thereafter, Melitta and her husband, Hugo, launched the company that still bears her name.

DON'T RAISE ANY DUST • Before you clean the ash out of your fireplace, sprinkle it with wet coffee grounds. It will be easier to remove, and the ash and dust won't pollute the atmosphere of the room.

KEEP WORMS ALIVE • A cup of used coffee grounds will keep your bait worms alive and wiggling all day long. Just mix the grounds into the soil in your bait box before you dump in the worms. They like coffee almost as much as we do, and the nutrients in the grounds will help them live longer.

KEEP CATS OUT OF THE GARDEN • Kitty won't think of your garden as a toilet anymore if you spread a pungent mixture of orange peels and used coffee grounds around your plants. The mix acts as great fertilizer, too.

DID YOU KNOW?

Coffee grows on trees that reach a height of up to 20 feet (6 m), but growers keep them pruned to about 7 feet (2 m) to simplify picking and to encourage heavy berry production. The first visible sign of a coffee tree's maturity is the appearance of small, white blossoms, which fill the air with a heady aroma reminiscent of jasmine and orange. The mature tree bears cherry-sized, oval berries, each with two coffee beans, flat sides together. A mature tree will produce 1 pound (450 g) of coffee per growing season. It takes 2,000 hand-picked Arabica coffee berries (4,000 beans) to make 1 pound (450 g) of roasted coffee.

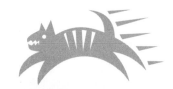

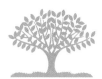

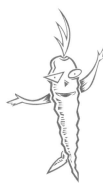

FERTILIZE YOUR PLANTS •
Don't throw out those old coffee grounds. They're chock-a-block full of nutrients that your acid-loving plants crave. Save them to fertilize rosebushes, azaleas, rhododendrons, evergreens, and camellias. It's better to use grounds from a drip coffeemaker than the boiled grounds from a percolator. The drip grounds are richer in nitrogen.

BOOST CARROT HARVEST
To increase your carrot harvest, mix the seeds with freshly ground coffee before sowing. Not only does the extra bulk make the tiny seeds easier to sow, but the coffee aroma may repel cutworms and other pests. As an added bonus, the grounds will help add nutrients to the soil as they decompose around the plants. You might also like to add a few radish seeds to the mix before sowing. The radishes will be up in a few days to mark the rows, and when you cultivate the radishes, you will be thinning the carrot seedlings and cultivating the soil at the same time.

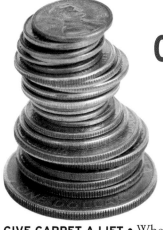

COINS

TEST TIRE TREAD • Let old Abe Lincoln's head tell you if it's time to replace the tires on your car. Insert an penny into the tread. If you can't cover the top of Honest Abe's head inside the tread, it's time for a trip to the tire store. Check tires regularly and you will avoid the danger and inconvenience of a flat tire on a busy road.

GIVE CARPET A LIFT • When you move a chair, couch, table, or bed, you can't help noticing the deep indentations in your carpet made by the legs. To fluff the carpet up again, simply hold a coin on its edge and scrape it against the flattened pile. If that doesn't pop it back up, hold a steam iron about 2 inches (5 cm) above the affected spot. When the area is damp, try fluffing again with the coin.

INSTANT MEASURE • If you need to measure something but don't have a ruler, just reach into your pocket and pull out a quarter. It measures exactly 1 inch (2.54 cm) in diameter. Just line up quarters to measure the length of a small object.

KEEP CUT FLOWERS FRESH • Your posies and other cut flowers will stay fresh longer if you add an old copper penny and a cube of sugar to the vase water.

MAKE A NOISEMAKER • Drop a few coins into an empty aluminium drink can, seal the top with duct tape and head for the stadium to root for the home team. Take your noisemaker with you when you walk the dog and use it as a training aid. When the dog is naughty, just shake the noisemaker.

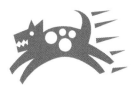

more COINS over →

DECORATE A HAIR CLIP • Use shiny old pennies or small, foreign coins to decorate a barrette for a little girl. Gather enough of the small coins to complete the project and arrange them as you like on the barrette's fastener and use a hot glue gun to attach them. Allow 24 hours to dry.

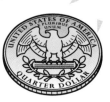

HANG DOORS PERFECTLY • Next time you hang an entry door, nickel-and-dime it to ensure proper clearance between the outside of the door and the inside of the frame. When the door is closed, the gap at the top should be the thickness of a nickel, and the gap at the sides should be that of a dime. If you do it properly, you will keep the door from binding and it won't let in drafts.

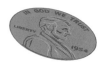

MAKE A PAPERWEIGHT • If you have ever traveled abroad, you have probably come home with a few odd-looking coins from foreign lands. Instead of leaving them lying around in a desk drawer, use them to make an interesting paperweight. Just put the coins into a small glass jar with a closable lid and cover the lid with decorative cloth or paper.

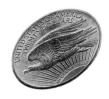

DID YOU KNOW?

Coins were first produced around 700 B.C. by Lydians, a people who lived in what is now Turkey. From there, they spread to ancient Greece and Rome. However, worldwide use of coins (and paper money) took centuries to occur. In early America, bartering remained the way to exchange goods and services. On April 2, 1792, after ratifying the U.S. Constitution, Congress passed the Mint Act, establishing the dollar as the official U.S. currency. The first U.S. coins were produced by the Philadelphia Mint in 1793.

SCIENCE **WORKS!**

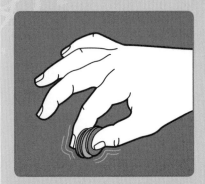

Scientists use optical illusions to show how the brain can be tricked. This simple experiment uses two coins, but you'll think you are seeing three.

Hold two coins on top of each other between your thumb and index finger. Quickly slide the coins back and forth and you will see a third coin!

How does it work? Scientists say that everything we see is actually light reflected from objects. Our eyes use the light to create images on our retinas, the light-sensitive linings at the back of our eyeballs. Because images don't disappear instantly, when something moves quickly you may see both an object and an after-image of it at the same time. Amazing!

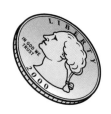

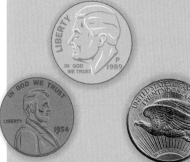

COLANDERS

PREVENT GREASE SPLATTERS • Sick of cleaning grease splatters on the stovetop after cooking your famous burgers? Prevent them by inverting a large metal colander over the frying pan. The holes will let heat escape but the colander will trap the splatters. However, be careful, as the metal colander will be hot—use an oven mitt or dishtowel to remove it.

HEAT A PASTA BOWL • Does your pasta get cold too fast after it's been served up? To keep it warmer longer, heat the serving bowl first. Place a colander in the bowl, pour the pasta and water into the colander and let the hot water stand in the bowl for a few seconds to heat it. Pour out the water, add the pasta and sauce, and you're ready to serve.

ORGANIZE BATH TOYS • Don't let the bathtub look like a messy toy box. After a bath, collect your child's small bath toys in a large colander and store it on the edge of the tub. The water will drain from the toys, keeping them ready for next time, and the bathtub will stay tidy.

USE AS A SAND TOY • Forget spending money on expensive sand toys for your budding archaeologist. A simple, inexpensive plastic colander is perfect for digging at the beach or in the sandbox.

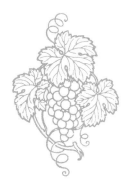

KEEP BERRIES AND GRAPES FRESH

Do your berries and grapes get moldy before you've had a chance to enjoy their sweet taste? To keep them fresh longer, store them in a colander–not a closed plastic container–in the refrigerator. The cold air will circulate through the holes in the colander, keeping them fresher for days.

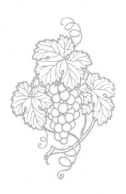

COLD CREAM

ERASE TEMPORARY TATTOOS • Kids love temporary tattoos, but getting them off can be a painful scrubbing job. To make removal easier, rub cold cream on the tatoo to loosen it, then gently rub it off with a washcloth.

MAKE FACE PAINT

Need a safe, easy recipe for children's face paint? Mix 1 teaspoon (5 ml) cornstarch, 1/2 teaspoon (2 ml) water, 1/2 teaspoon (2 ml) cold cream, and 2 drops of food coloring (depending on the costume) together. Use a small brush to paint designs on your child's face. This paint will come off easily with a bit of soap and water.

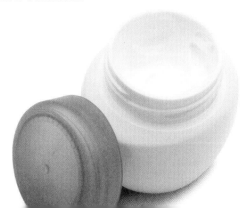

more COLD CREAM over →

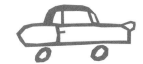
REMOVE BUMPER STICKERS

Does your bumper sticker still say "Bush for President"? Erase the past by rubbing cold cream on the sticker and letting it soak in. Once it does, you should be able to just peel it right off.

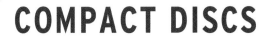

COMPACT DISCS

USE AS CHRISTMAS ORNAMENTS • Decorate your Christmas tree in style! Hang CDs, shiny side out, to create a flickering array of lights—or paint and decorate the label side to create inexpensive personalized ornaments. For a bit of variety you can cut the CDs into stars and other shapes with very sharp scissors. Drill a ¼-inch (6 mm) hole through the CD and thread ribbon through the hole to hang.

DECORATE A TEENAGER'S ROOM • Old CDs make inexpensive and quirky wall art for a teenager's room. Attach the CDs with thumbtacks and use them to create a border at the ceiling or halfway up the wall. Or let your teenager use them to frame his or her favorite posters.

CATCH CANDLE DRIPS • You should always use a candleholder specifically designed to catch melting wax. However, if one is not available, a CD is great in a pinch. Make sure it's a short candle that can stand on its own with a flat bottom. It should be slightly larger than the CD hole. Place the CD candleholder on a stable, heat-resistant surface and keep a watchful eye on it.

MAKE ARTISTIC BOWLS • Looking for a funky bowl? Place a CD in the oven on low heat over a metal bowl until it is soft. Wearing protective gloves, gently bend the CD into the desired shape. 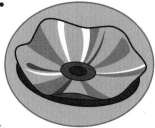 Seal the hole by gluing the bottom edge to another surface, such as a flat dish, using epoxy or PVC glue. Don't use the bowl for food.

Kids' Stuff

*U*se an old CD to make a picture frame for someone you love. You need a CD, a picture of you that is larger than the CD hole, a large bead, ribbon, and glue. Glue the picture in the middle of the CD on the shiny side. If you wish, decorate the CD with markers or stickers. Use a hot glue gun to attach the bead at the top of the CD, allow it to dry, and thread ribbon through the bead.

USE AS FOOTPATH OR DRIVEWAY REFLECTORS • Forget those ugly orange reflectors. Instead, drill small holes in a CD and screw it onto your mailbox post or a wooden stake and push it into the ground. Install several of them to light a nighttime path to your front door.

MAKE A DECORATIVE SUN CATCHER • Sun catchers are attractive to watch and all you need to make one is a couple of CDs. Glue two CDs together, shiny sides out, wrap wool or colored string through the hole and hang them in a window. The prism will make a beautiful light show.

CREATE A SPINNING TOP • Turn an old CD into a fun toy for the kids (and adults too!). With a craft knife, make two slits across from each other in the CD hole. Force a coin halfway through the hole and spin the CD on its edge.

MAKE A CD CLOCK • Old CDs can be functional. Turn a disc into a funky clock face for clockwork sold by arts-and-crafts stores. Paint and design one side of the CD and let it dry. Write on the painted surface or use stickers to create the numbers around its edge. Assemble the clockwork onto the CD.

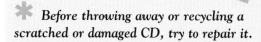

CD repair

✻ Before throwing away or recycling a scratched or damaged CD, try to repair it.

Firstly, clean it thoroughly with a lint-free cloth or mild soap and a little bit of water. Hold the CD by the edge to prevent getting fingerprints on it. Polish it from the middle to the edge, not in a circular motion. If your CD still skips, try fixing it with a little non-gel toothpaste. Dab toothpaste on the end of your finger and rub it lightly onto the entire CD. Use a damp paper towel to remove the toothpaste and dry it with a fresh paper towel. The fine abrasive in the toothpaste might smooth out the scratch. You might also want to use car wax on a scratch *(see page 105)*.

USE AS A TEMPLATE FOR A PERFECT CIRCLE

Need to draw a perfect circle? Forget tracing around cups or using cumbersome compasses. Every CD provides two circle sizes. You can trace around the inner hole or the outer circumference.

COVER WITH FELT AND USE AS COASTERS • CDs can help to prevent those unsightly stains from cups left on the table. Simply cut a round piece of felt or thin cork sheeting to fit over the CD and glue it onto the label side of the CD so that the shiny side will face up when you use the coaster.

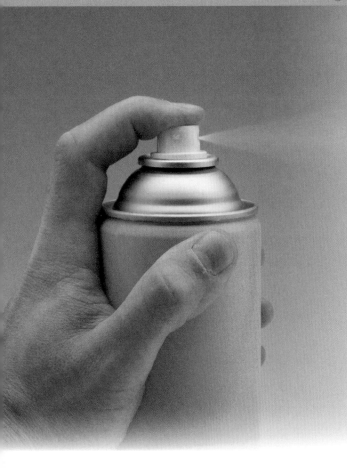

COOKING SPRAY

MAKE GRATING CHEESE EASY • Put less elbow grease into grating cheese by using a nonstick cooking spray on your cheese grater for smoother grating. The spray also makes for easier and faster cleanup.

PREVENT TOMATO SAUCE STAINS • To prevent tomato sauce from staining plastic containers, apply a light coating of nonstick cooking spray on the inside of a container before you pour in a tomato sauce.

PREVENT RICE AND PASTA FROM STICKING • Most cooks know that a little cooking oil in the boiling water will keep rice or pasta from sticking together when you drain it. However, if you run out of cooking oil, a squirt of cooking-oil spray will do the job just as well.

KEEP CAR WHEELS CLEAN • You know that fine black stuff that collects on the wheels of your car and is so hard to clean off? That's brake dust—it's produced every time you apply your brakes as the pads wear against the brake discs or cylinders. The next time you invest the elbow grease to get your wheels shiny, give them a light coating of cooking spray. The brake dust will wipe right off.

DE-BUG YOUR CAR • When those insects smash into your car at 55 mph (88 km) per hour, they really stick. Give the grille a squirt of nonstick cooking spray and you can just wipe away the insect debris.

CLEAN UP WAX • If you love candles but don't like the cleanup that comes with them, you'll love this trick. If you spray candles with cooking spray before lighting them (just a light coat!), the wax will come right off whatever surface you put them on later.

REMOVE PAINT AND GREASE • Forget smelly solvents to remove paint and grease from your hands. Instead, use cooking spray to do the job. Work it in well and rinse. Wash again with soap and water.

CURE DOOR SQUEAK
Heard that door squeak just one time too many? Hit the hinge with some nonstick cooking spray and say "bye-bye" to that annoying noise once and for all. Just be sure to you have paper towels handy to wipe up the drips.

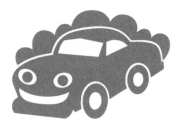

C

PREVENT GRASS FROM STICKING • Mowing the lawn should be easy, but cleaning stuck grass from the mower blades can be tedious. You can prevent grass from sticking to the blades and the underside of the housing by spraying them with cooking spray before you begin mowing.

PREVENT SNOW FROM STICKING • Shovelling snow is hard enough, but it can be more aggravating when the snow sticks to the shovel. Spray it with nonstick cooking spray before shovelling—the snow will slide right off the shovel.

QUICK CASTING • Pack a can of cooking spray with your gear when you go fishing. Spray it on your fishing line and the line will cast easier and farther.

GET RID OF SOAP SCUM • Say good-bye to your shower's soap scum! Spray that gunk with cooking spray and it will come off with just a swipe of a towel—and wash the surface with soap and water. This clever trick works because oil breaks down the lime deposits, making it easily removable.

SPEED-DRY NAIL POLISH

Need your nail polish to dry in a hurry? Spray it with a coat of olive oil cooking spray and let it dry. The spray is also a great moisturizer for your hands.

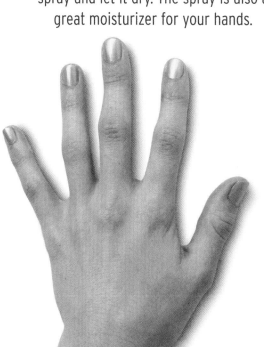

DID YOU KNOW?

The first patent for a nonstick cooking spray was issued in the United States in 1957 to Arthur Meyerhoff and his partner, Leon Rubin, who began marketing PAM ('Product of Arthur Meyerhoff') All Natural Cooking Spray in 1959. After appearing on local Chicago TV cooking shows in the early 1960s, the product developed a loyal following, and it quickly became a household word—and was copied all over the world.

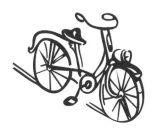

LUBRICATE A BICYCLE CHAIN • If your bike chain is a bit creaky and you don't have any lubricating oil handy, give it a shot of nonstick cooking spray instead. Don't use too much—the chain shouldn't look wet. Wipe off the excess with a clean rag.

SHINE YOUR FAUCETS • Using cooking spray on faucets and other fixtures throughout your house doesn't just clean them—it makes them sparkle!

FORM PERFECT PATTIES • Attention, carnivores! This one is a life-changer. Cooking oil is your best friend when you have to make burger patties or any sticky and somewhat spherical foods. Spray your hands generously with the oil and rub to coat them. From now on, you won't have to deal with remnants of those food mixtures getting stuck to your fingers.

CORKS

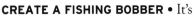

CREATE A FISHING BOBBER • It's an idea that's as old as Mark Twain's Tom Sawyer, but worth remembering. A cork makes a great substitute fishing bobber. Drive a staple into the top of the cork, then pull the staple out just a bit so you can slide your fishing line through it.

MAKE AN IMPROMPTU PINCUSHION • If you're looking for a place to store pins while sewing, save wine-bottle corks—they make great pincushions!

PREVENT POTTERY SCRATCHES • Your beautiful pottery can make ugly scratches on furniture. To save scratching tabletops, cut thin slices of cork and glue them to the bottom of your ceramic objects.

REPLACE SODA BOTTLE CAPS • If you've lost the cap to your soda bottle and need a replacement, just put a cork in it. Most wine corks will fit soda bottles perfectly.

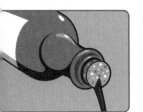

MAKE A POUR SPOUT • If you don't have one of those fancy metal pour spouts to control the flow from your oil or vinegar bottle, you can make your own by cutting out a wedge of the cork along its length. Use a craft knife to do the job. Stick the cork in the bottle and pour away. When you're through, cover the hole with a tab of masking tape.

USE AS FACE PAINT • Kids love to dress up as a hobo for Halloween or a costume party. To create that scruffy look, char the end of a piece of cork by holding it over a candle. Let it cool a for a minute or two, then rub it on the child's face.

BLOCK SUN GLARE • In the good old days of football and baseball, players would burn cork and rub it under their eyes to reduce glare from the sun and stadium lights. These days, they use commercial products to do the same, but you can still use cork to get the job done.

PREVENT SCRAPING-CHAIR NOISES • The sound of a chair scraping across your beautiful floor can make your skin crawl. Solve the problem by cutting cork into thin slices and attaching them to the bottom of the chair legs with a spot of wood glue.

FASTEN EARRINGS • Earring backs always get lost, and you can't always find a perfect-sized stand-in when you need it. Use a snippet of cork as a temporary substitute. Slice a small piece about the size of the backing and push it on. An eraser cut from the end of a pencil will also work.

CREATE A COOL BEAD CURTAIN • Want a creative, stylish beaded curtain for your child's or teenager's room? Just drill a hole through a series of corks and string them on a cord, along with beads and other decorations. Make as many strings as you need and tie them on a curtain rod.

DID YOU KNOW?

Cork, the bark of the cork oak, has been used to seal wine bottles and other vessels for more than 400 years. The bark has a unique honeycomb cell structure—each cell is sealed, filled with air and not connected to any other cell. This makes it waterproof and a poor conductor of heat and vibration. Plus, cork contains suberin, a natural waxy substance that makes it impermeable to liquids and gases and prevents the cork from rotting. No wonder it's still the material of choice for sealing your favorite cabernet.

CAUTION: Should you use a corkscrew to open a bottle of wine? Yes, but don't use it on a bottle of champagne! Pushing a corkscrew down into a bottle of champagne against the pressure of the carbonation can actually make the bottle explode. If possible, after transporting the champagne, wait a day before opening and let the carbonation settle a bit. Wrap the cork in a towel and twist the bottle, not the cork, slowly.

To open wine, use a traditional corkscrew that twists into the stopper. Peel off the top of the plastic or foil to expose the cork. Insert the corkscrew in the center, twist it straight down, and pull the cork straight out using even pressure.

PICTURE-PERFECT FRAMES • If you're always straightening picture frames on the wall, cut some small, flat pieces of cork—all the same thickness—and glue them to the back of the frame. The cork will grip the wall and stop it from sliding. It will also prevent the frame from marring the wall.

CORNSTARCH

DRY SHAMPOO • Fido needs a bath, but you just don't have time. Rub cornstarch into his coat and brush it out. The dry bath will fluff up his coat until it's bath time.

UNTANGLE KNOTS • Knots in string or shoelaces can be difficult to undo, but the solution is easy. Sprinkle the knot with a little cornstarch. It will then be easy to work the segments apart.

MAKE YOUR OWN PASTE • The next time the kids want to go wild with construction paper and paste, save money by making the paste yourself. Mix 3 teaspoons (15 ml) cornstarch for every 4 teaspoons

MASS-PRODUCE SOWING HOLES • Here's a clever trick for quickly getting your seeds sown in straight rows of evenly spaced holes. Mark out the spacing you need on a board. Drill drywall screws through the holes, using screws that will protrude about ¾ inch (2 cm) through the board. Twist wine corks onto the screws. Just press the board, corks down, into your garden bed and voila!—instant seed holes.

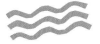

CREATE CRAFT STAMPS • You can use cork to create a personalized stamp. Carve the end of a cork into any shape or design you want. Use it with ink from a stamp pad to decorate note cards. Or let the kids dip carved corks in paint to create artwork.

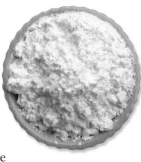

(20 ml) cold water. Stir until it reaches a paste consistency. It's great for applying with fingers, a wooden tongue depressor, or a popsicle stick. If you add food coloring, the paste can be used for painting objects.

MAKE FINGER PAINTS • This simple recipe will keep the kids happy for hours. Mix together ¼ cup (50 g) cornstarch and 2 cups (500 ml) cold water. Bring to a boil and continue boiling until the mixture becomes thick. Pour your product into several small containers and add food coloring to each container—you've just created a collection of homemade finger paints.

more CORNSTARCH over →

CLEAN STUFFED ANIMALS • To clean a stuffed toy animal, rub a bit of cornstarch on the toy, wait about 5 minutes, and brush it clean. Or place the stuffed animal (or a few small ones) into a bag. Sprinkle cornstarch into the bag, close it tightly and shake. Now brush the stuffed toy pets clean and dispose of the cornstarch and the bag.

SEPARATE MARSHMALLOWS

Ever buy a bag of marshmallows only to find them stuck together? Here's how to get them apart. Add at least 1 teaspoon (5 ml) cornstarch to the bag and shake. The cornstarch will absorb the extra moisture and force most of the marshmallows apart. Repackage the remaining marshmallows in a container and freeze them to avoid them sticking in the future.

LIFT A SCORCH MARK FROM CLOTHING • If you move an iron around a bit too slowly you could end up with a scorch mark on your favorite shirt. If this happens, wet the scorched area and cover it with cornstarch. Allow the cornstarch to dry, then brush it away along with the scorch mark.

REMOVE GREASE SPATTERS FROM WALLS • Even the most careful cook cannot avoid an occasional spatter. A busy kitchen takes some wear and tear but here's a handy remedy for that unsightly grease spot. Sprinkle cornstarch on a soft cloth, then rub the grease spot gently until it disappears.

DID YOU KNOW?

Cornstarch has been made into biodegradable packing 'peanuts' sold in bulk. If you receive an item shipped in this material, just toss the peanuts on the lawn. They'll dissolve with water, leaving no toxic waste. To test if the peanuts are made from cornstarch, wet one in the sink to see if it dissolves.

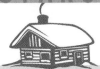

DOMESTIC BLISS!

SOAK UP FURNITURE POLISH RESIDUE • You've finished polishing your furniture, but there's still a bit left on the surface. Sprinkle cornstarch lightly on furniture after polishing, and wipe up the oil-and-cornstarch mixture. Buff the surface to a non-oily shine.

REMOVE INK STAINS FROM CARPET • Oh no, ink on the carpet! In this case a little spilt milk might save you from crying. Mix the milk with cornstarch to make a paste. Apply the paste to the ink stain. Allow the concoction to dry on the carpet for a few hours, brush off the dried residue, and vacuum it up.

GIVE CARPETS A FRESH SCENT • Before vacuuming a room, sprinkle a little cornstarch on your carpeting. Wait about half an hour and vacuum as usual.

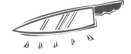

GET RID OF BLOODSTAINS

The quicker you act, the better. Whether it's on clothing or table linens, you can remove or reduce a bloodstain with this method. Make a paste of cornstarch mixed with cold water. Cover the spot with the cornstarch paste and rub it gently into the fabric. Now put the cloth in a sunny location to dry. Once dry, brush off the remaining residue. If the stain is not completely gone, repeat the process.

POLISH SILVER • If the sparkle has gone from your good silverware, make a paste by mixing cornstarch with water and, using a damp cloth, apply it to your silverware. Let it dry, then rub it off with cheesecloth or another soft cloth to reveal that old shine.

MAKE WINDOWS SPARKLE • Create your own streak-free window cleaning solution by mixing 2 tablespoons (30 ml) cornstarch with ½ cup (125 ml) ammonia and ½ cup (125 ml) white vinegar in a bucket containing 3 to 4 quarts (3–4 L) warm water.

Don't be put off by the milky concoction you create. Mix well and put the solution in a spray bottle. Spray on the windows and wipe with a warm-water rinse. Lastly, rub with a dry paper towel or lint-free cloth.

SAY GOOD RIDDANCE TO ROACHES • There's no delicate way to manage this problem. Make a mixture that is 50 percent plaster of Paris and 50 percent cornstarch. Spread the mixture in the crevices where cockroaches appear. It's a killer recipe.

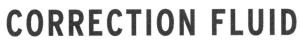

CORRECTION FLUID

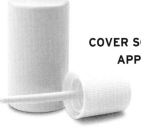

COVER SCRATCHES ON APPLIANCES • Daub small nicks on household appliances with correction fluid. Once it dries, cover your repair with clear nail polish for staying power. This works well on white china, too, but only for display. Now that correction fluid comes in a rainbow of colors, its uses go beyond white. You may easily find a match for your beige or yellow kitchen stove or refrigerator.

TOUCH UP A CEILING • Hide marks on white or beige ceilings with judiciously applied brush strokes of correction fluid. You can tone down the brightness, if you need to, by buffing the repaired area with a paper towel once it has dried.

ERASE SCUFFS • Need a quick fix for scuffed white shoes? Correction fluid will camouflage the offensive marks. On leather, buff gently once the fluid dries. No need to buff patent leather.

PAINT THE TOWN • Decorate your windows for any occasion. Paint snowflakes, flowers, or 'Welcome

DID YOU KNOW?

Correction fluid was invented in 1951 by Bette Nesmith Graham, mother of Michael Nesmith of the Monkees pop group. Graham was working as an executive secretary in Texas. She used water-based paint to correct mistakes and began supplying little bottles of it to other secretaries, calling it Mistake Out. Five years later, she improved the formula and changed the name to Liquid Paper. Despite its proven use, Graham was turned down when she tried to sell it to IBM, so she marketed it on her own. In the 1960s her invention began to generate a tidy profit; by 1979, when she sold the product to the Gillette Corp, she received $47.5 million plus a royalty on every bottle sold until 2000. Today, with the ease of correcting documents on a computer, correction fluid is no longer the office essential it once was.

Home' signs using correction fluid. Later, you can remove your art with nail polish remover, an ammonia solution, vinegar and water, or a commercial window cleaner. Or scrape it off with a single-edged razor blade in a holder made for removing paint from glass.

cotton balls
cotton balls
cotton balls
cotton balls
CRAYONS
CRAYONS

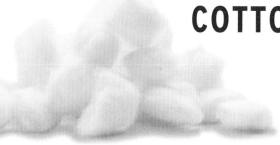

COTTON BALLS

DEODORIZE THE REFRIGERATOR • Sometimes the refrigerator just doesn't smell fresh. Dampen a cotton ball with vanilla extract and place it on a shelf near the back of the fridge. You'll find it acts as a deodorizer, offering its own pleasant scent.

SCENT THE ROOM • Saturate a cotton ball with your favorite cologne and drop it into the vacuum cleaner bag. Now, as you vacuum the scent will be expressed and gently permeate the room.

PROTECT LITTLE FINGERS • Pad the ends of drawer runners with a cotton ball. This will prevent the drawer from closing completely so children won't catch their fingers as the drawer slides shut.

FIGHT MILDEW • There are always hard-to-reach spots in the bathroom, usually around the fixtures, where mildew may breed in the grout between tiles. Forget about becoming a contortionist to return the sparkle to those areas. Soak a few cotton balls in bleach and place them in those difficult spots. Leave them to work their magic for a few hours. When you remove them, you'll find your job has been done. Finish by rinsing with warm water.

RESCUE YOUR RUBBER GLOVES • If your long, manicured nails sometimes puncture the fingertips of rubber dishwashing gloves, here's a solution you'll appreciate. Push a cotton ball down into the fingertips of your rubber gloves. The soft barrier should prolong the gloves' life and protect your fingernails from soapy water.

CRAYONS

USE AS A FLOOR FILLER • Crayons make great fill material for small gouges or holes in resilient flooring. Get out your crayon box and select a color that most closely matches the floor. Melt the crayon in the microwave over wax paper on medium power, a minute at a time until you have a pliant glob of color. Now, with a plastic knife or putty knife, fill the hole. Smooth it over with a rolling pin, a book, or some other flat object. You'll find the crayon cools down quickly. Now wax the floor, to provide a clear protective coating over your new fill.

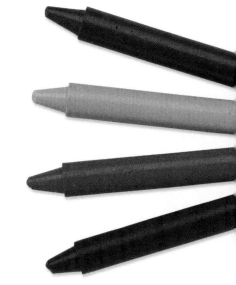

FILL FURNITURE SCRATCHES • Do your pets sometimes treat your furniture like—well, a scratching post? Don't despair. Use a crayon to cover scratches on wooden furniture. Choose the color most like the wood finish. Soften the crayon with a hair dryer or in the microwave on the defrost setting. Color over the scratches, then buff your repair job with a clean rag to restore the luster.

CARPET COVER-UP • Even the most careful among us manage to stain the carpet at some time or other. If you've tried to remove a stain and nothing works, here's a remedy you might be able to live with. Find a crayon that matches or will blend with your carpet. Soften the crayon a bit with a hair dryer or in the microwave on the defrost setting. Now color over the spot. Cover your repair with wax paper and gently iron the color in, keeping the iron on a low setting. Repeat as often as necessary.

COLORFUL DECORATION • Here's a fun project to do with the kids. Make a multicolored sun catcher by shaving crayons onto a 4 or 5-inch (10–12 cm) sheet of wax paper. Use a potato peeler or grater for this task. Place another sheet of wax paper over the top and press with a hot iron until the shavings melt together. Poke a hole near the top through the layers of wax and crayon while still warm. Once your ornament cools, peel away the papers and thread a ribbon through it so you can hang it in a window.

DID YOU KNOW?

Jazberry Jam and Mango Tango. They aren't ice cream flavors, they are recently introduced Crayola crayon colors. When Edwin Binney and C. Harold Smith introduced the first crayons safe for children to use in 1903, a box of eight sold for five cents and included colors with more pedestrian names, such as black, brown, blue, red, violet, orange, yellow, and green. Since then, the manufacturer of the famous Crayola crayons, Binney and Smith, has introduced more than 400 colors, retiring many along the way, so that currently there are 120 colors available.

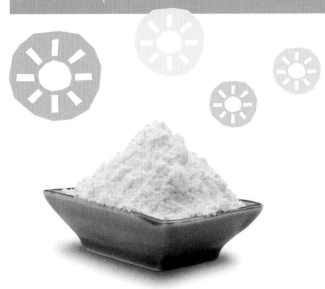

CREAM OF TARTAR

MAKE PLAY DOUGH FOR KIDS

Here's a recipe for play dough that's as good as the stuff you buy. Mix 2 tablespoons (30 ml) cream of tartar, 1 cup (250 g) salt, 4 cups (1 kg) plain (non-rising) flour and 1 to 2 tablespoons (15-30 ml) cooking oil. Stir well with a wooden spoon and slowly add 4 cups (1 L) water. Cook the mixture in a saucepan over medium heat, stirring occasionally until it thickens. It's ready when it forms a ball that is not sticky. Work in food coloring, if you like. Let it cool and watch the kids get creative. It dries out quicker than the commercial variety, so be sure to store it in an airtight container in the fridge.

TUB SCRUBBER • Let this simple solution of cream of tartar and hydrogen peroxide do the hard work of removing a bathtub stain for you. Fill a small, shallow cup or dish with cream of tartar and add hydrogen peroxide drop by drop until you have a thick paste. Apply to the stain and let it dry. When you remove the dried paste, you'll find that the stain is gone too.

BRIGHTEN COOKWARE • Discolored aluminium pots will sparkle again if you clean them with a mixture of 2 tablespoons (30 ml) cream of tartar dissolved into 4 cups (1 L) water. Bring the mixture to the boil inside the pot and boil for 10 minutes.

CURTAIN RINGS

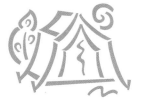

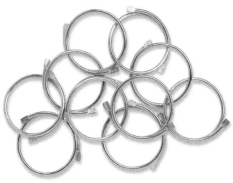

GET HOOKED • On a camping trip or a hike, when you don't want to carry a backpack, it's easy to lash a few items to your belt loop with the help of a curtain ring. Mountain climbers rely on expensive carabiners, which they use to hold items and to control ropes. But you don't need to carry along anything so heavy. Attach your sneakers to your sleeping bag with a metal curtain ring. Your gloves and water bottle can dangle from a metal shower curtain ring or a brass key ring.

KEEP CURIOSITY AT BAY • It's a natural stage of development, but not always one you want to encourage. Curious toddlers can't help poking around in your kitchen cupboards. If you've got a toddler visiting, lock up your accessible cupboards by clicking shower-curtain rings over the latches. And when the baby leaves, it's easy to remove the rings.

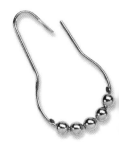

FOR THE DO-IT-YOURSELFERS

HOLD YOUR HAMMER • Sometimes you need three hands when you're doing household repair jobs. Attach a sturdy metal shower curtain ring to your belt and slip your hammer through it. Now you can climb a ladder or otherwise work with both hands and just grab the hammer when needed.

STORE NUTS AND WASHERS • Keep nuts and washers on metal shower curtain rings hung from a hook in your workshop. The ring's pear shape and latching action ensure secure storage. Put nuts and washers of similar size on their own rings so that you can find the right size quickly.

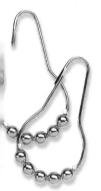

KEEP TRACK OF KIDS' GLOVES

'Where are my gloves, Mom?' 'Where did you leave them?' 'I dunno.' Something as simple as a curtain ring can help you do away with this dialogue. Drive a nail into the hallway wall or the back of the door. Hand your child a curtain ring and tell him or her to use it to clip their gloves together and hang them on the nail.

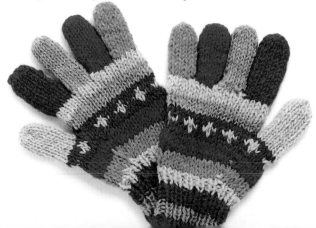

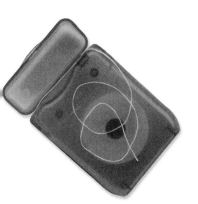

DENTAL FLOSS

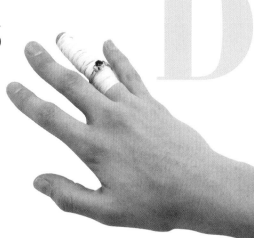

REMOVE A STUCK RING • Here's a simple way to slip off a ring that's stuck on your finger. Wrap the length of your finger from the ring to the nail tightly with dental floss (the flat, tape-style works well). Then slide the ring off over the floss 'carpet'.

LIFT COOKIES FROM A BAKING TRAY • Ever fought with a freshly baked cookie that wouldn't come off the pan? Crumbled cookies may taste just as good as those in one piece, but they definitely don't look as nice on the serving plate. Use dental floss to easily remove cookies from the cookie sheet. Hold a length of dental floss taut and slide it neatly between the cookie's bottom and the pan.

SLICE CAKE AND CHEESE • Use dental floss to cut cakes, especially delicate and sticky ones that tend to adhere to a knife. Just hold a length of floss taut over the cake and slice away, moving it slightly side to side as you cut through the cake. You can also use dental floss to cut small blocks of cheese cleanly.

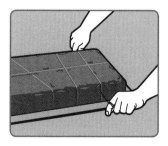

REPAIR OUTDOOR GEAR • Because dental floss is strong and resilient but slender, it's the ideal replacement for thread when you are repairing an umbrella, tent, or backpack. These items take a beating and sometimes get pinhole nicks. Sew up the small holes with floss. To fix larger gouges, sew back and forth over the holes until you have covered the space with a floss patch.

EXTRA-STRONG STRING FOR HANGING THINGS • Considering how thin it is, dental floss is strong stuff. Use it instead of string or wire to securely hang pictures, sun catchers, or wind chimes. Use it with a needle to thread together papers you want to attach or those you want to display, in clothesline fashion.

SECURE A BUTTON PERMANENTLY • Did that button fall off again? This time, sew it back on with dental floss—it's much stronger than thread, which makes it perfect for reinstalling buttons on coats, jackets, and heavy shirts.

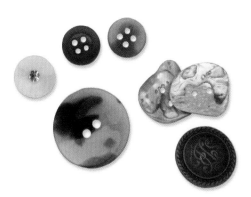

SEPARATE PHOTOS • Sometimes photos get stuck to each other and it seems the only way to separate them is to ruin them. Try working a length of dental floss between the pictures to gently pry them apart.

DENTURE TABLETS

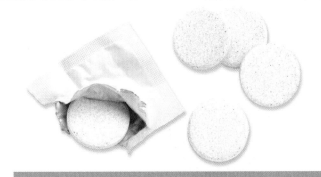

RE-IGNITE YOUR DIAMOND'S SPARKLE • Has your diamond ring lost its sparkle? Drop a denture tablet into a glass containing a cup of water. Follow that with your ring or diamond earrings. Let it sit for a few minutes, then remove your jewelry and rinse to reveal the old sparkle and shine.

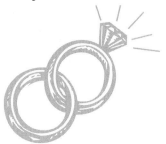

DID YOU KNOW?

Bleaching agents are a common component of denture tablets, providing the chemical action that helps the tablets remove plaque and to whiten and bleach away stains. This is what makes them so very useful for cleaning toilets, coffeemakers, jewelry, and enamel cookware, among other things.

GET RID OF MINERAL DEPOSITS ON GLASS • Fresh flowers often leave a ring on your glass vases that seems impossible to remove no matter how hard you scrub. Here's the answer. Fill the vase with water and drop in a denture tablet. When the fizzing has stopped, all of the mineral deposits will be gone. Use the same method to clean thermos bottles, cruets, glasses, and wine decanters.

CLEAN A COFFEEMAKER

Hard water leaves mineral deposits in the tank of your electric drip coffee maker that not only slow the perking but also affects the taste of your brew. Denture tablets will fizz away these deposits and give the tank a bacterial cleaning, too. The tablets were designed to clean and disinfect dentures, and they'll do the same job on your coffeemaker. Drop 2 denture tablets in the tank, fill it with water, and run the coffeemaker. Discard that potful of water and follow up with one or two rinse cycles with clean water.

CLEAN YOUR TOILET • Looking for a way to make the toilet sparkle again? Porcelain fixtures respond to the cleaning agent in denture tablets. Here's a solution that does the job in the twinkling of an eye. Drop a denture tablet in the bowl, wait about 20 minutes, and flush. That's it!

CLEAN ENAMEL COOKWARE • Stains on enamel cookware are a natural for the denture tablet cleaning solution. Fill the pot or pan with warm water and drop in a tablet or two, depending on its size. Wait a bit—once the fizzing has stopped, your cookware will be clean.

UNCLOG A DRAIN • Slow drain got you down? Reach for the denture tablets. Drop a couple of tablets into the drain and run water until the problem clears. For a more stubborn clog, drop 3 tablets down the sink, follow that with 1 cup (250 ml) white vinegar and wait a few minutes. Now run hot water in the drain until the clog is gone.

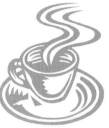

DISPOSABLE DIAPERS

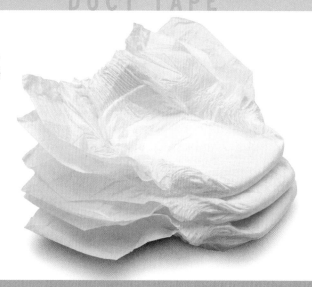

MAKE A HEATING PAD • Use a disposable diaper's high level of absorbency to your advantage to create a soft, pliant heating pad. Moisten a disposable diaper and place it in the microwave on medium-high for about 2 minutes. Check that it's not too hot for comfort and apply to aching muscles.

KEEP A PLANT WATERED • Before potting a plant, place a clean disposable diaper in the bottom of the flowerpot–absorbent side up. It will absorb water that would otherwise drain out the bottom and will keep the plant from drying out too fast. And you won't have to water as often.

PAD A PACKAGE • If you have disposable diapers on hand, wrap delicate items in the diapers or insert them as padding before sealing the box containing breakables. Diapers cost more than regular protective packaging wrap, but in a pinch they are a great standby, and you can be assured your gift will arrive in one piece.

DID YOU KNOW?

Looking for an alternative to messy cloth diapers, American mother Marion Donovan first created a plastic covering for diapers. She made her prototype from a shower curtain and later parachute fabric. Manufacturers weren't interested, but when she created her own company and introduced the product in 1949 at the prestigious department store, Saks Fifth Avenue in New York City, it was an instant success. Donovan soon added disposable absorbent material to create the first disposable diaper and, in 1951, sold her company for a cool $1 million.

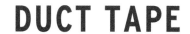

38 USES!

DUCT TAPE

around the house

● ● ●

TEMPORARILY HEM YOUR PANTS • You've found a terrific pair of jeans, but the length isn't right. You expect a little shrinkage anyway, so why spend time hemming? Besides, thick denim jeans are difficult to sew through. Fake the hem with a judiciously placed strip of duct tape. The new hem should last through a few washes, too.

REMOVE LINT ON CLOTHING • You're all set to go out for the night and suddenly you notice pet hairs on your outfit. Grab the duct tape and in no time, you'll be ready to go. Wrap your hand with a length of duct tape, sticky side out. Then roll the sticky tape against your clothing in a rocking motion until every last hair has been picked up. Don't wipe, since that may affect the nap of the fabric on your clothes.

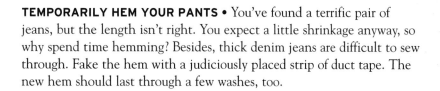

more DUCT TAPE over →

MAKE A BANDAGE IN A PINCH • If you've got a bad scrape, here's how to protect it until you get a proper bandage. Fold tissue paper or paper towel to cover the wound and cover this with duct tape. It may not be attractive, but it works in a jam.

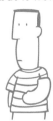

RESEAL BAGS OF CHIPS • Tired of stale potato chips? To keep a half-finished bag fresh, fold up the top and seal it tightly with a piece of duct tape.

PROTECT YOUR WALLET • Old wallets may lose their resiliency but are otherwise useful. Cover your old wallet with duct tape; reinforce between sections and it's as good as new.

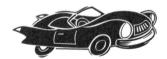

MAKE A BUMPER STICKER • Got something to say? Make your own bumper sticker. Cut a length of duct tape, attach it to your bumper, and with a fine point marker, pen your message.

REPAIR A VACUUM HOSE • Has your vacuum hose cracked and developed a leak? It doesn't spell the end of your vacuum. Repair the broken hose with duct tape. Your vacuum will last until the motor gives out.

HANG CHRISTMAS LIGHTS • Festive holiday lights are fun in season, but a real drag when it's time for them to come down. Use duct tape to hang your lights and the removal job will be much easier. Tear duct tape into thin strips. At intervals, wrap strips around the wire and tape the strand to the gutters or wherever you hang your lights.

KEEP A SECRET CAR KEY

You'll never get locked out of your car again if you attach an extra key to the undercarriage with duct tape.

CATCH ANNOYING FLIES • You've just checked into a rustic cabin on the lake and you're ready to start your vacation. Everything would be perfect if only the flying insects were not part of the deal. Grab your roll of duct tape and roll off a few foot-long (30 cm) strips. Hang them from the rafters as flypaper. Soon you'll be rid of the flies and you can roll up the tape to toss it in the garbage.

REPLACE A SHOWER CURTAIN EYELET • How many times have you ripped through a shower curtain eyelet? You can repair them with duct tape. Once the curtain is dry, cut a rectangular piece and fold it from front to back over the torn hole. Slit the tape with a craft knife, razor blade, or scissors, and push the shower curtain ring back into place.

REPAIR A PICTURE FRAME

Many people enjoy displaying family photos in easel-type frames on mantels and side tables throughout the house. Sometimes the fold-out leg that holds a frame upright pulls away from the back of the frame and your photo won't stand up properly. Don't despair! Just use duct tape to reattach the broken leg to the frame back.

for the kids

MAKE FANCY DRESS COSTUMES • Want to be the Tin Man for Halloween? How about a robot? These are just two ideas that work naturally with the classic silver duct tape. Make a basic costume from brown paper grocery bags, with openings in the back so the child can easily put on and take off the costume.

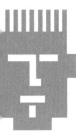

Cover this pattern with rows of duct tape. For the legs, cover an old pair of pants, again giving your little robot or Tin Man an easy way to remove the outfit for toilet breaks. Duct tape (and electrical tape) now comes in several colors, so let your imagination lead your creativity.

MAKE A TOY SWORD • Got a couple of would-be swashbucklers around the house? Make toy swords for the junior Errol Flynns by sketching a kid-sized sword on a piece of cardboard. Use two pieces if you haven't got one thick enough. Be sure to make a handle the child's hand can fit around comfortably once it's been increased in thickness by several layers of duct tape. Wrap the entire blade shape in silver duct tape and the handle in black tape.

MAKE PLAY RINGS AND BRACELETS • Make rings by tearing duct tape into strips about ½-inch (1 cm) wide, then folding the strips in half lengthwise— sticky sides together. Continue to put more strips over the first one until the ring is thick enough to stand on its own. You can adjust the size with scissors and tape the ends closed. To make a stone for the ring, cover a small item such as a pebble and attach it to the ring. Make a bracelet by winding duct tape around a stiff paper pattern.

MAKE HAND PUPPETS • Duct tape is great for puppet making. Use a small paper lunch bag as the base for the body of your puppet. Cover the bag with overlapping rows of duct tape. Make armholes through which your fingers will poke out. Create a head from a tape-covered ball of wadded paper and fix buttons or beads in place for eyes and mouth.

for the do-it-yourselfer

SHORT-TERM CAR HOSE FIX • Until you can get to your mechanic, duct tape makes a strong and dependable temporary fix for broken water hoses on your car. But don't wait too long; duct tape can only withstand temperatures up to 200°F (93°C). Also, don't use it to repair a leak in your car's fuel line— the gasoline will dissolve the adhesive.

MAKE A TEMPORARY ROOF SHINGLE • If you've lost a wooden roof shingle, make a temporary replacement by wrapping duct tape in strips across a piece of ¼-inch (6-mm) plywood you've cut to size. Wedge the makeshift shingle in place to fill the space. It will close the gap and repel water until you get around to repairing the roof.

MAKE A QUICK FIX FOR A TOILET SEAT • You're giving a party and someone taps you on the shoulder to tell you the toilet seat has broken. You don't have to make a mad dash to the home-improvement store. Grab the duct tape and carefully wrap the break for a neat repair. The party can go on and your guests will thank you.

MEND A SCREEN • Have those insects found the tiny tear in your window or door screen? Block their entrance until you get around to fixing it permanently by covering the hole with duct tape.

more DUCT TAPE over →

FIX A HOLE IN YOUR SIDING • Has stormy weather damaged your vinyl siding? A broken tree limb tossed by the storm, hailstones, or even an errant baseball can rip your siding. Patch tears in vinyl siding with strips of duct tape. If possible, choose tape in a color that matches your siding and apply it when the surface is dry. Smooth your repair by hand or with a rolling pin, then paint it to match, if necessary. The patch should last at least a season or two.

TAPE A BROKEN WINDOW • Before removing broken window glass, crisscross the broken pane with duct tape to hold it all together. This will ensure a shard doesn't fall out and cut you.

REPAIR A GARBAGE CAN • Plastic garbage cans often split or crack along the sides. But don't toss out the can with the garbage. Repair the tear with duct tape. It's strong enough to withstand the abuses a garbage can take, and is easy to manipulate on the curved or ridged surface of the can. Put tape over the crack both outside and inside the can.

REPLACE LAWN-CHAIR WEBBING

Summertime is here and you go to the shed to get out the lawn furniture only to discover that the webbing on your favorite backyard chair has worn through. Don't throw it out! Colorful duct tape makes a great, sturdy replacement webbing. Cut strips twice as long as you need. Double the tape, putting sticky sides together, so that you have backing facing out on both sides. Then screw it in place using the screws on the chair.

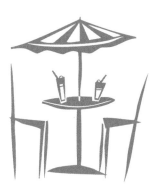

for sports and outdoor gear

REPAIR YOUR SKI PANTS • When ski pants get ripped and the wind whips into the nylon outer layer, don't pay for a new pair if you have a roll of duct tape handy. Just slip a piece of tape inside the rip, sticky side out, and carefully press both sides of the rip together. The repair will be barely detectable.

REPAIR YOUR SKI GLOVES • When ski-glove seams tear open, duct tape is the perfect solution to mend the rips because it's waterproof, incredibly adhesive, strong, and can easily be torn into strips of any width. Make your repair lengthwise or around the fingers, and get back out on the slopes.

TIGHTEN SHIN GUARDS • Hockey players need a little extra protection, so use duct tape to attach shin guards firmly in place. When all your equipment is on, including socks, split the duct tape to the width appropriate for your size—children might need narrower strips than adults—and start wrapping around your shin guard to keep it tight to your leg.

EXTEND THE LIFE OF SKATEBOARD SHOES • Kids who perform fantastic feats on their skateboards find their shoes wear out very quickly because a lot of the jumps involve sliding the toe or side of the foot along the board. They wear holes in new shoes fast. Protect their feet and prolong the life of their shoes by putting a layer or two of duct tape on the area that scrapes along the board.

ADD LIFE TO A HOCKEY STICK • Hockey sticks take a beating. If yours is showing its age, breathe a little more life into it by wrapping the bottom of the stick with duct tape. Replace the tape as often as needed.

REPAIR A TENT • You open your tent at the campsite and oops—a little tear. Not a problem as long as you've brought your trusty roll of duct tape along. Cover the hole with a patch and for double protection mirror the patch inside the tent. You'll keep biting insects and rainy weather where they both belong.

ADD EXTRA INSULATION • Make your winter boots a little bit warmer by taping the innersoles with duct tape, silver-side up. The shiny tape will reflect the warmth of your feet back into your boots.

STAY AFLOAT • If you're out for a paddle and you discover a small hole in your canoe, you'll be saved if you thought to pack duct tape in your supply kit. Pull the canoe out of the water, dry the area around the hole, and apply a duct tape patch to the outside of the canoe. You're ready to shove off again.

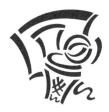

MAKE AN EMERGENCY SHOELACE

When you're enjoying a game of driveway hoops and you bust a sneaker lace, ask for a brief time-out while you grab the duct tape from the garage. Cut off a piece of tape that's as long as you need and rip off twice the width you need. Fold the tape in half along its length, sticky side in. Thread your new lace onto your sneaker, tie it up, and you're ready for your next jump shot.

WATERPROOF FOOTWEAR • Need a waterproof pair of shoes for fishing, gardening, or pushing off a canoe into the water? Cover an old pair of sneakers with duct tape, overlapping the edges of each row. When you get to the corners, cut little V's in the edges of the tape so that you can lap the tape smoothly around the corner.

PROTECT YOUR GAS-BOTTLE HOSE • For some reason, mice and rats love to chew on rubber, and one of their favorite snacks is often the rubber hose that connects the portable gas bottle to your barbecue. Protect the hose by wrapping it in duct tape.

PATCH A HOLE IN YOUR POOL'S LINER • Duct tape will repair a hole in your swimming pool liner well enough to stand up to water for at least a season. Just be sure to cover the area thoroughly.

more DUCT TAPE over →

DID YOU KNOW?

The people at 3M's product information service handle a lot of calls about duct tape.

Three of the most commonly asked questions are:
1 Can duct tape be used for removing warts?
2 Can it be used to secure the duct from the household dryer to the outdoors?
3 Is it waterproof?

The official answers:
1 Duct tape is not recommended for removing warts, because it hasn't been scientifically tested.
2 The company does not recommend using duct tape for the dryer duct, because the temperatures may exceed 200°F (93 °C), the maximum temperature duct tape can withstand.
3 The backing of the duct tape is waterproof, but the adhesive is not. Duct tape will hold up to water for a while, but eventually the adhesive will give out.

PROTECT YOURSELF FROM TICKS • When you're out on a hike, on your way to your favorite fishing hole, or just weeding in the garden, protect your ankles from those annoyingly persistent ticks. Wrap duct tape around your pant cuffs to seal them out. This is a handy way to keep pant legs out of your bicycle chain, too!

CREATE A CLOTHESLINE • If you're out in the wilderness on a camping trip or have pitched a tent in your own backyard and you need a clothesline, you can use duct tape. Twist a long piece of duct tape into a rope and tie it between two trees for a clothesline. It makes a great jump rope as well or a basic rope sturdy enough to lash two items together. You can even use your 'rope' to pull a child's wagon.

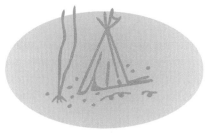

DUSTPANS

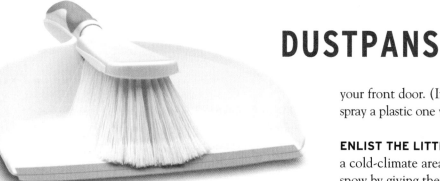

DECORATE YOUR DOOR FOR AUTUMN • Gather dried autumn foliage, such as branches with red and orange berries and other decorative leaves. Tie them together as a bouquet with a rubber band or tape. Spread them out in a fan shape and cover the binding with a ribbon. Now set this against a copper dustpan. Use super glue or a glue gun to attach your bouquet to the pan. Hang this homage to autumn on your front door. (If you don't have a copper dustpan, spray a plastic one with copper-colored metallic paint.

ENLIST THE LITTLEST SHOVELER • If you live in a cold-climate area, get the kids to help you shovel snow by giving them a dustpan to use as a shovel.

USE AS A SAND TOY • Pack a clean dustpan with your beach toys. It's a great sand scoop and will really help the castle builders with their task.

SPEED TOY CLEANUP • Picking up all those little toys gets pretty boring. Scoop them up with a dustpan and then deposit them in the toy bin. It's a real-time saver, not to mention back-saver.

EARRINGS

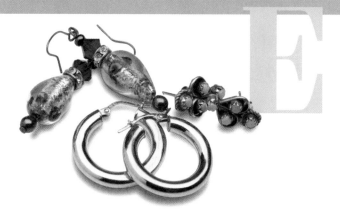

USE AS A BULLETIN BOARD TACK • Lend a little personal style to your bulletin board. Use mateless pierced earrings to tack up pictures, notes, souvenirs, and clippings.

CREATE A BROOCH • Got a batch of mateless pierced earrings collecting dust in a box? Use wire cutters to snip off the stems and get creative. Arrange the earrings on a swatch of cardboard or foam core, and secure them with a drop from a hot glue gun. Add a pin backing and you have a new brooch. Or use the same method to jazz up a plain picture frame.

MAKE A MAGNET • Give your fridge some glitz. Use wire cutters to cut the stem off an orphan earring and glue it to a magnet. What a great way to emphasize how pleased you are with that perfect school report when you stick it on the refrigerator!

CLIP YOUR SCARF • Did you lose one of your favorite earrings? Oh well, at least you can still work the survivor into the picture by using it to secure a scarf. Just tie the scarf as you normally would, then clip or pierce it at the center with the earring.

DECORATE YOUR CHRISTMAS TREE • Scatter clip-on earrings around the boughs of your Christmas tree as eye-catching accents to your larger tree decorations. Or use them as the main adornment on a small tree or wreath.

MAKE AN INSTANT BUTTON

Drats! You're dressed to go out and you discover a button is missing. No need to reinvent your whole outfit. Just dip into your collection of clip-on earrings. Clip the earring on the button side of the clothing to create a new 'button' and button as usual with the buttonhole. If there's time, move the top button on that blouse to replace the lost one and use the earring at the top of the blouse.

DID YOU KNOW?

People have been wearing–and probably losing–earrings for nearly 5,000 years. According to historians who have studied jewelry, the tiny baubles were probably introduced in western Asia in about 3000 BC. The oldest earrings date to 2500 BC and were found in Iraq. The popularity of earrings over time has grown or receded, depending on hairstyles and clothing trends. The clip-on earring was introduced in the 1930s, and by the 1950s, fashion-conscious women simply did not pierce their ears. But 20 years later, pierced ears were back.

EGG CARTONS

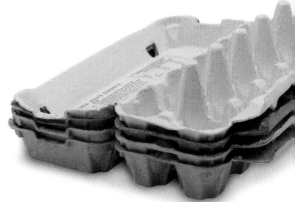

USE FOR STORING AND ORGANIZING • With a dozen handy compartments, egg cartons are a natural for storing and organizing small items. Here are some ideas to get you going. You're sure to come up with more of your own.

■ Instead of emptying all that loose change in your pocket into a jar for later sorting, cut off a four-section piece of an egg carton and leave it on your dresser or in a handy spot somewhere else. Sort your quarters, dimes, nickels, and pennies as you pull them out of your pockets. (Dump dollars in a larger container, such as a jar, or put them in a piggy bank.)

■ Organize buttons, safety pins, threads, sewing-machine bobbins, and fasteners on your sewing table.

■ Organize washers, tacks, small nuts and bolts, and screws on your workbench. Or use cartons to keep disassembled parts in sequence.

■ Keep small Christmas ornaments from being crushed in stackable egg cartons, with individual ornaments stored in their own compartment.

START SEEDLINGS • An egg carton can become the perfect nursery for your seeds. (Use a cardboard egg carton, not a polystyrene one.) Fill each cell in the carton with soil and plant a few seeds in each one. Once the seeds have sprouted, divide the carton into individual cells and plant, cardboard cells and all.

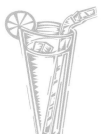

MAKE ICE • Making a lot of ice for a picnic or party? Use the bottom halves of clean polystyrene egg cartons as auxiliary ice trays.

REINFORCE A GARBAGE BAG • Yuck! You pull the plastic garbage bag out of the kitchen can and messy, smelly gunk drips out. Next time, put an opened empty egg carton at the bottom of the garbage bag to prevent tears and punctures.

GOLF BALL CADDY • An egg carton in your golf bag is a great way to keep golf balls that have been cleaned ready for teeing off.

START A FIRE • Fill a cardboard egg carton with briquettes (and a bit of leftover candle wax if it's handy), place in your barbecue, and light. Egg cartons can also be filled with kindling, such as small bits of wood and paper, and used as a fire starter in a fireplace or a woodstove.

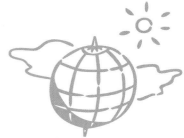

CREATE SHIPPABLE HOMEMADE GOODIES

Here's a great way to brighten the day of a soldier, student, or any faraway friend or loved one. Cover an egg carton with bright wrapping paper. Line the individual cells with shredded paper or shredded coconut. Nestle homemade treats inside each cell. Include the carton in your next care package or birthday gift, and rest assured the treats will arrive intact.

eggs
EGGS EGGS electrical tape electrical tape

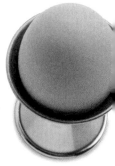

EGGS

MAKE A FACIAL • Who has the time or money to spend at the local day spa to have someone tell you how awful your skin looks? Instead, head to the fridge and grab an egg. If you have dry skin, separate the egg and beat the yolk. Oily skin takes egg white to which a bit of lemon or honey can be added. For normal skin, use the whole egg. Apply the beaten egg, relax, wait 30 minutes, and rinse. You'll love the look of your fresh, new face.

USE AS GLUE • Out of regular white glue? Egg whites can act as a glue substitute when gluing paper or light cardboard together.

ADD TO COMPOST • Eggshells are a great addition to your compost because they're rich in calcium —a nutrient that helps plants to reach their maximum growth. Crushing them before you put them in your compost pile will help them break down faster.

WATER YOUR PLANTS • After boiling eggs, don't pour the water down the drain. Instead, let it cool, and water plants with the nutrient-rich water.

START SEEDS • To plant seeds in eggshells, first place the eggshell halves in the carton, fill each with soil, and press seeds inside. The seeds will draw extra nutrients from the eggshells. Once the seedlings are about 3 inches (8 cm) tall, they are ready to be transplanted. Remove them from the shell first, crush the eggshells, and put them in your compost pile or plant them with your seedlings in the garden.

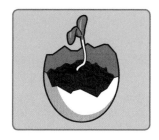

ELECTRICAL TAPE

STOP ANTS IN THEIR TRACKS • Is an army of ants marching towards the cookie jar on your countertop or some sweet prize in your pantry? Create a 'moat' around the object by surrounding it with vinyl plastic electrical tape placed sticky side up.

MAKE A LINT-LIFTER • To lift lint and pet hair off clothing and upholstery, you don't need a special lint remover. Just wrap your hand with electrical tape, sticky side out.

COVER CASTORS • Prevent your furniture from leaving marks on your wood or vinyl floor by wrapping the furniture's castor wheels with electrical tape.

CLEAN A COMB • To remove the gunk that builds up between the teeth of your comb, press a strip of electrical tape along the comb's length and lift it off. Then dip the comb in a solution of alcohol and water, or ammonia and water, to sanitize it. Let dry.

HANG GLUE AND CAULK TUBES • Got an ungainly heap of glue and caulk tubes on your workbench? Cut a strip of electrical or duct tape several inches long and fold it over the bottom of each tube, leaving a flap at the end. Punch a hole in the flap with a paper hole punch and hang the tube on a nail or hook. You'll free up bench space, and you'll be able to find the right tube fast.

more ELECTRICAL TAPE over →

 147

FOR BOOKWORMS!

REINFORCE BOOK BINDING • Electrical tape is perfect for repairing broken book binding. Using colored tape of a suitable color (matching or contrasting the cover so that it looks appealing), run the tape down the length of the spine and cut shorter pieces to run perpendicular to that if you need extra reinforcement.

COVER A BOOK • Use electrical tape in any color to create a durable book cover for a textbook or a paperback that you carry to the beach. Make a pattern for the cover on a sheet of newspaper. Fit the pattern to your book, and cover the pattern, one row at a time, with electrical tape, overlapping the rows. The resulting removable cover will be waterproof and sturdy.

MAKE BICYCLE STREAMERS • Add cool streamers to children's bicycle handlebars. Make them using electrical tape in various colors. Cut the tape into strips about ½ inch (1 cm) wide by 10 inches (25 cm) long. Fold each strip in half, sticky sides together. Once you have about half a dozen for each side, stick them into the end of the handlebar and secure them with electrical tape. Be sure your child can still have a good grip on the handlebars.

SAFELY REMOVE BROKEN WINDOW GLASS • Removing a window sash to fix a broken pane of glass can be dangerous. There's always the possibility that a sharp shard will fall out and cut you. To prevent this, crisscross both sides of the broken pane with electrical tape before removing the sash. And don't forget to wear heavy leather gloves to protect your hands when you pull the glass shards out of the frame.

WRAP CHRISTMAS PRESENTS • Here's a novel way to wrap a special gift. Don't bother with the paper; go straight for the tape. Press electrical tape directly on the gift box. Make designs or cover in stripes, then add decorative touches by cutting shapes, letters, and motifs from tape to attach to the 'wrapped' surface.

REPAIR A TAILLIGHT • If someone has backed into your car (or you got a bit to close to that cement wall) and smashed the taillight, here's a quick fix that will last until you have time to get it repaired. Depending on where the cracks lie, use yellow or red electrical tape to hold the remaining parts together.

REPAIR OUTDOOR CUSHIONS • Don't let a little rip in the cushions of your outdoor furniture bother you. Repair the tear with closely matched electrical tape and it will hold up for several seasons.

EMERY BOARDS

SAND DEEP CREVICES • If you are refinishing an elaborate piece of wood such as turned table legs or chair spindles, use emery boards to gently smooth those hard-to-reach crevices before applying stain or finish. These filelike nail sanders are easy to handle and provide a choice of two sanding grits.

SAVE YOUR SUEDE • Did somebody step on your blue suede shoes? Or worse, spill some wine on them? Don't check into Heartbreak Hotel, just try rubbing the stain lightly with an emery board, then hold the shoe over steam from a kettle or saucepan to remove the stain. This works for suede clothing, too.

REMOVE DIRT FROM A PENCIL ERASER

Do you have a fussy student who doesn't like dirt on the eraser end of their pencil? Take an emery board and rub lightly over the eraser until the dirt has been filed off.

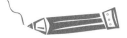

PREPARE SEEDS FOR PLANTING • You can use an old emery board to remove the hard coating on seeds before you plant them. This will speed sprouting and help them absorb moisture.

ENVELOPES

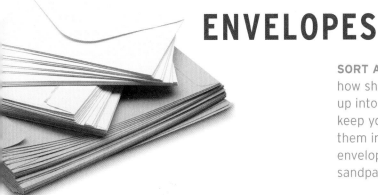

SORT AND STORE SANDPAPER • You know how sheets of sandpaper love to curl themselves up into useless tubes? Prevent that problem and keep your sandpaper sheets organized by storing them in standard letter-size cardboard mailing envelopes. Use one envelope for each sheet of sandpaper and record the grit on the envelope.

SHRED OLD RECEIPTS FASTER • The best way to get rid of receipts that may have your credit card number or other personal information in them is to shred them. But feeding tiny receipts into a shredder is tedious. Instead, place all the old receipts into a few used envelopes and shred the envelopes.

MAKE A SMALL FUNNEL • You save money by buying your spices in bulk and you want to transfer them to smaller bottles for use in the kitchen, but you don't have a small funnel to do the job. Make a couple of disposable funnels from an envelope. Seal the envelope, cut it in half diagonally and snip off one corner on each half. Now you have two funnels for pouring spices into your smaller jars.

MAKE BOOKMARKS • Recycle envelopes by making them into handy bookmarks of different sizes. Cut off the gummed flap and one end of the envelope and slip the remainder over the corner of the page where you stopped reading for a quick placeholder that doesn't damage your book. They're a great homemade addition to a book given as a present.

MAKE FILE FOLDERS • Don't let papers get disorganized just because you run out of file folders. Cut the short ends off a light cardboard mailing envelope. Turn it inside out so you have blank cardboard on the outside. Cut a ¾-inch (2-cm) wide strip lengthwise off the top of one side. The other edge becomes the place where you label your file.

EPSOM SALT

SOFTEN TOWELS • Soak bath towels overnight in a bucket of warm water with ½ cup (125 g) Epsom salt. The next day, wring out and tumble dry for soft-as-new towels.

CLEAN BATHROOM TILES • Are the tiles in your bathroom getting that grungy look? Time to bring in the Epsom salt. Mix it in equal parts with dishwashing liquid, then dab it on the offending area and start scrubbing. The Epsom salt works with the detergent to scrub and dissolve the grime.

REGENERATE A CAR BATTERY • Does your car battery sound as if it won't turn over? Worried you'll be stuck next time you try to start your car? Try this potion: Dissolve 2 tablespoons (30 ml) Epsom salt in warm water and add it to each battery cell.

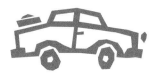

GET RID OF BLACKHEADS • Here's a sure-fire way to dislodge blackheads. Mix 1 teaspoon (5 ml) Epsom salt and 3 drops of iodine in ½ cup (125 ml) boiling water. When the mixture cools enough to stick your finger into it, apply it to blackheads with a cotton ball. Repeat this three or four times, reheating the solution if necessary. Gently remove the blackheads and dab the area with an alcohol-based astringent.

FROST YOUR WINDOWS FOR CHRISTMAS • If you are dreaming of a white Christmas, at least you can make your windows look frosty. Mix Epsom salt with stale beer until the salt stops dissolving. Apply the mixture to your windows with a sponge. For a realistic look, sweep the sponge in an arc at the bottom corners. When the mixture dries, the windows will look frosted.

FOR THOSE WITH GREEN FINGERS …

DETER SLUGS • Are you tired of visiting your garden at night only to find the place crawling with slimy slugs? Sprinkle Epsom salt where they glide and say goodbye to the slugs.

MAKE YOUR GRASS GREENER • How green is your garden? If the answer is not green enough, Epsom salt, which adds magnesium and iron to the soil, may be the answer. All you need to do is add 2 tablespoons (30 ml) to 1 gallon (4 L) water, spread it on your lawn and water the grass with plain water to make sure the mixture soaks in.

FERTILIZE TOMATOES AND OTHER PLANTS • Want those Big Boys to be big? Add Epsom salt as a fertilizer. Each week, for every 1 foot (30 cm) height of your tomato plant, add 1 tablespoon (15 ml). Your tomatoes will be the envy of the neighborhood. Epsom salt is also a good fertilizer for houseplants, roses, gardenias, other flowers, and trees.

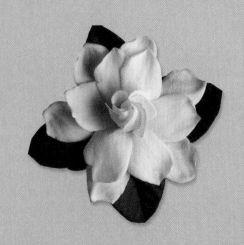

Kids' Stuff

Here are two fun winter-inspired projects using Epsom salt.

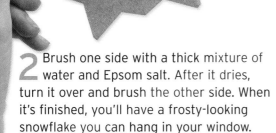

1 Make decorative snowflakes by folding a piece of blue paper several times and snipping shapes into the resulting piece of paper. Unfold your snowflake.

2 Brush one side with a thick mixture of water and Epsom salt. After it dries, turn it over and brush the other side. When it's finished, you'll have a frosty-looking snowflake you can hang in your window.

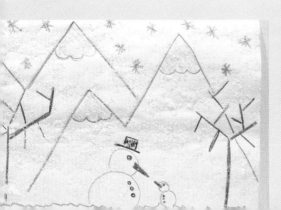

SNOW FUN! • To make a snowy scene, use crayons to draw a picture on construction paper. Mix equal parts Epsom salt and boiling water. Let it cool, then use a wide artist's paintbrush to paint the picture. When it dries, 'snow' crystals will appear.

FABRIC SOFTENER

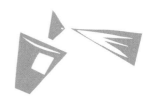

STOP DUST CLINGING TO YOUR TV • Are you frustrated to see dust fly back onto your television screen, or other plastic surfaces, right after cleaning them? To eliminate the static cling that attracts dust, simply dampen your dust rag with fabric softener straight from the bottle and dust as usual.

REMOVE OLD WALLPAPER • Removing old wallpaper is a cinch with fabric softener. stir 1 capful of liquid softener into 1 quart (1 L) water and sponge the solution onto the wallpaper. Let it soak in for 20 minutes, and scrape the paper from the wall. If the wallpaper has a water-resistant coating, score it with a wire-bristled brush before treating it with the fabric softener solution.

CLEAN NOW, NOT LATER • Clean glass tables, shower doors and other hard surfaces, and repel dust with liquid fabric softener. Mix 1 part softener into 4 parts water and store in a spray bottle, such as an empty dishwashing liquid bottle. Apply a little solution to a clean cloth, wipe the surface, and polish with a dry cloth.

UNTANGLE AND CONDITION HAIR • Liquid fabric softener diluted in water and applied after shampooing can untangle and condition both fine, flyaway hair, and curly, coarse hair. Experiment with the amount of conditioner to match it to the texture of your hair, using a weaker solution for fine hair and a stronger solution for coarse, curly hair. Comb through your hair and rinse.

REMOVE HAIR-SPRAY RESIDUE • Dried-on over-spray from hair spray can be tough to remove from walls and vanities, but even a buildup of residue is no match for a solution of 1 part liquid fabric softener to 2 parts water. Stir to blend, pour into a spray bottle, spritz the surface, and polish it with a dry cloth.

ABOLISH CARPET SHOCK

To eliminate static shock when you walk across a carpet, spray the carpet with a fabric softener solution. Dilute 1 cup (250 ml) softener with 10 cups (2.5 L) water, fill a spray bottle and lightly spray the carpet. Don't saturate it and damage the carpet backing. Spray in the evening and let dry overnight before walking on it. The effect should last for several weeks.

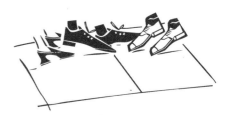

MAKE YOUR OWN FABRIC SOFTENER SHEETS • Fabric softener sheets are convenient to use, but they're no bargain when compared to the price of liquid softeners. You can make your own dryer sheets and save money. Just moisten a washcloth with 1 teaspoon (5 ml) liquid softener and toss it into the dryer with your next dryer load.

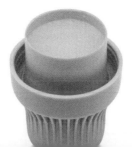

REMOVE HARD-WATER STAINS • Hard-water stains on windows can be difficult to remove. To speed up the process, dab full-strength liquid fabric softener on the stains and let it soak for 10 minutes. Then wipe the softener and stain off the glass with a damp cloth and rinse thoroughly.

FLOAT AWAY BAKED-ON GRIME • Forget scrubbing. Instead, soak burned-on foods from casseroles with liquid fabric softener. Fill the casserole dish with water, add a squirt of liquid fabric softener, and soak for an hour or until the residue wipes easily away.

DID YOU KNOW?

How does fabric softener reduce cling as well as soften clothes? The secret is in the electrical charges. Positively charged chemical lubricants in the fabric softener are attracted to your load of negatively charged clothes, softening the fabric. The softened fabrics create less friction, and less static, as they rub against each other in the dryer, and because fabric softener attracts moisture, the slightly damp surface of the fabrics makes them electrical conductors. As a result, the electrical charges travel through them instead of staying on the surface to cause static cling and sparks as you pull the clothing from the dryer.

KEEP PAINTBRUSHES PLIABLE

After using a paintbrush, clean the bristles thoroughly and rinse them in a coffee can full of water with a drop of liquid fabric softener mixed in. After rinsing, wipe the bristles dry and store the brush as usual.

FABRIC SOFTENER SHEETS

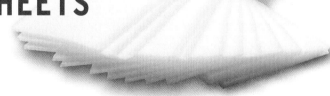

PICK UP PET HAIR • Pet hair can get a pretty tenacious grip on furniture and clothing. But a used fabric softener sheet will suck that fur right off the fabric with a couple of swipes. Just toss the fuzzy wipe into the garbage.

END CAR ODORS • Has that new-car smell gradually turned into that old-car stench? Tuck a fresh fabric softener sheet under each car seat to counteract musty odors and cigarette smells.

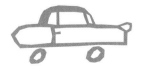

FRESHEN DRAWERS

There's no need to buy scented drawer-liner paper. Give your dresser drawers a fresh-air fragrance by tucking a new dryer fabric softener sheet under existing drawer liners or just tape one to the back of each drawer.

more FABRIC SOFTENER SHEETS over →

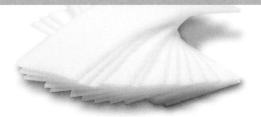

FRESHEN UP HAMPERS & WASTEBASKETS

There's still plenty of life left in used fabric softener sheets. Toss one into the bottom of a laundry basket or wastebasket to counteract odors.

LIFT BURNED-ON CASSEROLE RESIDUE • Those sheets will soften more than fabric. The next time food gets burned onto your casserole dish, save the elbow grease. Instead fill the dish with hot water and toss in three or four used softener sheets. Soak overnight, remove the sheets, and you'll have no trouble washing away the residue. Rinse well.

REPEL DUST FROM ELECTRICAL APPLIANCES • Because television and PC screens are electrically charged, they actually attract dust, making dusting them a never-ending chore, but not if you dust them with used fabric softener sheets. These sheets are designed to reduce static cling, so they remove the dust and keep it from resettling for several days.

DO AWAY WITH DOGGY ODOR • If man's best friend comes in from the rain and smells like a, well, wet dog, wipe him down with a used fabric softener sheet, and he'll smell as fresh as a daisy.

> **CAUTION:** People with allergies or chemical sensitivities may develop rashes or skin irritations when they come into contact with laundry that's been treated with some commercial fabric softeners or fabric softener sheets. If you are sensitive to softeners, you can still soften your laundry by substituting 1/4 cup (50 ml) white vinegar or the same amount of your favorite hair conditioner to your washing machine's last rinse cycle for softer, fresher-smelling laundry.

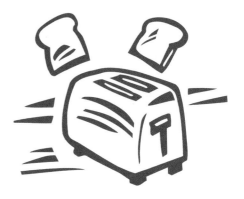

BUFF CHROME TO A BRILLIANT SHINE

After chrome is cleaned, it can still look streaky and dull, but whether it's your toaster or the hub caps on your car, you can easily buff up the shine with a used dryer fabric softener sheet.

USE AS A SAFE MOSQUITO REPELLENT • For a safe mosquito repellent, look no further than the laundry. Save used dryer fabric softener sheets and pin or tie one to your clothing when you go outdoors to help repel mosquitoes.

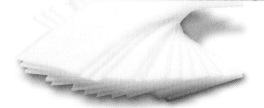

DO AWAY WITH STATIC CLING • You'll never be embarrassed by static cling again if you keep a used fabric softener sheet in your purse or dresser drawer. When faced with static, dampen the sheet and rub it over your pantyhose to put an end to clinging skirts.

KEEP DUST OFF BLINDS • Cleaning venetian blinds is a tedious job, so make the results last by wiping them down with a used fabric softener sheet to repel dust. Just wipe them with another sheet whenever the effect wears off.

USE AS INCONSPICUOUS AIR FRESHENERS • You don't need to spend hard-earned money on those expensive plug-in air fresheners. Just tuck a few fabric softener sheets into closets, behind curtains, and under chairs.

USE A DRYER SHEET AS A TACK CLOTH • Sticky tack cloths are designed to pick up all traces of sawdust on a woodworking project before you paint or varnish it, but they are expensive and not always easy to find at the hardware store. If you're in the middle of a project without a tack cloth, substitute an unused fabric softener sheet; it will attract sawdust and hold it like a magnet.

CONSOLIDATE SHEETS AND MAKE THEM SMELL FRESH • To improve your sheet storage, put each sheet set into one of its matching pillowcases, then tuck a new fabric softener sheet into the packet for a fresh fragrance.

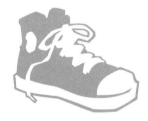

TAME LOCKER-ROOM AND SNEAKER SMELLS • Deodorizing sneakers and gym bags calls for strong stuff. Tuck a new fabric softener sheet into each shoe and leave overnight to neutralize odors (just remember to pull them out before wearing them). Drop a dryer sheet into the bottom of a gym bag and leave it there until your nose lets you know it's time to renew it.

WIPE SOAP SCUM FROM SHOWER DOORS • If you're tired of having to clean those scummy shower doors, give it up! It's easy to wipe the soap scum away with a used dryer fabric softener sheet. A sparkling clean glass shower door is just a swipe away.

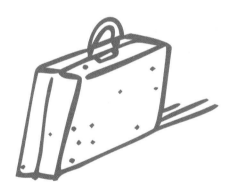

PREVENT MUSTY ODORS IN SUITCASES

Place a single, unused fabric softener sheet into an empty suitcase or other piece of luggage before storing. The bag will smell great the next time you use it.

more FABRIC SOFTENER SHEETS over →

ABOLISH TANGLED SEWING THREAD • To put an end to tangled thread, keep an unused fabric softener sheet in your sewing kit. After threading the needle, insert it into the sheet and pull all of the thread through to give it a nonstick coating.

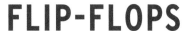

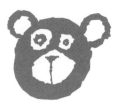

RENEW GRUBBY STUFFED TOYS • Wash fake-fur stuffed animals in the washing machine on gentle cycle and put them into the dryer, along with a pair of old tennis shoes and a fabric softener sheet. They will come out fluffy with silky-soft fur.

FLIP-FLOPS

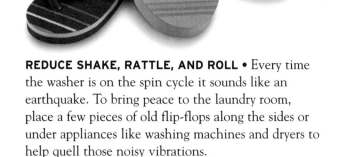

USE FOR PACKING OR STUFFING • Recycled flip-flops make excellent material for packing breakable items. Place them as is on the top and bottom of a box or shred them and use like Styrofoam peanuts. They can also be shredded for stuffing in cushions.

REMOVE PET HAIR • Slip a flip-flop on your hand and rub carpets and rugs in the direction of the pile. Pet hair will form into balls that can then be vacuumed up. This works well on upholstery, too, including car seats.

KEEP A DOOR OPENED • Cut a wedge of rubber from an old flip-flop and use it to keep a door in the open position on a breezy day.

MAKE A BATHTUB BOAT • Keep the kids amused at bathtime by putting those old flip-flops to good use. Remove the side straps and carefully pull out the toe holder. Make a sail out of colored paper and attach it to a small dowel or pencil. Use a hot-glue gun to seal the dowel into the hole. "Anchors aweigh!"

REDUCE SHAKE, RATTLE, AND ROLL • Every time the washer is on the spin cycle it sounds like an earthquake. To bring peace to the laundry room, place a few pieces of old flip-flops along the sides or under appliances like washing machines and dryers to help quell those noisy vibrations.

PREVENT RATTLING WINDOWS • Can't sleep whenever the wind blows? If your older-style windows rattle in their frames whenever it's windy, cut slivers of rubber from an old flip-flop and wedge them between the window and the frame.

KEEP FURNITURE STEADY
Stop the wobbles in a wonky table by cutting a piece of an old flip-flop to the shape of the offending leg and gluing it underneath.

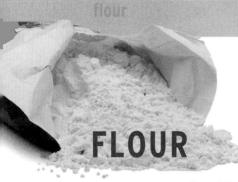

FLOUR

REPEL ANTS WITH FLOUR • Sprinkle a line of flour along the backs of pantry shelves and wherever you see ants entering the house. Repelled by the flour, ants won't cross over the line.

SAFE PASTE FOR CHILDREN'S CRAFTS • Look no further than your kitchen canister for an inexpensive, nontoxic paste that is ideal for children's paper craft projects, such as papier-mâché and scrapbooking. To make the paste, add 3 cups (750 ml) cold water to a saucepan and blend in 1 cup (250 g) plain flour. Stirring constantly, bring the mixture to the boil. Reduce the heat and simmer, stirring until smooth and thick. Cool and pour into a plastic squeeze bottle to use. This simple paste will keep for weeks in the refrigerator and cleans up easily with soap and water.

POLISH BRASS AND COPPER • No need to go out and buy cleaner for your brass and silver. You can whip up your own at much less cost. Just combine equal parts of flour, salt, and vinegar, then mix into a paste. Spread the paste onto the metal, let it dry, and buff it off with a clean, dry cloth.

DID YOU KNOW?

Ever wondered why the word *flour* is pronounced exactly like the word *flower*? Well, you may be surprised to learn that *flour* is actually derived from the French word for flower, which is *fleur*. The French use the word to describe the most desirable, or floury (flowery) and protein-rich, part of a grain after processing removes the hull. And, because much of our food terminology comes from the French, we still bake and make sauces with the flower of grains, such as wheat, which we call flour.

MAKE MODELING CLAY • Keep the kids busy on a rainy day with modeling clay—they can even help you make the stuff. Knead together 3 cups (750 g) plain flour, ¼ cup (50 g) salt, 1 cup (250 ml) water, 1 tablespoon (15 ml) vegetable oil and 1 or 2 drops food coloring. If the mixture is sticky, add more flour; if too stiff, add more water. When the 'clay' is sufficiently pliable, store it in a zip-lock plastic bag.

BRING BACK LUSTER TO A DULL SINK • To buff your stainless steel sink back to a warm glow, sprinkle flour over it and rub lightly with a soft, dry cloth. Then rinse the sink to restore its shine.

 FRESHEN PLAYING CARDS

After a few games, cards can accumulate a patina of snack residue and hand oil, but you can restore them with some plain flour in a paper bag. Drop the cards into the bag with enough flour to cover, shake vigorously, and remove the cards. The flour will absorb the oils, and it can be easily knocked off the cards by giving them a vigorous shuffle.

FLOWERPOTS

CONTAINER FOR BAKING BREAD • Take a new, clean, medium-sized clay flowerpot, soak it in water for about 20 minutes and lightly grease the inside with butter. Place your bread dough, prepared as usual, in the pot and bake. The clay pot will give your bread a crusty outside and keep the inside moist.

CREATE A FIREWOOD CONTAINER • Who needs an expensive metal or brass rack to hold firewood by the fireplace? Spare yourself the expense and put an extra-large, empty ceramic or clay flowerpot beside the hearth. It's a perfect—and cheap—place to keep kindling and small logs ready for when the weather outside gets frightful.

UNWIND WOOL WITHOUT KNOTTING • Knitting a sweater will take ages to finish if you're constantly stopping to untangle the wool. To prevent this, place your ball of wool under an upturned flowerpot and thread the end through the drain hole.

CREATE AN AQUARIUM FISH CAVE • Some fish love to lurk in shadowy corners of their aquariums, keeping themselves safe from imagined predators. Place a mini flowerpot on its side on the aquarium floor to create a cave for lurking fish.

KILL FIRE ANTS • If fire ants are plaguing your garden or patio and you're tired of getting stung by the tiny attackers, a flowerpot can help you solve the problem. Place the flowerpot upside down over the ant hill. Pour boiling water through the drain hole and you'll be burning down their house.

SAVE POTTING MIX WHEN PLANTING SHALLOW-ROOTED PLANTS • The plants you want to put in that beautiful, new, deep flowerpot you ordered for your patio have a shallow root system and you don't want to go to the bother—and expense—of filling that huge pot completely with potting mix. So what do you do? One easy solution is to find another smaller flowerpot that will fit upside down in the base of the deeper pot and occupy a lot of that empty space. After you insert it, fill around it with potting mix before putting in your plants.

KEEP SOIL IN A FLOWERPOT • Soil from your house plant won't slip-slide away if you place broken clay flowerpot shards in the bottom of the pot before replanting. When watering your plants, you'll find that the water drains out, but not the soil.

DID YOU KNOW?

For thousands of years people have been plopping plants into pots to transport a native plant to a new land or to bring an exotic plant home. In 1495 B.C., Egyptian queen Hatshepsut sent workers to Somalia to bring back incense trees in pots. And in 1787 Captain Bligh reportedly had more than 1,000 breadfruit plants in clay pots aboard the H.M.S. *Bounty*. The plants were destined for the West Indies, where they were to be grown as food for the slaves.

FOAM FOOD TRAYS

MAKE KNEE PADS FOR GARDENING • If you find gardening is a pain in the knees when you work in and around your little patch of green, tape a couple of foam food trays to your knees. Or attach them to your legs using the top halves of old tube socks. The trays give you extra padding while you pull out weeds and fertilize your plants.

RELEASE YOUR INNERSOLES • If your tired old dogs need a little padding, grab a couple of clean meat trays and cut them to fit inside the soles of your shoes or boots. You'll have happy feet and some extra cushioning for free.

PRODUCE A DISPOSABLE SERVING DISH • Wash a disposable foam food tray with soap and water, cover it entirely with foil, and load it up with food. Use these serving dishes to deliver goodies to the church potluck, bake sale, or a sick neighbor and you'll have no worries about losing your own platters.

PROVIDE AN ART PALETTE • Create a paint palette for your budding Picasso. A thoroughly cleaned and dried food tray is the perfect place for kids to squirt their tempera or oil paints. Are they experimenting with watercolors? Use two trays: Put watercolor paint in one and water in the other. At the end of the art session, you can just throw them away.

PROTECT PICTURES IN THE MAIL

Why buy expensive padded envelopes to send photographs to loved ones? Cut foam trays slightly smaller than your mailing envelope. Insert your photographs between the trays, place in the envelope and mail. The photos will arrive without creases or bends.

FREEZER

ELIMINATE UNPOPPED POPCORN • Don't you just hate the hard kernels of popcorn that are left at the bottom of the bowl? Eliminate the popcorn duds by keeping your unpopped supply in the freezer.

REMOVE WAX FROM CANDLESTICKS • Give silver candlesticks a new life by placing them in the freezer, and you can pick off the accumulated wax drippings. **WARNING: Don't do this if your candlesticks are made from more than one type of metal. The metals can expand and contract at different rates and damage the candlesticks.**

EXTEND CANDLE LIFE • Place candles in the freezer for at least 2 hours before burning. This way, they will last longer when they're burning.

UNSTICK PHOTOS • If you pull stuck-together photos apart, your pictures will be ruined. Instead, stick them in the freezer for about 20 minutes, then use a butter knife to very carefully separate the photos. If they don't come free, place them back in the freezer. This works for envelopes and stamps, too.

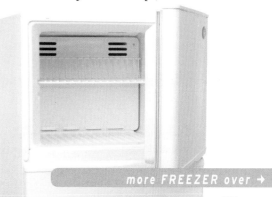

more FREEZER over →

REMOVE ODORS • Got a musty-smelling book or a plastic container with a fish odor? Place them in the freezer overnight. By morning they'll be fresh again. It works with almost any other small item that has a bad smell you want to get rid of.

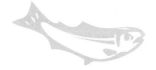

CLEAN A POT • If your favorite pot has been left on the stove too long, you have a burned-on mess to contend with. All you have to do is place the pot in the freezer for a couple of hours. When the burned-on food freezes, it will be easier to remove.

EXTEND BATTERY LIFE • We all know batteries are expensive, but if you buy them in bulk, you might be able to save a lot of money in the long run. Storing unused NiMH and NiCd batteries (often used in electronics) in the freezer will extend their life by about 90%. Storing alkaline batteries in the freezer, on the other hand, will only extend their life by about 5%, so make sure you are freezing the right kind of battery. When you're ready to use them, just make sure you bring them to room temperature first!

REMOVE GUM FROM YOUR SHOE • Stepped in gum? You could try scraping it off but here's an easy way to remove it. Stick a small piece of paper over the gum and place the shoe in the freezer for 1 to 2 hours. Take the shoe out, peel the paper off, and the gum should peel off with the paper! If there's any residue left, a simple scrape with a knife should do the trick.

SHARPEN EYELINER LIKE A PRO • Before you sharpen your pencil eyeliner, stick it in the freezer for 10-15 minutes. You'll find that when you sharpen it, the point will make your line much more precise.

Freezer tactics

Here are some inventive ways to get the most out of your freezer or your refrigerator's freezer compartment.

● To prevent spoilage, keep your freezer at 0°F (-18°C). To check the temperature, stick a freezer thermometer (available at hardware stores) in between two frozen food containers.

● A full freezer runs the compressor less often and stays colder longer, which is good to remember next time there's a blackout.

● Because the shelves on a freezer door are exposed to the outside air when the fridge is opened, they are a bit warmer than the freezer interior, making them ideal for storing items such as bread and coffee.

● When defrosting your freezer, place a large towel or sheet on the bottom. Water drips onto it, making the cleanup much easier.

● The next time you defrost your freezer, apply a thin coating of petroleum jelly to the walls to keep frost from sticking to them.

KEEP NATURAL BEAUTY PRODUCTS FRESH • All-natural beauty products have become popular for a number of reasons. The problem is that preservatives and additives in un-natural products are what keeps them fresh longer! If you buy a natural product, you could keep it in the fridge and it might last a little longer. For natural beauty products bought in bulk or ones that you use occasionally (like a unique shade of lipstick), putting them in the freezer will extend their lifetime much longer.

STORE EGGS IN THE FREEZER • When the grocery store has a sale on fresh eggs, here's an easy way to take advantage of it. Crack whole eggs into a ziplock bag and freeze it flat. For baking, freeze yolks and whites separately in their own ice cube trays. Thaw them in the refrigerator and they'll be ready to use.

FUNNELS

TABLETOP CHRISTMAS TREE DECORATION • Looking for a little something special to enhance your holiday table? Hit the flea markets and pick up different sizes of old metal funnels. Stack them with the opening of the largest one for your base, and decreasing sizes going to the top of your "tree." Decorate by hot-gluing colorful ball ornaments on the outside of the funnels and topping it off with a star.

RUSTIC CANDLESTICKS • Are you planning an outdoor brunch or dinner but you don't want to use your good candlesticks? A few metal funnels will do the job and add a rustic look your al fresco table. For a snug fit in the spout, just shave the edge of the candles.

MAKE A STRING DISPENSER • Don't get yourself tied up in knots over tangled string. Nail a large funnel to the wall, with the stem pointing down. Place a ball of string in the funnel and thread the end through the funnel's stem and you have an instant knot-free string dispenser.

SEPARATING EGGS • Here's an egg-ceptional method for handling a potentially messy kitchen job. Try a funnel. Crack the whole egg into the funnel. The white will slide out of the spout into another container, while the yolk stays in the funnel. Of course, you have to be careful not to break the yolk when you're cracking the egg!

Kids' Stuff

Here's a fun science experiment to perform with your kids that will teach them about air flow. Light a candle and point the wide end of the funnel at the candle. Ask the kids to blow it out by blowing through the small end of the funnel. Hard as they try, they won't have much luck. It's a neat way to demonstrate how the speed of air slows when it's blown through a wide opening.

MAKE A PENDANT LIGHT FIXTURE • Hanging fixtures are perfect for adding task lighting to a countertop or kitchen island. Select a metal funnel (or more) in a size that works for the space and hang upside down. You can find wiring kits at hardware or home improvement stores. Run wire up through the spout through a chain, cut to the length you need. Be sure to get professional help if you plan on installing the pendant in the ceiling.

MAKE A KIDS' TELEPHONE • Just because you choke every time you open your phone bill doesn't mean the kids have to, too. Use two small plastic funnels to make them a durable string telephone. For each funnel, tie a button to one end of a length of string and thread it through the large end of the funnel. Tie another button at the bottom of the spout to keep the string in place and the kids can start yakking!

MAKE A NEW HANGING PLANTER • Is it time to swap out that old hanging-basket planter that has seen better days? A big metal funnel could make an inexpensive replacement next time you decide to repot with new flowers. Punch a few holes with a screwdriver along the wide end of the funnel for attaching hanging wire or chain. Add small piece of sponge inside to cover the hole and fill with fresh soil and new plants.

GARDEN HOSE

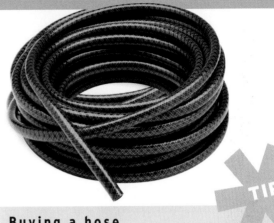

MAKE A DECOY TO SCARE BIRDS • If flocks of annoying, messy birds are invading your backyard, try replicating their natural predator to keep them away. Cut a short length of hose, lay it in your grass—poised like a snake—and the birds will steer clear.

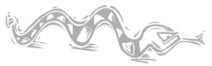

STABILIZE A TREE • A short length of old garden hose is a good way to tie a young tree to its stake. You'll find that the hose is flexible enough to bend when the tree does, but at the same time, it's strong enough to keep the tree tied to its stake until it can stand on its own. Also, the hose will not damage the bark of the young tree as it grows.

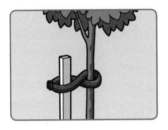

CAPTURE EARWIGS • Pesky garden earwigs will find their final resting place in that leaky old hose. Cut the hose into 12-foot (30-cm) lengths, making sure the inside is completely dry. Place the hose segments where you have seen earwigs crawling around and leave them overnight. By the morning the hoses should be filled with the earwigs and ready for disposal. One method is to dunk the hoses in a bucket of soapy water.

UNCLOG A DOWNSPOUT • When leaves and debris clog downspouts and gutters, turn to your garden hose to get things flowing again. Push the hose up the downspout and poke through the blockage. You don't even have to turn the hose on, because the water in the gutters will flush out the dam.

Buying a hose

It's just a garden-variety hose, right? Nothing special. Actually, there are a few important points to keep in mind when you buy this basic but important outdoor tool.

● To determine how long a hose you need, measure the distance from the faucet to the farthest point in your yard. Add several feet (meters) for watering around corners to avoid aggravating kinks that cut water pressure.

● Vinyl and rubber hoses are generally more sturdy and weather resistant than ones made of cheaper forms of plastic. If a hose flattens when you step on it, it is not up to gardening duties.

● Buy a hose with a lifetime warranty; only good-quality garden hoses have one.

COVER SWING SET CHAINS • To avoid kids getting hurt on a backyard swing, put a length of old hose over each chain to protect little hands from getting pinched on the swing chain. If you have access to one end of the chains, just slip the chain through the hose. Otherwise, slit the hose down the middle and slip it over the chains. Close the slit hose with a few wraps of duct or electrical tape.

MAKE A PLAY PHONE • Transform your old garden hose into a fun new telephone for the kids. Cut any length, stick a funnel at each end, and attach it with glue or tape. Now the kids can talk for as long as they like, with no roaming charges.

PROTECT YOUR HANDSAW AND ICE SKATE BLADES • Keep your handsaw blade sharp and safe by protecting it with a length of garden hose. Just cut a piece of hose to the length you need, slit it along its length and slip it over the teeth. This is also a good way to protect the blades of your ice skates and your cooking knives when you pack them for a camping trip.

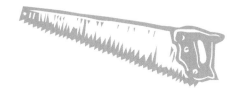

GLOVES

GRIP A STUBBORN JAR LID • It's annoying when you can't open a jar of peanut butter or olives. If the lid just won't come loose, put on some rubber gloves—you'll get a better grip to unscrew the top.

MAKE AN ICE PACK • If you need an ice pack in a hurry, fill a kitchen rubber glove with ice. Close the wrist with a rubber band to contain water from the melting ice and apply it to the body part. When you're finished, turn the glove inside out to dry.

PAPER-SORTING FINGER • Don't fancy licking your finger when you riffle through a stack of papers or dollar bills? Cut off the index finger from an old rubber glove and you'll have an ideal sheath for your finger the next time you have to quickly sort through some papers.

MAKE STRONG RUBBER BANDS • If you need some extra-strong rubber bands, cut up old rubber gloves. Make horizontal cuts in the finger sections for small rubber bands and in the body of the glove for large ones.

MAKE A PAINT CAN GRIP • You don't want a heavy paint can to slip and spill. And those thin wire handles can really cut into your hand. Get a better grip by cutting a short length of hose. Slit it down the middle and slip it on the paint can handle.

MAKE A SANDER FOR CURVES • If you've got a tight concave surface to sand—a piece of cove molding, for example—grab a 10-inch (25-cm) length of garden hose. Split open the hose lengthwise and insert one edge of the sandpaper. Wrap it around the hose, cut it to fit and insert the other end in the slit. Firmly close the slit with a bit of duct tape.

REMOVE CAT HAIR • Here's a quick and easy way to remove cat hair from upholstery. Put on a rubber glove and wet it. When you rub it against fabric, the cat hair will stick to the glove. If you are worried about getting the upholstery slightly damp, test it in an inconspicuous area first.

USE LATEX GLOVES FOR EXTRA INSULATION • If you've got a good pair of gloves or mittens, but your hands still get cold while shoveling snow or doing other outdoor activities in cold weather, try slipping on a pair of latex surgical gloves underneath your usual mittens or gloves. The rubber is a fantastic insulator, so your hands will stay warm—and dry, too.

CLEAN YOUR KNICKKNACKS • Need to dust that collection of glass animals or other delicate items? Put on some fabric gloves—the softer the better—to clean your knickknacks thoroughly.

DUST A CHANDELIER • If your chandelier has become a haven for spiderwebs and dust, try this surefire dusting tip. Soak some old fabric gloves in window cleaner. Slip them on and wipe off the lighting fixture. You'll beam at the results.

GLYCERINE

MAKE YOUR OWN SOAP • Homemade soap is a great gift and cinch to make if you have glycerine soap base and a microwave. Here's how. Cut the glycerine soap base, usually sold in blocks, into 2-inch (5-cm) cubes. Using a microwave set on half-power, zap several cubes in a glass container for 30 seconds at a time—checking and stirring as needed—until the glycerine melts. Add drops of colored dye or scents at this point, if you wish. Pour the melted glycerine into soap or chocolate molds. If you don't have any molds, fill the bottom 3/4 inch (2 cm) of a polystyrene cup. Let it harden for 30 minutes.

CLEAN A FREEZER SPILL • Spilled sticky foods at the bottom of your freezer don't have a chance against glycerine. Unstick the spill and wipe it clean with a rag dabbed with glycerine, a natural solvent.

REMOVE TAR STAINS • It's not impossible to remove a tar or mustard stain if you use glycerine. Rub glycerine into the spot and leave it for about an hour and, with paper towels, gently remove the spot using a blot-and-lift motion. You may need to do this several times.

DID YOU KNOW?

Glycerine is a clear, colorless thick liquid that is a by-product of the soap-making process, in which lye is combined with animal or vegetable fat. Commercial soap makers remove the glycerine when they make soap so that they can use it in more profitable lotions and creams. Glycerine works well in lotions because it is essentially a moisturizing material that dissolves in alcohol or water. Glycerine is also used to make nitroglycerine and candy and to preserve fruit and laboratory specimens. Look for glycerine at your local pharmacy or in the hand lotion aisle of your supermarket. Solid glycerine soap base is available from specialty craft stores that carry a range of soap-making products.

MAKE NEW LIQUID SOAP • Wondering what to do with those little leftover slivers of soap? Add a bit of glycerine and crush them together with some warm water. Pour the mixture into a pump bottle. You'll have liquid soap on the cheap.

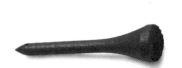

GOLF GEAR

MAKE A GOLF-TEE TIE RACK • If your ties are scattered around the closet, try using golf tees to get them organized. Sand and paint a length of particle board. Drill 1/8-inch (3-mm) holes every 2 inches (5 cm). Dip the tip of each tee in yellow carpenter's glue and tap it into a hole. Hang the tie rack on the closet wall or inside the door. It's a perfect gift for the golfer in your life.

AERATE YOUR LAWN • Kill two birds with one stone by wearing golf shoes to aerate your lawn while you mow. The grip that a golf shoe gives you is also a good idea if you have to push the mower uphill.

FILL STRIPPED SCREW HOLES • If you're replacing a rusty door hinge when you discover that a screw won't grip because its hole has gotten too big, dip the tip of a golf tee in yellow carpenter's glue and tap the tee into the hole. Cut the tee flush with the door frame surface using a craft knife. When it's dry, drill a new pilot hole for the screw in that spot.

HAIR CONDITIONER

TAKE OFF MAKEUP • Put your face first. Why buy expensive makeup removers when a perfectly good substitute sits in your shower stall? Hair conditioner quickly and easily removes makeup for much less money than name-brand makeup removers.

UNSTICK A RING • Grandma's antique ring just got stuck on your middle finger. Now what? Grab a bottle of hair conditioner and slick down the finger. The ring should slide right off.

PROTECT YOUR SHOES IN FOUL WEATHER • Here's a way to protect your shoes during winter. Lather your shoes or boots with hair conditioner to protect them from winter's harsh elements. It's a good leather conditioner, too.

LUBRICATE A ZIPPER • You're racing out the door, throwing on your jacket and the zipper gets stuck, so you yank and pull until it finally zips up. A dab of hair conditioner rubbed along the zipper teeth can help you avoid that problem in future.

SMOOTH SHAVE-IRRITATED LEGS • After you shave your legs, they may feel rough and irritated. Rub on hair conditioner; it acts like a lotion and can soothe the hurt away.

MAKE A SHOWER CURTAIN SLIDE SMOOTHLY • Tired of pulling on the shower curtain? Instead of closing smoothly, does it stutter along the curtain rod, letting the shower spray water on the floor? Rub the shower-curtain rod with hair conditioner and the curtain will glide across it.

CLEAN AND SHINE YOUR HOUSEPLANTS • Do your houseplants need a good dusting? Feel like your peace lily could use a makeover? Put a bit of hair conditioner on a soft cloth and rub the plant leaves to remove dust and add shine to the leaves.

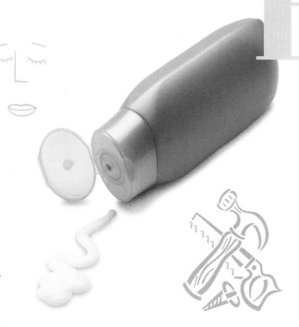

PREVENT RUST ON TOOLS

Every good do-it-yourselfer knows how important it is to take care of the tools in your toolbox. One way to condition them and keep rust from invading is to rub them down with some inexpensive hair conditioner.

OIL SKATE WHEELS • Do your child's skateboard wheels whine? Or are the kids complaining about their in-line and roller skates sticking? Try rubbing hair conditioner on the axles of the wheels, and they'll be back on the block with their rehabilitated equipment in no time.

SHINE STAINLESS STEEL • Apply hair conditioner to your faucets, golf clubs, chrome fixtures, or anything else that needs a shine. Rub it off with a soft cloth and you'll be impressed with the gleam.

more HAIR CONDITIONER over →

DID YOU KNOW?

Hair conditioner has been around for about 50 years. While researching ways to help World War II burn victims, Swiss chemists developed a compound that improved the health of hair. In the 1950s, other scientists developing fabric softeners found that the same material could soften hair.

Despite our efforts to keep hair healthy with hair conditioner, we still lose on average between 50 and 100 strands a day. For most of us, thankfully, there are still many more strands left. People with blond hair have an average of 140,000 strands of hair, brown-haired people, 100,000 and redheads, 90,000.

CLEAN SILK GARMENTS • Do you dare to ignore that "dry clean only" label on your silk shirt? Here's a low-cost alternative to sending it out. Fill the sink with water (warm water for whites and cold water for colors). Add 1 tablespoon (15 ml) hair conditioner. Immerse the shirt in the water and let it sit for a few minutes. Pull it out, rinse, and hang it up to dry. The conditioner keeps the shirt feeling silky smooth.

HAIR SPRAY

EXTERMINATE HOUSEFLIES • When an annoying, buzzing housefly outstays its welcome after a day or so, make it bite the dust with a squirt of hair spray. Take aim and fire, and watch the fly drop. But make sure the hair spray is water soluble so that if any spray hits the wall, you'll be able to wipe it clean. Works on wasps and bees, too.

REMOVE LIPSTICK FROM FABRIC • Has someone been kissing your shirts? Apply hair spray to the lipstick stain and let it sit for a few minutes. Wipe off the hair spray and the stain should come off with it. Wash your shirts as usual.

REDUCE RUNS IN PANTYHOSE • Often those bothersome runs in your pantyhose or stockings start at the toes. Head off a running disaster by spraying hair spray on the toes of a new pair of pantyhose. The spray strengthens the threads and makes them last longer.

PRESERVE A CHRISTMAS WREATH • When you buy a fresh pine wreath at your local florist, it's fresh, green and lush, but by the time a week has gone past, it's starting to shed needles and look a bit dry. To make it last longer, spritz it all over with hair spray as soon as you get the fresh wreath home. The hair spray traps the moisture in the needles.

PROTECT CHILDREN'S ARTWORK • Picture this: Your preschooler has just returned home with a priceless work of art demanding that it find a place on the refrigerator door. Before you stick it up, preserve the creation with hair spray, to help it last longer. This works especially well on chalk pictures, keeping them from being smudged so easily.

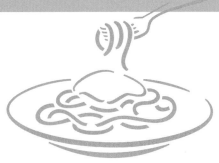

KEEP RECIPE CARDS SPLATTER-FREE • Don't let the spaghetti sauce on the stove splatter on your favorite recipe card. A good coating of hair spray will prevent the card from being ruined by kitchen eruptions. With the protection, they wipe off easily.

PRESERVE YOUR SHOES' SHINE • After you've lovingly polished your shoes to give them the just-from-the-store look, lightly spray them with hair spray. The shoe polish won't rub off as easily with this protective coating.

KEEP CURTAINS DIRT-FREE • Did you just buy new curtains or have your old ones cleaned? Want to keep that like-new look for a while? The trick is to apply several coats of hair spray, letting each coat dry thoroughly before the next one.

REMOVE INK MARKS ON GARMENTS • If a toddler just went wild with a ballpoint pen on your white upholstery or your new shirt, squirt the stain with hair spray and the pen marks should come right off.

DID YOU KNOW?

Hair spray has been around for a long time. Here are some great moments in its history:

■ A Norwegian inventor developed the technology that became the aerosol can in the early 1900s. What would hair spray be without aerosol cans?

■ L'Oréal introduced its hair spray, called Elnett, in 1960. The next year Alberto VO5 introduced its own version of what was to become a classic.

■ In 1964 hair spray surpassed lipstick as women's most popular cosmetic aid. Must have been all those beehive hairdos.

■ As Marge Simpson knows, hair spray makes possible the bumper sticker that reads "The Higher the Hair, the Closer to God."

■ In 1984, the hair spray on Michael Jackson was in the news when his hair suddenly ignited while he was rehearsing a commercial for Pepsi.

EXTEND THE LIFE OF CUT FLOWERS

A bouquet of cut flowers is such a beautiful thing, you want to do whatever you can to postpone wilting. Just as it preserves your hairstyle, a spritz of hair spray can preserve your cut flowers. Stand about 1 foot (30 cm) away from the bouquet and give them a quick spray, just on the undersides of the leaves and petals.

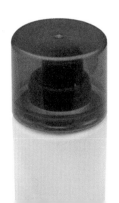

HYDROGEN PEROXIDE

REMOVE STAINS OF AN UNKNOWN ORIGIN • Can't tell what a stain is, but still want to try removing it? Try this surefire mixture. Mix 1 teaspoon (5 ml) 3% hydrogen peroxide with a little cream of tartar or a dab of non-gel toothpaste. Rub the paste on the stain with a soft cloth and rinse. The stain should be gone.

REMOVE GRASS STAINS • If grass stains are ruining your kids' clothes, hydrogen peroxide may bring relief. Mix a few drops of ammonia with just 1 teaspoon (5 ml) 3% hydrogen peroxide. Rub on the stain. As soon as it disappears, rinse and launder.

CAUTION: Hydrogen peroxide is considered corrosive—even in the relatively weak 3% solution sold as a household antiseptic. Never put it in or anywhere near your eyes or around your nose. And don't ever swallow it or try to set it on fire, either.

REMOVE MILDEW • Mildew is a bathroom's enemy, and a sign that you need to bring out the tough ammunition—a bottle of 3% hydrogen peroxide. Don't water it down. Just it attack directly by pouring the peroxide on the offending area, and wiping it clean. Mildew surrender.

REMOVE FRESH BLOODSTAINS FROM FABRIC • Apply 3% hydrogen peroxide directly to the fresh bloodstain on your clothing, rinse with fresh water, and launder as usual.

DID YOU KNOW?

Hydrogen peroxide (H_2O_2) was discovered in 1818. The most common household use for it is as an antiseptic and bleaching agent. (It's the key ingredient in most teeth-whitening kits and all-fabric oxygen bleaches, for example.) Textile manufacturers use higher concentrations of hydrogen peroxide to bleach fabric. During World War II, hydrogen peroxide solutions fueled torpedoes and rockets.

SANITIZE YOUR CUTTING BOARD

Hydrogen peroxide is a sure-fire bacteria-killer–just the ally you need to fight the proliferation of bacteria on your cutting board, especially after you've cut chicken or other meat. To kill the germs on a cutting board, use a paper towel to wipe the board down with vinegar, then use another paper towel to wipe it with hydrogen peroxide. Ordinary 3% peroxide is fine.

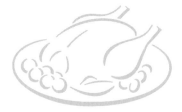

REMOVE WINE STAINS • Hydrogen peroxide works well to remove wine stains from clothing, so don't worry if you spill some while you quaff.

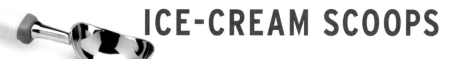

ICE-CREAM SCOOPS

SCOOP MEATBALLS AND COOKIE DOUGH • If you want uniform-sized meatballs every time, use an ice-cream scoop to measure out the perfect balls. This method works well for cookies, too. Dip the scoop in the dough and plop the ball on the cookie sheet. You'll end up with cookies all the same size— no tiffs over which one is the largest.

MAKE BUTTER BALLS • At your next large family dinner, scoop out big globes of butter or margarine to serve to your guests. A smaller scoop or melon baller can create individual-sized balls of butter.

CREATE SAND CASTLES • On your next trip to the beach, throw an ice-cream scoop into the bag. Your kids will have a fun tool for making their sand castles down by the water. The scoop allows them to make interesting rounded shapes with the sand.

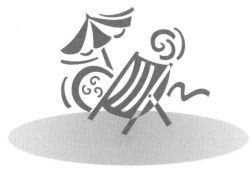

PLANT SEEDS • If you're out in the garden faced with a plot of earth that needs seeding, turn to your kitchen drawer for help. An ice-cream scoop will make equal-sized planting holes for the seeds for your future harvest.

REPOT A HOUSEPLANT • Does dirt scatter everywhere when you repot your houseplants? An ice-cream scoop is a perfect way to add potting mix to the new pot without making a mess.

DID YOU KNOW?

Spade, dipper, spatula, or spoon—the styles of ice-cream scoop you can buy are almost as varied as the flavors of ice cream you'll put in them. One web site lists 168 choices of the device! Here's some more dish on ice-cream scoops that you might not know:

■ A scoop introduced during the Depression, called the slicer, helped ice-cream parlor owners scoop out the same amount of ice cream every time, so as not to give away any extra.

■ Many ways have been developed to help the ice cream pop out of a scoop. Some scoops split apart; others have a wire scraper to nudge the stuff out. Still others have antifreeze in the handle or a button on the back to make it pop out.

■ Some ice-cream scoops, also called molds, can imprint symbols and logos on the ice cream.

PRE-SCOOP ICE CREAM

If you're tiring of constantly being bugged by your kids for a scoop of ice cream, try this tip. Scoop several scoops of ice cream onto a wax paper-lined cookie sheet, spaced apart. Place the tray with the scoops back in your freezer to re-harden. Remove the scoops from the paper and pile them up in a ziplock plastic bag. The next time the kids want a scoop of strawberry ice cream, they can help themselves.

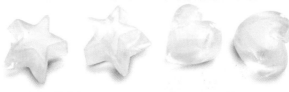

ICE CUBES

WATER HANGING PLANTS AND CHRISTMAS TREES • If you're constantly reaching for the step stool to water hard-to-reach hanging plants, ice cubes can help. Just toss several cubes into the pots. The ice melts and waters the plants and does it without causing a sudden downpour from the drain hole. This is also a good way to water your Christmas tree, whose base may be hard to reach with a watering can.

REMOVE DENTS IN CARPETING • If you've recently rearranged the furniture in your living room, you know that heavy pieces can leave ugly indents in your carpet. Use ice cubes to remove them. Put an ice cube on the spot where the chair leg stood. Let it melt, then brush up the dent.

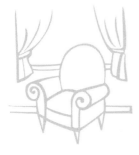

SMOOTH CAULKING SEAMS • You're caulking around the bathtub, but the sticky caulk compound keeps adhering to your finger as you try to smooth it. If you don't do something about it, the finished job will look pretty awful. Solve the problem by running an ice cube along the caulking line. This forms the caulking into a nice even bead and the caulk will never stick to the ice cube.

HELP IRON OUT WRINKLES

So your ready-to-wear shirt is full of wrinkles and there's no time to wash it again. Turn on the iron and wrap an ice cube in a soft cloth. Rub over the wrinkle just before you iron and the shirt will smooth out.

FOR THE FOODIES

MAKE CREAMY SALAD DRESSING • Do you want to make your homemade salad dressing as smooth and even as the bottled variety? Try this. Put all the dressing ingredients in a jar with a lid, and add a single ice cube. Close the lid and shake vigorously. Spoon out the ice cube and serve. Your guests will be impressed by how creamy your salad dressing is.

STOP SAUCES FROM CURDLING • Imagine this: Your snooty neighbors are over for a Sunday brunch featuring eggs Benedict. But when you mixed butter and egg yolks with lemon juice to make hollandaise sauce for the dish, it curdled. What do you do? Place an ice cube in the saucepan, stir and watch the sauce turn back into a silky masterpiece.

DE-FAT SOUPS AND STEWS • Want to get as much fat as possible out of your homemade soup or stew as quickly as possible? Fill a metal ladle with ice cubes and skim the bottom of the ladle over the top of the liquid in the soup pot. Fat will collect on the ladle.

REHEAT RICE • Does your leftover rice dry out when you reheat it in the microwave? Try this. Put an ice cube on top of the rice when you put it in the microwave. The ice cube will melt as the rice reheats, giving the rice much-needed moisture to keep it fluffy and even textured.

MASK THE TASTE OF MEDICINE • No matter what flavor your local pharmacist offers in children's medicine, kids often don't like the taste. Have them suck on an ice cube before taking the medicine. This numbs the tastebuds and allows the medicine to go down, without the spoonful of sugar.

PLUCK A SPLINTER • Removing a splinter from the hand of a screaming, squirming toddler would have to be one of life's more difficult challenges. So, before you start jabbing with that needle, grab an ice cube and numb the area. This should make splinter removal more painless and quicker.

PREVENT BLISTERING FROM A BURN •
If you or someone in your family burns themselves, apply an ice cube directly to the burn area to stop it from blistering.

REMOVE GUM FROM CLOTHING • If you're just about to walk out the door when your child points to the chewing gum stuck to his or her pants, keep your cool and grab an ice cube. Rub the ice on the gum to harden it, then scrape it off with a spoon.

PROVIDE COOLER WATER FOR YOUR PETS • Imagine wearing a fur coat in the middle of summer. Your rabbits, hamsters, and guinea pigs will appreciate it if you place a few cubes in their water dish to cool the water down. This is also a good tip for a cat who's spent the hot morning lounging in the sun, or a dog who's just had a long romp in the park.

DID YOU KNOW?

Here are some cold, hard facts about ice cubes.

■ To make clear ice cubes, use distilled water and boil it first. It's the air in the water that causes ice cubes to turn cloudy when frozen.
■ A British Columbian company sells fake ice cubes that glow and blink in your drink.
■ Those aren't ice cubes in that inviting drink in the print advertisement, because they'd never last under hot studio lights. They're plastic or glass.

ICE CUBE TRAYS

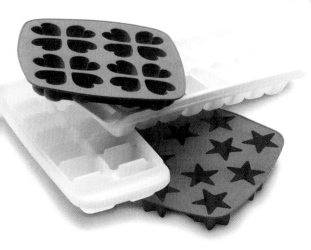

DIVIDE A DRAWER • If your junk drawer is an unsightly mess, insert a plastic ice cube tray for easy, low-cost organization. One 'cube' can hold paper clips; the next, rubber bands; another, stamps. It's another small way to bring order to your life.

ORGANIZE YOUR WORKBENCH • If you're looking through your toolbox for that perfect-sized fastener that you know you have somewhere, here's the answer to your problem. An ice cube tray can help you organize and store small parts you may need at one time or another, such as screws, nails, bolts, and other diminutive hardware.

more ICE CUBE TRAYS over →

KEEP PARTS IN SEQUENCE • You're disassembling your latest gadget that has lots of small parts and

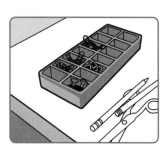

worry that you'll never be able to get them back together again in the correct sequence. Use an old plastic ice cube tray to help keep the small parts in the right order until you get around to reassembling it. If you really want to be organized, mark the sequence by putting a number on a piece of masking tape in each compartment. The bottom half of an egg carton will also do the trick.

A PAINTER'S PALETTE • Your child, a budding Picasso, requires a palette to mix colors. A plastic ice cube tray provides a perfect sturdy container for holding and mixing small amounts of paints and watercolors.

FREEZE EXTRA EGGS • Are you overstocked on bargain-priced eggs? Freeze them for future baking projects. Medium eggs are just the right size to freeze in plastic ice cube trays with one egg in each cell and no spillover. After they freeze, pop them out into a resealable plastic bag. Defrost as many as you need when the time comes.

FREEZE FOODS IN HANDY CUBES • An ice cube tray is a great way to freeze small amounts of many different kinds of food for later use. The idea is to freeze the food in the tray's cells, pop out the frozen cubes and put them in a labelled ziplock plastic bag for future use. Here are a few ideas to start off:

■ If you've grown plenty of basil, but your family can't eat pesto as quickly as you're making it, make a big batch of pesto (without the cheese) and freeze it in ice cube trays. Later, when you're ready to enjoy summer's bounty in the middle of winter, defrost the pesto ice cubes, add cheese, and toss with pasta.

■ There's only so much sweet potato your growing baby will eat at one sitting. Freeze the rest of it in trays for a future high chair meal.

■ If a recipe calls for ½ cup (125 g) chopped celery, but you have an entire head of celery and no plans to use it soon, just chop it all, place it in an ice cube tray, add a little water and freeze. The next time you need chopped celery, it's at your fingertips. This works well for onions, carrots, or any other vegetable you'd use for casseroles and soups.

■ Are you always throwing out leftover parsley? Just chop it up, put it in an ice cube tray with a little water, and freeze it for future use. This method works well with other fresh herbs, too.

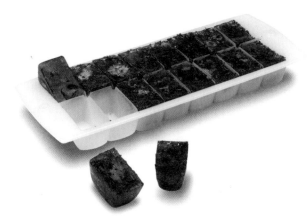

■ There's a bit of chicken soup left in the bottom of the pot. It's too little for another meal, but you hate to throw it out. Freeze the leftovers, and the next time you make soup or another dish that needs some chicken stock, just grab a cube or two.

■ If you are cooking a homemade stock, make an extra-large batch and freeze the excess in ice cube trays. You'll have stock ice cubes to add instant flavor to risotto and casseroles whenever you need it. You can do the same with leftover canned stock.

■ Here's what to do with that half-drunk bottle of red or white wine. Freeze the wine into cubes that can be used later in pasta sauce, casseroles, or stews.

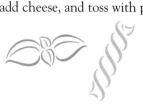

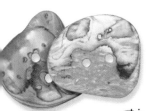

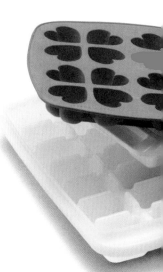

Kids' Stuff

This is a great summer holiday project. Collect a bunch of small objects around your house: buttons, beads, tiny toys. Then get an ice cube tray and place one or more of the items in each tray cube. Fill the tray with water. Cut a length of wool (long enough to make a comfortable necklace, bracelet or anklet). Lay the wool in the ice cube tray, making sure it hits every cube and is submerged properly, then put the tray in the freezer. When frozen, pop out and tie on the jewelry. The kids will cool off when their creation starts to melt!

ICE SCRAPERS

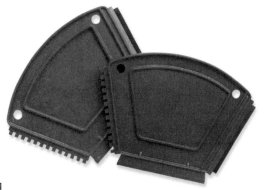

REMOVE SPLATTERED PAINT • If you just painted your bathroom and have got paint splatters all over your acrylic bathtub, use an ice scraper to remove them without scratching the tub surface. You can use ice scrapers to remove paint specks from any other nonmetallic surfaces.

SMOOTH WOOD FILLER • Do you have small gouges in your wood floors and want to use wood filler to make them smooth again? An ice scraper can help you do the job properly. Once you've packed wood filler into a hole, the ice scraper is the perfect tool to smooth and level it.

REMOVE WAX FROM SKIS • Every experienced skier knows that old wax buildup on skis can slow you down. An ice scraper can swiftly and neatly take off that old wax and prepare your skis for the next coat.

SCRAPE OUT YOUR FREEZER • Your windshield isn't the only place ice and frost build up. If the frost is building up in your freezer and you want to delay the defrosting job for a while, head out to the car and borrow the scraper.

CLEAN UP BREAD DOUGH • No matter how much flour you put on your work surface, some of that sticky bread dough always seems to stick to it. A clean ice scraper is just the tool for skimming the sticky stuff off the countertop. In a pinch, a plastic scraper can also substitute for a spatula for nonstick pans.

JAR LIDS

MAKE SAFETY REFLECTORS • Is your driveway difficult to maneuver after dark? With some scrap wood and jar lids you can make inexpensive reflectors to guide drivers. Spray the lids with reflective paint, screw them to the sides of stakes cut from the scrap wood, and drive the stakes into the ground. Voila! No more dinged bumper bars or flattened flowers!

SAVE HALF-EATEN FRUIT • Got half a peach or apple you'd like to save for later? Wrap a jar lid in plastic wrap or waxed paper and put the fruit, cut side down, on it in the refrigerator. A bit of lemon juice on the cut surface of the fruit will help prevent discoloration. And why throw out the contents of a partially consumed glass of milk or juice? Just cover it with a lid and refrigerate to keep it smelling and tasting fresh.

CUT BISCUITS • Yum, homemade biscuits! Lids with deep rims or canning jar bands (the part with the cut-out center) make impromptu biscuit and scone cutters. Use different-sized lids for Dad, Mom, and baby biscuits. Dip the bottom edge of the lid in flour to keep it from sticking when you press it into the dough. Avoid lid rims that are rolled inward; the dough can get stuck inside and be hard to extract.

CREATE A SPOON REST • Place a jar lid on the stove or the countertop next to the stove while cooking. After stirring a saucepan, rest the spoon on the lid and there'll be less to clean up later.

CATCH DRIPS UNDER A HONEY JAR • Honey is delicious, but it can be a sticky mess. At the table, place the honey jar on a plastic lid to stop drips from getting on the table. Store it that way, too, and your pantry shelf will stay cleaner.

Kids' Stuff

You've probably got a collection of magnets and children's artwork on the fridge door. Combine the two and you've got something both useful and beautiful. Set out a bunch of fun materials—paints, glue, fabrics, family photos, googly eyes, glitter, pompoms, or even just paper and felt-tipped pens—and let your children decorate several jar lids. Glue some strong magnets from a hardware shop on the backs (a hot glue gun works well) and stick them on!

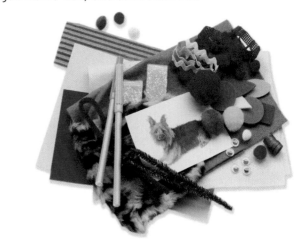

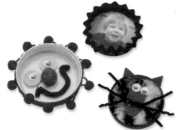

1 With an assortment of craft materials at the ready, let the kids go crazy decorating the painted jar lids.

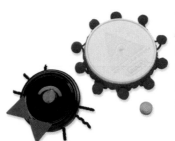

2 After the glued-on bits and pieces have dried, stick a magnet on the back of each decorated lid. Allow to dry thoroughly.

MAKE COASTERS TO PROTECT FURNITURE •
Wet drinking glasses and hot coffee mugs can do
a lot of damage to wooden furniture finishes. The
simple solution is to keep plenty of coasters on hand.
Glue rounds of felt or cork to both sides of a jar lid
(especially flat canning jar lids, which shouldn't
be reused for canning, anyway), and keep a stack
wherever cups and glasses accumulate in your
house. Your furniture will thank you!

USE AS SAUCERS FOR POTTED PLANTS • Lids
with a rim are perfect for catching excess water under
small potted plants and, unlike your ceramic saucers,
if they get encrusted with minerals you won't mind
throwing them out.

JARS

WATERPROOF CAMPING STORAGE • When you're
boating or camping, keeping things like matches and
paper money dry can be a challenge. Store items that
you don't want to get wet in clear jars with screw
tops that can't pop off. Even if you're backpacking,
plastic peanut butter jars are light enough not to
weigh you down, plus they provide more protection
for crushable items than a ziplock plastic bag.

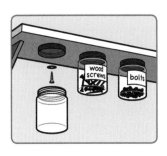

**CREATE WORKSHOP
STORAGE •** Don't let
workshop hardware
get mixed up. Keep all
your nails, screws, nuts,
and bolts organized by
screwing jar lids to the
underside of a wood or
melamine shelf. (Make
sure the screw won't poke through the top of the
shelf.) Then put each type of hardware in its own jar
and screw each jar onto its lid. You'll keep everything
off the benches, and by using clear jars you can find
what you need at a glance. This system works well for
storing seeds in the potting shed, too.

ORGANIZE YOUR DESK • Corral those paper
clips and other small office items that clutter
up your desk, by putting them in jar lids with
deep rims. Jar lids work well to hold loose
change or earrings on your dressing table or chest
of drawers, too. A quick coat of matte spray paint
and an acrylic sealant will make them more
attractive and water-resistant.

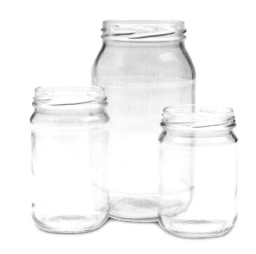

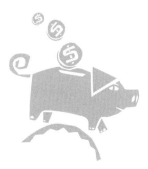

MAKE A
PIGGY BANK

Encourage thriftiness in
your child by making a
piggy bank out of any
jar with a metal lid. Take
the lid off the jar, place
it on a flat work surface,
such as a cutting board, and tap a screwdriver
with a hammer to carefully punch a slot hole in
the center. Use the hammer or a rasp to smooth
the rough edges on the underside of the slot to
protect from scratches. Decorate with paints for
a fun rainy-day project.

more JARS over →

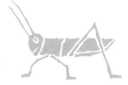

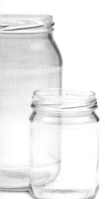

COLLECT INSECTS • Help your children observe nature by gently collecting beetles and other interesting insects in clear jars. Punch a few small airholes in the lids for ventilation. Don't make the holes too large or your insects will escape! And don't forget to let the creepy crawlies go after you've admired them.

CUT OUT COOKIES • Just about any clean, empty wide-mouthed jar is just the right size for cutting cookies out of any rolled cookie dough.

BRING ALONG BABY'S TREATS • Dry cereal can be a nutritious snack for your baby. And there's no need to bring the whole box when you leave the house. Pack individual servings in clean, dry, baby food jars. If they spill, the mess is minimal.

MAKE BABY-FOOD PORTIONS • Take advantage of the fact that baby food jars are already the perfect size for baby's portions. Clean them thoroughly before reuse, and fill them with anything from pureed carrots to vanilla pudding. Attach a spoon with a rubber band, and you've got a perfect take-along meal when you travel with your little one.

USE JARS TO DRY GLOVES OR MITTENS

If you live in a cold-climate area and shoveling snow is just part of the winter routine, no doubt you'll be wearing gloves or mittens. To help your gloves or mittens dry out after working in the snow, pull each one over the bottom of an empty jar, then stand the jar upside down on a radiator or hot-air vent. Warm air will fill the jar and radiate out to dry the damp gloves in a flash.

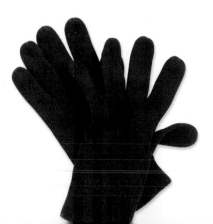

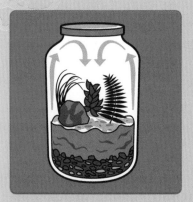

SCIENCE **WORKS!**

Turn a large wide-mouthed jar into a miniature biosphere.

Clean the jar and lid, then place a handful of pebbles and charcoal chips along the bottom. Add several trowelfuls of slightly damp, sterilized potting mix. Select a few plants that like similar conditions (such as ferns and mosses, which both like moderate light and moisture). Add a few colorful stones, seashells, or a piece of driftwood. Add water to make the terrarium humid. Tighten the lid and place the jar in dim light for two days. Then display in bright light but not direct sunlight. You shouldn't need to add water—it cycles from the plants to the soil and back again.

It's important to use sterilized soil to avoid introducing unwanted organisms. The charcoal chips filter the water as it recycles within the terrarium.

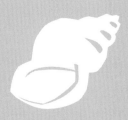

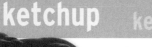
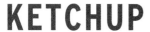

KETCHUP

MAKE COPPER POTS GLEAM • When copper pots and pans—or decorative molds—get tarnished, brighten them with ketchup. It's cheaper than commercial tarnish removers and safe to apply without gloves. Coat the copper surface with a thin layer of ketchup straight from the bottle. Let sit for 5 to 30 minutes. Acids in ketchup react with the tarnish and remove it. Rinse and dry.

GET RID OF CHLORINE GREEN • If chlorine from swimming pools is turning your blond tresses green, eliminate the problem with a ketchup shampoo. In the shower, massage ketchup generously into your hair. Leave it in for 15 minutes and wash it out with baby shampoo. The green tinge—and the chlorine ordor—should both be gone.

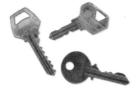

KEYS

MAKE FISHING SINKERS • Old, unused keys make great weights for your fishing line. Since they already have a hole in them, attaching them to the line is a cinch. Whenever you come across an unidentified key, toss it into your tackle box.

MAKE A PLUMB BOB • If you are getting ready to hang wallpaper, you'll need to draw a perfectly vertical line on the wall to get you started. Take a length of cord or string and tie a key or two to one end. You'll have a plumb bob that will give you a true vertical.

WEIGH DOWN CURTAINS • If your curtains aren't hanging properly, slip a few old keys into the hems. If you are worried about them falling out, tack them in place with a few stitches through the holes in the keys. Keep cords on blinds from tangling by attaching keys to their ends.

DID YOU KNOW?

Ketchup originated in the Far East as a salty fish sauce and probably comes from China or Malasia. Brought to the West, by the 1700s it included a variety of sauces. You can still find banana, mushroom, and other ketchups. Tomato ketchup is actually a relative newcomer. First sold in 1837, it is found in more than 90 percent of homes in North America. What would your charbroiled hamburger be without ketchup?

KEEP IT SPARKLING!

Use ketchup to polish your silver jewelry. If a ring or bracelet has a smooth surface, dunk it in a small bowl of ketchup for a few minutes. If it has a detailed surface, use a toothbrush and work ketchup into the crevices. Don't leave ketchup on any longer than necessary. Rinse and dry thoroughly.

KOOL-AID

MAKE PLAY MAKE-UP LIP GLOSS •
Make some tasty lip gloss for little girls playing dress-up. Let the girls pick their favorite presweetened Kool-Aid flavor. Blend a package of the drink mix with 3 tablespoons (45 ml) solid vegetable shortening and microwave for 1 minute. Transfer to a small plastic container and refrigerate overnight.

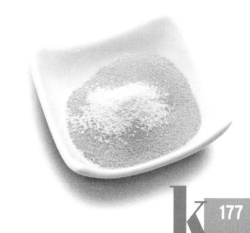

LADDERS

MAKE DISPLAY SHELVING • Convert a short wooden stepladder to shelving for displaying plants and collectibles. It's as easy as one, two, three:

1 • Remove the folding metal spreader that holds the front and rear legs of the ladder together. Then position the ladder's rear legs upright against the wall and attach two 1 x 2 cleats to fix the distance between the front and rear legs. Position the cleats so that their tops are level with the top of a rung.

2 • Each shelf will be supported at front by an existing rung. To support the back of each shelf, attach a cleat between the rear legs, positioning it at the same level as a rung.

3 • Cut plywood or boards to fit as shelves and screw them to the rungs and cleats. Now screw the centermost rear cleat to the wall and you're done.

CONSTRUCT A RUSTIC INDOOR TRELLIS

Give your vines and trailing plants something to climb on. Using wall anchors, attach vinyl-covered hooks to your wall and hang a straight ladder (or a segment of one) from the hooks, positioning the ladder's legs on the floor a few inches from the wall. It's easy to train potted plants to grow up and around this rustic support. It looks nice on a porch, too.

DISPLAY QUILTS AND MORE • Don't let your fancy stitching languish in the linen closet. For that homespun feel, a ladder is a great way to display lacework, crochet, quilts, and throws. To prevent rough surfaces from damaging delicate fabrics, smooth wooden rungs with sandpaper or metal rungs with steel wool if necessary.

MAKE A TEMPORARY TABLE • The big family picnic is a summer staple, but where to put all the food? You can cook up a makeshift table in no time by placing a straight ladder across two sawhorses. Top it with plywood and cover it with a tablecloth. The ladder will provide strength to support your buffet, as well as any guests who might lean on it.

MAKE A POT RACK • Accessorize your country kitchen with a pot rack made from a sawed-off section of a wooden straight ladder with thin, round rungs. Sand the cut ends smooth, then tie two pieces of sturdy rope to the rungs at either end. To suspend your pot rack, screw four large metal eye hooks into the ceiling, going into the joists, then tie the other ends of the ropes to them. Hang some S-hooks from the rungs to hold your kitchenware. Leave the rack unfinished if you want a rustic look or paint or stain it if you want a more finished look.

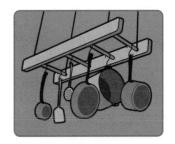

IN THE GARDEN ...

CREATE A GARDEN FOCAL POINT • Got some old wooden straight ladders around that you no longer trust? Show your whimsical side by using them to create a decorative garden archway. Cut two sections of old ladder to the desired height

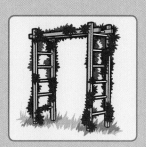

and position them opposite one another along a path. Screw the legs of each one to two strong posts sunk deep in the soil. Cut a third ladder section to fit across the top of the two others and tie it to them using supple grapevine, young willow twigs, or heavy jute twine. Festoon your archway with fun and fanciful stuff, such as old tools, or let climbing plants clamber up and over it. It also works well as the entry to an enclosed area.

PLOP IT DOWN AND PLANT IT • When a ladder is truly on its last legs, it can still be of service lying down. On the ground, a straight ladder or the front part of a stepladder makes a shallow planter with ready-made sections that look attractive filled with annuals, herbs, or salad greens. After a couple of years of contact with soil, a wooden ladder will decompose, so don't plan to use it again.

LEMONS

around the house

ELIMINATE FIREPLACE ODOR • There's nothing cosier on a cold winter night than a warm fire burning in the fireplace—unless the fire happens to smell horrible. Next time you have a fire that sends a stench into the room, try throwing a few lemon peels into the flames. Or simply burn some lemon peels along with your firewood as a preventive measure.

GET RID OF TOUGH STAINS ON MARBLE • You probably think of marble as stone, but it is really petrified calcium (also known as old seashells). That explains why it is so porous and easily stained and damaged. Those stains can be hard to remove, but here is a simple method that should do the trick. Cut a lemon in half, dip the exposed flesh into some table salt, and rub it vigorously on the stain.

MAKE A ROOM SCENT/HUMIDIFIER • Freshen and moisturize the air in your home on dry winter days. Make your own room scent that also doubles as a humidifier. If you have a wood-burning stove, place an enamelled cast-iron pot or bowl on top, fill with water, and add lemon (and/or orange) peels, cinnamon sticks, cloves, and apple skins. If you don't have a wood-burning stove, use your stovetop instead and just simmer the water periodically.

NEUTRALIZE LITTER BOX ODOR • To neutralize foul-smelling cat litter box odors or freshen the air in your bathroom, just cut a couple of lemons in half. Place them, cut side up, in a dish in the room and the air will soon smell lemon-fresh.

more LEMONS over →

DEODORIZE A HUMIDIFIER • When your humidifier starts to smell awful, simply deodorize it. Just pour 3 or 4 teaspoons (15–20 ml) lemon juice in the water. It will not only remove the bad odor but replace it with a lemon-fresh fragrance. Repeat every couple of weeks to keep the odor from returning.

CLEAN TARNISHED BRASS • Say goodbye to tarnish on brass, copper, or stainless steel. Make a paste of lemon juice and salt (or substitute baking soda or cream of tartar for the salt) and coat the affected area. Leave it on for about 5 minutes. Wash in warm water, rinse and polish dry. Use the same mixture to clean metal kitchen sinks, too. Apply the paste, scrub gently, and rinse.

POLISH CHROME • Get rid of mineral deposits and polish chrome faucets and other tarnished chrome by simply rubbing lemon rind over the chrome and watching it shine! Rinse well and dry with a soft cloth.

in the kitchen ● ● ●

PREVENT POTATOES FROM TURNING BROWN • Potatoes and cauliflower tend to turn brown when boiling, especially when you're having friends for dinner. You can make sure the white vegetables stay white by squeezing a teaspoon of fresh lemon juice into the cooking water.

FRESHEN THE FRIDGE • Remove refrigerator odors with ease by dabbing a cotton ball or sponge in lemon juice and leaving it in the fridge for several hours. And make sure you toss out any malodorous items that might be causing the bad smell.

KEEP RICE FROM STICKING • To keep your rice from sticking together in a gluggy mass, add a spoonful of lemon juice to the boiling water when cooking. When the rice is done, let it cool for a few minutes, then fluff with a fork before serving.

BRIGHTEN DULL ALUMINIUM • Make those dull pots and pans sparkle, inside and out. All you need to do is rub the cut side of half a lemon all over them and buff with a soft cloth.

FRESHEN CUTTING BOARDS • No wonder your kitchen cutting board smells! After all, you use it to chop onions, crush garlic, cut raw and cooked meat and chicken, and prepare fish. To get rid of the smell and help sanitize it, rub it all over with the cut side of half a lemon or wash it in undiluted lemon juice straight from the bottle.

KEEP GUACAMOLE GREEN

You've been making guacamole all day long for the big party, and you don't want it to turn brown on top before the guests arrive. The solution? Sprinkle a liberal amount of fresh lemon juice over it and it will stay fresh and green. The flavor of the lemon juice is a natural complement to the avocados in the guacamole. Make the fruit salad hours in advance, too. Just squeeze some lemon juice on the apple slices, and they'll stay snowy white.

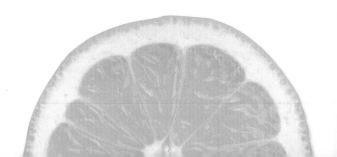

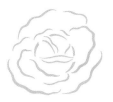

Kids' Stuff

Kids love to send and receive secret messages, and what better way to do it than by writing them in invisible ink? All they need is lemon juice (freshly squeezed or bottled) to use as ink, a cotton swab to write with, and a sheet of white paper to write on. When the ink is dry and they are ready to read the invisible message, have them hold the paper up to bright sunlight or a light bulb. The heat will cause the writing to darken to a pale brown and the message can be read! Just make sure they don't overdo the heating and ignite the paper.

MAKE SOGGY LETTUCE CRISP AGAIN • Don't toss that soggy lettuce into the garbage. With the help of a bit of lemon juice, you can toss it in a salad instead. Add the juice of half a lemon to a bowl of cold water, put the soggy lettuce in it, and refrigerate for about an hour. Make sure the leaves are completely dry before putting them in salads or sandwiches.

KEEP INSECTS OUT OF THE KITCHEN • You don't need insecticides or ant traps to ant-proof your kitchen. Just give it the lemon treatment. First squirt some lemon juice on door thresholds and windowsills. Then squeeze lemon juice into any holes or cracks where the ants are getting in. Finally, scatter small slices of lemon peel around the outdoor entrance. The ants will get the message that they aren't welcome. Lemons are also effective against roaches and fleas. Simply mix the juice of 4 lemons (along with the rinds) with 2 quarts (2 L) water, wash your floors with it, and watch the fleas and roaches flee. They hate the smell.

CLEAN YOUR MICROWAVE • Is the inside of your microwave caked with bits of hardened food? You can give it a good cleaning without scratching the surface with harsh cleansers or using a lot of elbow grease. Just mix 3 tablespoons (45 ml) lemon juice into 1½ cups (375 ml) water in a microwave-safe bowl. Microwave on *High* for 5 to 10 minutes, allowing the steam to condense on the inside walls and ceiling of the oven. Then just wipe away the softened food with a clean rag.

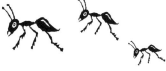

in the laundry

BLEACH DELICATE FABRICS • Ordinary chlorine bleach can cause the iron in water to precipitate out into fabrics, leaving additional stains. For a mild, stain-free bleach, soak your delicates in a mixture of lemon juice and baking soda for at least half an hour before washing.

REMOVE UNSIGHTLY UNDERARM STAINS • Remove those yellowing underarm stains from shirts and blouses by simply scrubbing them with a mixture of equal parts lemon juice (or white vinegar) and water.

BOOST LAUNDRY DETERGENT • To remove rust and mineral discolorations from cotton T-shirts and underpants, pour 1 cup (250 ml) lemon juice into the washing machine during the wash cycle. The natural bleaching action of the juice will zap the stains and leave your clothes smelling fresh.

more LEMONS over →

RID CLOTHES OF MILDEW • You unpack the clothes you've stored for the season and discover that some of the garments are stained with mildew. To get rid of mildew on clothes, make a paste of lemon juice and salt, rub it on the affected area, and dry the clothes in sunlight. Repeat the process until the stain is gone. This works well for rust stains on clothes, too.

WHITEN CLOTHES • Diluted or straight, lemon juice is a safe and effective fabric whitener when added to your wash water. Your clothes will also come out smelling lemony fresh.

for health and beauty

LIGHTEN AGE SPOTS • Before buying expensive medicated creams to lighten unsightly liver spots and freckles, try this. Apply lemon juice directly to the area, let it sit for 15 minutes and rinse your skin clean. Lemon juice is a safe and effective skin-lightening agent.

CREATE BLOND HIGHLIGHTS • For blond highlights worthy of the finest beauty salon, add ¼ cup (50 ml) lemon juice to ¾ cup (175 ml) water. Rinse your hair with the mixture and sit in the sun until your hair dries. Lemon juice is a natural bleach. (Put on plenty of sunscreen before you sit out in the sun.) To maximize the effect, repeat once daily up to a week.

CLEAN AND WHITEN NAILS • Pamper your nails without the help of a manicurist. Add the juice of ½ lemon to 1 cup (250 ml) warm water and soak your fingertips in the mixture for 5 minutes. After pushing back the cuticles, rub some lemon peel back and forth against the nail.

CLEANSE YOUR FACE • Clean and exfoliate your face by washing it with lemon juice. You can also dab lemon juice on blackheads to draw them out during the day. Your skin should improve after several days of using this treatment.

TIP

Before you squeeze

❋ *To get the most juice out of fresh lemons, bring them to room temperature and roll them under your palm on the kitchen counter before squeezing. This breaks down the connective tissue and juice-cell walls, releasing more liquid when you squeeze the lemon.*

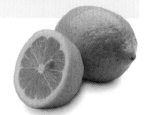

FRESHEN YOUR BREATH

Make an impromptu mouthwash using lemon juice straight from the bottle. Rinse with the juice and swallow it for longer-lasting fresh breath. The citric acid in the juice alters the pH level in your mouth, killing the bacteria that cause bad breath. Rinse after a few minutes, because long-term exposure to the acid in lemon juice can erode tooth enamel.

DID YOU KNOW?

With all due respect to the old song, a lemon tree actually isn't very pretty—and its flower isn't sweet either. The tree's straggly branches bear little resemblance to an orange tree's dense foliage, and its purplish flowers lack the pleasant fragrance of orange blossoms. Yes, the fruit of the 'poor lemon' is sour—thanks to its high citric acid content—but it is hardly 'impossible to eat'. Sailors have been sucking on vitamin C-rich lemons for hundreds of years to prevent scurvy. To this day, the British navy requires ships to carry enough lemons so that every sailor can have 2 tablespoons (30 ml) of juice daily.

SCIENCE **WORKS!**

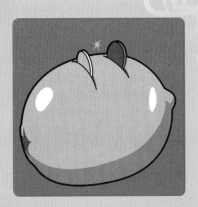

Turn a lemon into a battery! It won't start your car, but you will be able to feel the current with your tongue.

Roll the lemon on a flat surface to 'activate' the juices and cut two small slices in the lemon about 1/2 inch (1.25 cm) apart. Place a penny into one slot and a dime in the other. Now touch your tongue to the penny and the dime at the same time. You'll feel a slight electric tingle. Here's how it works. The acid in the lemon reacts differently with each of the two metals. One coin contains positive electric charges, while the other contains negative charges. The charges create current. Your tongue conducts the charges, causing a small amount of electricity to flow.

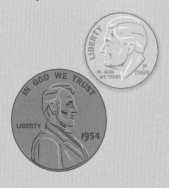

TREAT FLAKY DANDRUFF • If itchy, scaly dandruff has you scratching your head, relief may be no further away than your refrigerator. Just massage 2 tablespoons (30 ml) lemon juice into your scalp and rinse with water. Then stir 1 teaspoon (5 ml) lemon juice into 1 cup (250 ml) water and rinse your hair with it. Repeat once a day until your dandruff disappears. No more itchy scalp, and your hair will smell lemony fresh.

SOFTEN DRY, SCALY ELBOWS • It's bad enough when elbows are dry and itchy, but unfortunately they look terrible, too. Your elbows will look and feel better after a few treatments with this regimen. Mix baking soda and lemon juice to make an abrasive paste. Then rub the paste into your elbows for a soothing, smoothing, and exfoliating treatment.

REMOVE BERRY STAINS • It's always fun to pick your own berries, but your fingers are inevitably stained with berry juice that won't come off with soap and water. Try washing your hands with undiluted lemon juice. Wait a few minutes and wash with warm, soapy water. Repeat if necessary until the stain is completely gone.

DISINFECT CUTS AND SCRAPES • Stop bleeding and disinfect minor cuts and scrapes by pouring a few drops of lemon juice directly on the cut or applying the juice with a cotton ball and holding it firmly in place for 1 minute.

SOOTHE POISON IVY RASH • You won't need an ocean of calamine lotion the next time poison ivy comes a-creeping. Just apply full-strength lemon juice directly to the affected area to soothe itching and alleviate the rash.

RELIEVE ROUGH HANDS AND SORE FEET • You don't have to take extreme measures to soothe your extremities. If you have rough hands or sore feet, rinse them in a mixture of equal parts lemon juice and water, massage with olive oil, and pat dry with a soft cloth.

REMOVE WARTS • If you've tried countless remedies to get rid of your warts and nothing seems to work, next time, try this. Apply a dab of lemon juice directly to the wart, using a cotton ball. Repeat for several days until the acids in the lemon juice dissolve the wart completely.

LIGHTER FLUID

WIPE AWAY RUST • Rust marks on stainless steel will come off in a jiffy. Just pour a little lighter fluid on a clean rag and rub the rust spot away. Use another rag to wipe away any remaining fluid.

GET CHEWING GUM OUT OF HAIR • It happens to the best of us, not to mention the kids. Gum in the hair is a pain in the neck to remove. Here is an easy solution that really works. Apply a few drops of lighter fluid directly to the sticky area, wait a few seconds and comb or wipe away the gum. The solvents in the fluid break down the gum, making it easy to remove from many surfaces besides hair.

REMOVE LABELS WITH EASE • Lighter fluid will remove labels and adhesives from almost any surface. Use it to quickly and easily remove the tape from new appliances or to take stickers off book covers.

CAUTION: Lighter fluid is inexpensive, easy to find (look for a small plastic bottle next to the larger bottles of barbecue starter), and it has many surprising uses. But it is also highly flammable and can be hazardous to your health if inhaled or ingested. Always use lighter fluid in a well-ventilated area. Do not smoke around it or use it near an open flame.

REMOVE HEEL MARKS FROM FLOORS • You don't have to scrub to remove those black heel marks on the kitchen floor. Just pour a bit of lighter fluid on a paper towel and the marks will wipe right off.

GET RID OF COOKING-OIL STAINS ON CLOTHES • When cooking-oil stains won't wash out of clothes, try pouring a little lighter fluid directly on the stain before washing it the next time. The stain will come out in the wash.

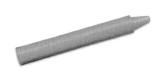

TAKE OUT CRAYON MARKS

Did the kids leave their mark with crayons on your walls during that last visit? No problem. Dab some lighter fluid on a clean rag and wipe until the marks vanish.

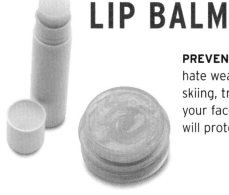

LIP BALM

PREVENT WINDBURN • You love to ski, but you hate wearing a ski mask. Next time you go snow skiing, try rubbing lip balm, such as ChapStick, on your face before you hit the slopes. The lip balm will protect your skin from windburn.

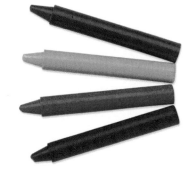

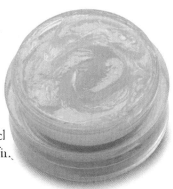

REMOVE A STUCK RING • No need to pull and tug on your poor beleaguered finger to try to remove that stuck ring. Simply coat the fin... wriggle the ring loose.

GROOM WILD EYEBROWS • You can use lip balm as a styling wax to groom unruly moustaches, eyebrows, or other wild hairs that may need taming.

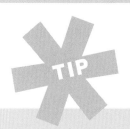

TIP

Lip balm and lipstick

* *During the dry winter months you may be tempted to apply a layer of lip balm before you put on your lipstick to protect from chapping.*

Beauty experts say this is not a good idea because the lip balm could interfere with the adherence of the lipstick. Instead of using lip balm during the day, experts recommend that you switch to a moisturizing lipstick for daytime and use lip balm for moisturizing your lips before you go to bed.

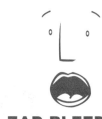

ZAP BLEEDING FROM SHAVING CUTS
OUCH!!!
You just cut yourself shaving and you don't have any time to spare. Just dab a bit of lip balm directly on the nick and the bleeding from most shaving cuts will quickly stop.

LUBRICATE A ZIPPER • Rub a small amount of inexpensive lip balm up and down the teeth of a sticky or stuck zipper then zip and unzip it a few times. This will act as a lubricant to make the zipper work smoothly.

SIMPLIFY CARPENTRY • Rub some lip balm over nails and screws being drilled or pounded into wood. The lip balm will help them slide in a little easier.

LUBRICATE TRACKS FOR SLIDING THINGS • Apply inexpensive lip balm to the tracks of drawers and windows or the ridges on a medicine cabinet to make opening and shutting easier.

KEEP A LIGHTBULB FROM STICKING

Outdoor lightbulbs are exposed to the elements so they often get stuck in the socket and become hard to remove. Before screwing a lightbulb into an outdoor socket, coat the threads on the bulb with a bit of lip balm. This will prevent sticking and make it easier to remove when it's time to change a burned-out bulb.

MAGAZINES

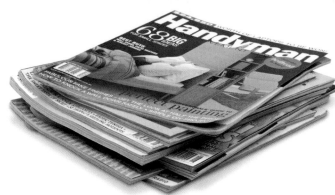

NO-COST GIFT WRAP • Cut out colorful magazine advertisements and use them to make interesting wrapping paper for small gifts.

KEEP WET BOOTS IN SHAPE • Roll up a couple of old magazines and use them as boot trees inside a pair of damp boots. The magazines will help the boots maintain their shape as they dry.

USE IN KIDS' CRAFT PROJECTS • Save up your old magazines for use in rainy-day craft projects with the kids. Let them go through the magazines to find pictures and words to use in collages. You can suggest themes for the collages to give them some ideas.

LINE DRAWERS • Pages from large magazines with heavy, coated paper make fantastic liners for small dressing table and desk drawers. Look for advertisements with especially colorful designs or pictures, cut out the pages, and place them inside the drawer. Press around the edges to define where to trim each page for a perfect fit.

MAGNETS

CLEAN UP A NAIL SPILL • Keep a strong magnet on your workbench. Next time you spill a jar of small items like nails, screws, tacks, or washers, save time and energy and let the magnet help pick them up for you.

PREVENT A FROZEN CAR LOCK • Here's a great way to use fridge magnets during the cold of winter. Place them over the outside door locks of your car overnight and they will keep the locks from freezing.

KEEP DESK DRAWERS NEAT • Are your paper clips all over the place? Place a magnet in your office desk drawer to keep the paper clips together.

STORE A BROOM IN A HANDY PLACE • Why run to the hall cupboard every time you need to sweep the kitchen? Instead, just use a screw to attach a magnet about halfway down the broom handle. Then store the broom attached to the side of your refrigerator between the fridge and the wall, where it will remain hidden until you are ready to use it.

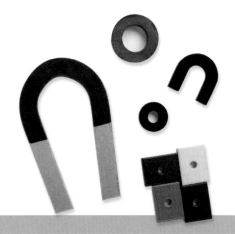

DID YOU KNOW?

Ancient Chinese and Greeks discovered that certain rare stones, called lodestones, seem to magically attract bits of iron and always pointed in the same direction when allowed to swing freely. Man-made magnets come in many shapes and sizes, but every magnet has a north pole and a south pole. If you break a magnet into pieces, each piece, no matter how small, will have a north and south pole. The magnetic field, which every magnet creates, has long been used to harness energy, although scientists still don't know exactly what it is!

MARGARINE TUBS

CORRAL THOSE ODDS AND ENDS • Loose drawing pins in every room? Odd bolts and nails in a broken cup? Stray superball under the couch? These are just some of the items waiting to be organized into your empty plastic margarine tubs. Get your board game going faster and easier by storing the loose pieces in a tub until the next time they're needed. And if you've sorted out all the sky pieces for a puzzle, keep them separate and safe in their own tub. With or without their lids, a few clean margarine tubs can do wonders for a junk drawer in need of organization.

MAKE A BABY FOOTPRINT PAPERWEIGHT • Make an enduring impression of your baby's foot, using quick-drying modeling clay—which comes in lots of great colors. Put enough clay in a margarine tub to hold a good impression. Put a thin layer of petroleum jelly on baby's foot and press it firmly into the clay. Let the clay dry as directed, then flex the tub away from the edges until the clay comes free. Years from now you'll be able to show little Johnny that his size 13s were once smaller than the palm of your hand! You can also preserve your pet's paw print the same way.

MAKE INDIVIDUAL ICE CREAM PORTIONS • Small margarine tubs are just the right size for a quick ice cream snack. And when it comes home from the supermarket, a half-gallon (2 L) of ice cream is the perfect consistency to dispense into the tubs. No more time-consuming getting out the bowls, the scoop, and waiting for the ice cream to soften up enough to dish out. Everyone can get their own and they all have equal portions—just by going to the freezer and pulling out a tub.

USE AS A PAINT CONTAINER • Want to touch up the little spots here and there in the living room, but don't want to lug around several quarts of paint? Pour a little paint into a margarine tub to carry as you make your inspection. Hold it in a nest of paper towels to catch any possible drips. The tubs with lids are also perfect for storing that little bit of leftover paint for future touch-ups.

MOLD GELATIN DESSERTS • Don't buy a fancy mold for your next birthday party or barbecue. Use a large margarine tub as the mold for a gelatin or mousse centerpiece. For individual fun gelatin dessert molds, use the smaller tubs and put a surprise gummy bear or mini-marshmallow face on the top, which will show through from the bottom when the mold is inverted. The flexible tubs are easy to squeeze to release the dessert.

FREEZE MEASURED PORTIONS • Reuse your clean, sturdy margarine and other plastic containers for freezing measured portions of soups and stocks, and to break up leftovers into single servings. A 2-pound (1 kg) container, for example, stores the perfect amount of sauce for a pound (500 g) of pasta. Before freezing, allow the food to cool just enough so that the amount of condensation is reduced.

GIVE KIDS SOME LUNCH BOX VARIETY

As a break from the usual sandwich, put some fruit salad, rice mix, or other interesting fare in one or two recycled margarine tubs for your child's lunch. The tubs are easy to open and will keep the food from getting crushed.

more MARGARINE TUBS over →

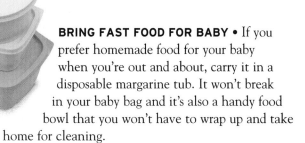

BRING FAST FOOD FOR BABY • If you prefer homemade food for your baby when you're out and about, carry it in a disposable margarine tub. It won't break in your baby bag and it's also a handy food bowl that you won't have to wrap up and take home for cleaning.

TRAVEL LIGHT WITH YOUR PET • Lightweight, disposable margarine tubs make the perfect pet food containers and double as food and water bowls. And those dog biscuits won't get crushed if you put them in a plastic tub. If your pet is vacationing at a friend's house, make things a little easier for the caregiver by putting one serving in each container, to be used and discarded as needed.

MAKE A PIGGY BANK • Use a tall tub as a homemade piggy bank for small children. Cut out a piece of paper that will fit wrapped around the side, tape it in place, and encourage the child to decorate it with flair. Then cut a slit in the top and start saving!

CREATE CHEAP SEED STARTERS • Starting your seeds indoors is supposed to save you money, so don't spend your savings on lots of big seed trays. Take a margarine tub, poke a few holes in the bottom, add moistened seed-starting mix and sow your seeds following packet instructions. Use permanent marker on the side of the tub to help you remember what you've sown and use the tub's lid as a drip saucer. Small tubs are space savers as well, especially if you want to start only one or two of each type of plant.

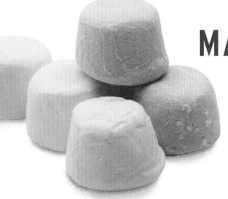

MARSHMALLOWS

SEPARATE TOES WHEN APPLYING NAIL POLISH

Get the comfort of a salon treatment when giving yourself a home pedicure. Just place marshmallows between your toes to separate them before you apply the nail polish.

DID YOU KNOW?

The ancient Egyptians made the first known sweet marshmallows–a honey-based concoction that is flavored and thickened with the sap of the root of the marshmallow plant (*Althaea officinalis*). Marshmallow grows in salt marshes and on banks of large bodies of water. Its sap was used to make sweet marshmallows and medicine until the mid-1800s. Today's commercial marshmallows are a mixture of corn syrup or sugar, gelatin, gum arabic, and flavoring.

KEEP BROWN SUGAR SOFT • Ever notice how brown sugar seems to harden overnight once you've opened the bag? Next time you open a bag of brown sugar, add a few marshmallows to the bag before closing it. The marshmallows will add enough moisture to keep the sugar soft for weeks.

STOP ICE-CREAM DRIPS • Here's an easy way to keep a leaky ice cream cone from staining your clothes. Just place a large marshmallow in the bottom of the cone before you add the ice cream.

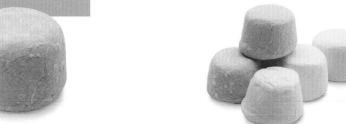

KEEP WAX FROM BIRTHDAY CAKES • If one of your birthday wishes is to keep candle wax off the icing on the cake, try this trick. Push each candle into a marshmallow and position the marshmallow on top of the icing. The wax will melt onto the marshmallow, which you can then discard. Meanwhile, colorful marshmallows will add a festive look to the cake.

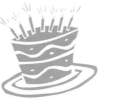

MAKE IMPROMPTU CUPCAKE TOPPING • If you're already mixing up the batter for the cupcakes when you realize you're out of icing, it's not going to be a problem if you have some marshmallows on hand. Just pop a marshmallow on top of each cupcake for about a minute or so before they come out of the oven. They will make a delicious, instant, gooey topping.

MASKING TAPE

LABEL FOODS AND SCHOOL SUPPLIES • You don't need to buy labels or a fancy machine that makes them. Use inexpensive masking tape instead to mark food containers and freezer bags before putting them in the refrigerator or freezer. And don't forget to write the date! You can also use masking tape to conveniently mark kids' schoolbooks and supplies.

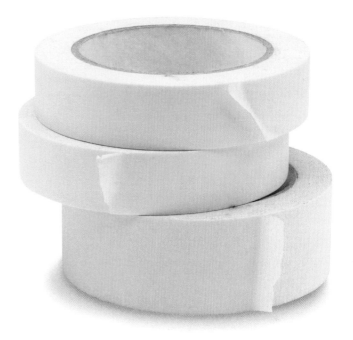

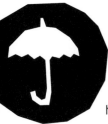

FIX A BROKEN UMBRELLA RIB • If a strong wind breaks a rib on your umbrella, it's easy to fix it. Use a piece of masking tape and a length of wire cut from a coat hanger to make a splint.

REUSE A VACUUM CLEANER BAG • Save money by using a vacuum cleaner bag twice. When the bag is full, don't empty it the usual way through the hole in the front. Take out the bag and cut a slit down the middle of the back. After you empty the bag, hold the cut edges together, fold them closed and seal them with masking tape. Your bag is ready to be used again. Be careful not to overfill during the second use.

KEEP A PAINT CAN NEAT

To prevent paint from filling the groove at the top of a paint can, simply cover the rim of the can with masking tape.

HANG PARTY STREAMERS • Use masking tape instead of transparent tape to put up streamers and balloons for your next party. The masking tape won't leave a residue on the wall like transparent tape does. And always remember to remove the masking tape within a day or two, because if you wait too long, it could take paint off the wall when it comes off.

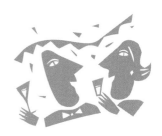

more MASKING TAPE over →

MAKE A ROAD FOR TOY CARS • Make a highway for those tiny toy cars that small children love to play with. Just tape two strips of masking tape to a floor or tabletop. Add a little handmade cardboard stop sign or two and they're off to the races. Carefully guiding a toy car along the taped roadway is more than just fun for small children. It also helps them improve their fine motor control, which is essential for skills they will need later on, such as writing.

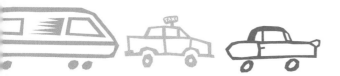

MAYONNAISE

CONDITION YOUR HAIR • Hold the mayo—and massage it into your hair and scalp instead, just as you would any fine conditioner! Cover your head with a shower cap, wait several minutes, and shampoo. The mayonnaise will moisturize your hair and give it a lustrous sheen.

GIVE YOURSELF A FACIAL • Why waste money on expensive creams when you can treat yourself to a soothing facial with whole-egg mayonnaise from your own refrigerator? Gently spread the mayonnaise over your face and leave it on for about 20 minutes. Then wipe it off and rinse with cool water. Your face will feel clean and smooth.

STRENGTHEN YOUR FINGERNAILS • To add some oomph to your fingernails, just plunge them into a bowl of mayonnaise every so often. Keep them bathed in the mayo for about 5 minutes, and wash thoroughly with warm water.

RELIEVE SUNBURN PAIN • If you happen to forget to put on sunscreen, you can treat dry, sunburned skin by slathering mayonnaise liberally over the affected area. The mayonnaise will relieve the pain as well as moisturize the skin.

REMOVE DEAD SKIN • Soften and remove dead skin from elbows and feet by rubbing mayonnaise over the dry, rough tissue, leaving it on for 10 minutes, then wiping it off with a damp cloth.

MAKE PLANT LEAVES SHINY • Professional florists use this trick to keep houseplant leaves shiny and clean. You can do the same thing at home. Just rub a bit of mayonnaise on the leaves with a paper towel and they will stay bright and shiny for weeks and weeks at a time.

SAFE WAY TO KILL HEAD LICE

Many dermatologists now recommend using mayonnaise to kill and remove head lice from kids instead of toxic over-the-counter preparations. What's more, lice are becoming more resistant to such chemical treatments. To treat head lice with mayonnaise, massage a liberal amount into the hair and scalp before bedtime. Cover with a shower cap to maximize the effect. Shampoo in the morning and use a fine-toothed comb to remove any lice and nits. To completely eradicate the infestation, repeat treatment in 7 to 10 days.

MAYONNAISE FOR MOTORISTS!

REMOVE BUMPER STICKERS • Time to get rid of that old political bumper sticker on your car? Instead of attacking it with a razor and risk scratching the bumper, rub some mayonnaise over the entire sticker and let it sit for several minutes before wiping it off. The mayonnaise will dissolve the glue.

GET TAR OFF YOUR CAR • To get road tar or plant sap off your car easily without damaging the paint, slather some mayonnaise over the affected area, let it sit for several minutes, and wipe it away with a clean, soft rag.

REMOVE CRAYON MARKS • If you find crayon marks on your wooden furniture, here's a simple way to remove them that requires hardly any elbow grease. Simply rub some mayonnaise on the crayon marks and let it soak in for several minutes. Then wipe the surface clean with a damp cloth.

CLEAN PIANO KEYS • If the keys on your piano are starting to yellow, just wipe the ivories with a bit of mayonnaise applied with a soft cloth. Wait a few minutes, wipe with a damp cloth and buff. The piano keys will look like new.

MILK

MAKE FROZEN FISH TASTE FRESH • If you want fish from your freezer to taste like it was freshly caught, try this trick. Place the frozen fish in a bath of milk until it thaws. The milk will make it taste fresher.

BOOST CORN-ON-THE-COB FLAVOR • Here's a simple way to make corn on the cob taste sweeter and fresher. Just add ¼ cup (50 g) powdered milk to the pot of boiling water before you toss in the corn.

POLISH SILVERWARE • Tarnished silverware will look like new with a little help from some sour milk. If you don't have any sour milk on hand, you can make some by adding vinegar to fresh milk. Then simply soak the silver in the milk for half an hour to loosen the tarnish; wash in warm, soapy water and buff with a soft cloth.

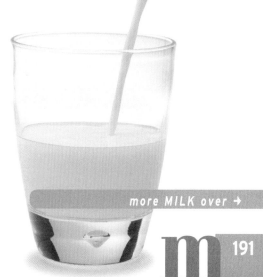

more MILK over →

SOOTHE SUNBURN AND INSECT BITES • If your skin feels like it's burning up from sun exposure or itchy insect bites are driving you crazy, try milk paste for soothing relief. Mix 1 part powdered milk with 2 parts water and a pinch or two of salt. Dab it on the burn or bite. Enzymes in the milk powder will help relieve sunburn pain and help neutralize the insect-bite venom.

SOFTEN SKIN • Treat yourself to a luxurious foamy milk bath. Toss ½ cup (125 g) powdered milk into the tub as it fills. Milk acts as a natural skin softener.

GIVE YOURSELF A FACIAL • Here's another way to give yourself a fancy spa facial at home. Make a mask by mixing ¼ cup (50 g) powdered milk with enough water to form a thick paste. Coat your face with the mixture, let it dry completely, and rinse with warm water. Your face will feel fresh and rejuvenated.

CLEAN & SOFTEN DIRTY HANDS

Working in the garden usually results in stained and gritty hands, and regular soap just won't get it off, but this will. Make a paste of rolled oats and milk and rub it vigorously on your hands. The stains will be gone and the oats-and-milk mixture will soften and soothe your skin.

MAKE QUICK MAKEUP REMOVER • When you run out of makeup remover, use powdered milk instead. Mix 3 tablespoons (45 ml) of powdered milk with $^1/_3$ cup (75 ml) warm water in a jar and shake well. Add more water or powder as needed to achieve the consistency of heavy cream. Apply your makeshift makeup remover with a washcloth. When you're done, wipe it off and rinse with water.

REMOVE INK STAINS FROM CLOTHES • Remove ink stains from colored clothes with an overnight milk bath. Soak the garment in milk overnight and machine wash as usual the next day.

CLEAN PATENT LEATHER • Make your patent-leather bags or shoes look like new again. Just dab on a little milk, let it dry, and buff with a soft cloth.

REPAIR CRACKED CHINA

Before you throw out that cracked plate from your grandmother's old china set, try mending it with milk. Place the plate in a pan, cover it with milk (fresh or reconstituted powdered milk), and bring to a boil. As soon as it starts to boil, lower the heat, and simmer for about 45 minutes. The protein in the milk will miraculously mend most fine cracks.

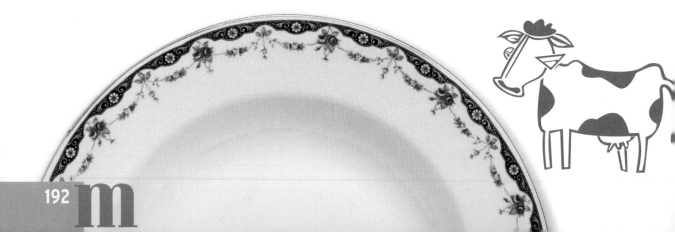

MILK CARTONS

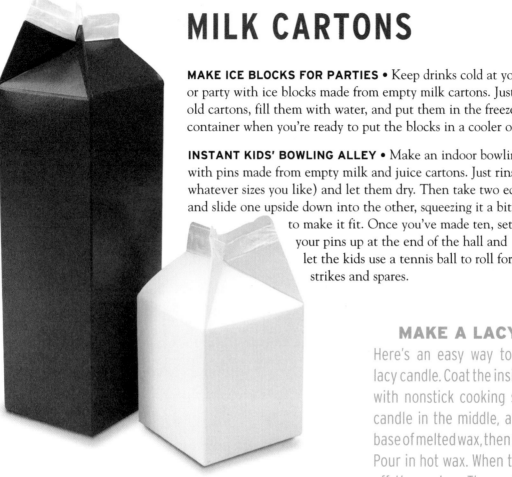

MAKE ICE BLOCKS FOR PARTIES • Keep drinks cold at your next barbecue or party with ice blocks made from empty milk cartons. Just rinse out the old cartons, fill them with water, and put them in the freezer. Peel away the container when you're ready to put the blocks in a cooler or punch bowl.

INSTANT KIDS' BOWLING ALLEY • Make an indoor bowling alley for children with pins made from empty milk and juice cartons. Just rinse the cartons (use whatever sizes you like) and let them dry. Then take two equal-sized cartons and slide one upside down into the other, squeezing it a bit to make it fit. Once you've made ten, set your pins up at the end of the hall and let the kids use a tennis ball to roll for strikes and spares.

MAKE A LACY CANDLE

Here's an easy way to make a delicate, lacy candle. Coat the inside of a milk carton with nonstick cooking spray, put a taper candle in the middle, anchoring it with a base of melted wax, then fill it with ice cubes. Pour in hot wax. When the wax cools, peel off the carton. The melting ice will form beautiful, lacy voids in the wax.

DID YOU KNOW?

John Van Wormer, a U.S. toy factory owner, didn't cry over spilt milk when he dropped a bottle of the stuff on the floor one morning in 1915. Instead, he was inspired to patent a paper-based milk carton he named Pure-Pak. It took him 10 years to perfect a machine that coated the paper with wax and sealed the carton with animal glues. Those early waxy containers bore little resemblance to today's milk cartons. In 1987, Elopak, a Norwegian company, bought the Pure-Pak license. Today, some 30 billion Pure-Pak cartons are sold annually around the world.

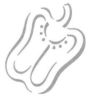

MAKE SEED STARTERS • Milk cartons are the perfect size to use for seed starters. Simply cut off the top half of a carton, punch holes in the bottom, then fill with potting mix, and sow the seeds according to instructions on the seed packet.

more MILK CARTONS over →

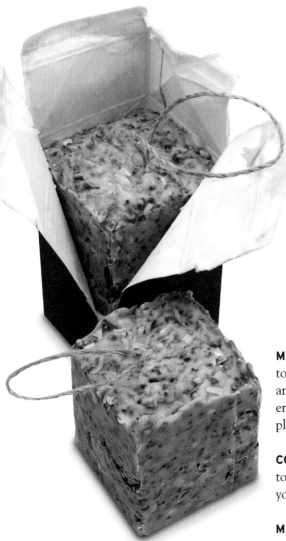

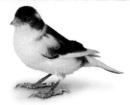

FEED BIRDS IN WINTER

To make a wintertime treat for feathered visitors, combine melted suet and birdseed in an empty milk carton. Suet is beef fat you can get from a butcher. To render it, chop or grind the fat, heat it over a low flame until it melts. Strain it through cheesecloth into the carton and insert a loop of string into the mixture while it's melted. After it hardens, tear away the carton and tie your chunk of bird food to a branch. Don't do this if the temperature gets above about 70°F (20°C) or the suet will turn rancid and melt.

MAKE VEGETABLE GARDEN COLLARS • Use empty milk cartons to discourage grubs and cutworms from attacking your young tomato and pepper plants. Just cut off the tops and bottoms of the containers, and when the ground is soft, push them into the soil around the plants when you set them out.

COLLECT FOOD SCRAPS FOR COMPOST • Keep an empty milk carton handy near the kitchen sink and use it to collect food scraps for your compost heap.

MAKE A DISPOSABLE PAINT HOLDER • If you have a small paint project and you don't want to save the leftover paint (or lug a heavy can), an empty milk carton can help. Just cut off the top of the carton and pour in the amount of paint you need. When the job is finished, throw the carton into the trash, leftover paint and all.

MOTHBALLS

RINSE WOOLENS FOR STORAGE

It is a good idea to store woolens with mothballs to ward off moths. To give your favorite sweaters even more protection, dissolve a few motballs in the final rinse when you wash them before storage.

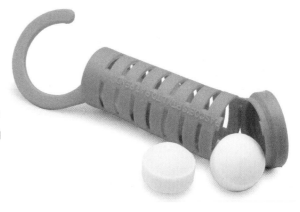

SCIENCE **WORKS!**

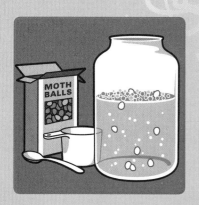

Make mothballs dance while giving the kids a basic science lesson at the same time.

Just fill a glass jar about ²/₃ full with water. Add about ¼ to ⅓ cup (50–75 ml) vinegar and 2 teaspoons (10 ml) baking soda. Stir gently, then toss in a few mothballs and watch them bounce up and down. The vinegar and baking soda create carbon dioxide bubbles, which cling to the irregular surfaces of the mothballs. When enough bubbles accumulate to lift the weight of a mothball, it rises to the surface of the water. There, some of the bubbles escape into the air and the mothball sinks to the bottom of the jar to start the cycle again. The effect will last longer if the container is sealed.

KILL INSECTS ON POTTED PLANTS • To get rid of insects on a potted plant, put the plant in a clear plastic bag, such as a garbage bag, add a few mothballs, and seal it for a week. When you take the plant out of the bag, your plant will be insect-free and the moths will stay away.

REPEL MICE FROM THE GARAGE OR SHED • Don't let mice spend their winter vacation in your garage. Place a few mothballs around the garage and the mice will seek other quarters. To keep mice out of your garden shed or greenhouse, put mothballs around the base of wrapped or covered plants.

KEEP DOGS AND CATS AWAY FROM THE GARDEN • Don't throw out old mothballs. Scatter them around your gardens and flowerbeds to keep cats, dogs, and rodents away. Animals hate the smell.

KEEP BATS AT BAY • Bats won't invade your belfry (or attic) if you scatter a few mothballs around. Add some mothballs to the boxes you store in the attic and silverfish will stay away, too.

MOUSE PADS

PAD UNDER TABLE LEGS • When you get a new mouse pad for your computer, don't throw out the old one. Use it to make pads for table legs and chairs to prevent them from scratching wood and other hard-surface floors. Just cut the foam-and-cloth pad into small pieces and superglue each piece to the bottom of a leg.

MAKE KNEEPADS FOR THE GARDEN • Old computer mouse pads are just the right size to cushion your knees when you're working in the garden. Kneel on them loose as is or attach them directly to your pant legs with duct tape.

MAKE A PAD FOR HOUSEPLANTS • Keep potted-plant containers from scratching or damaging your hard floors by placing the pot on top of an old mouse pad and your floor will remain scratch-free. Use four pads for large pots.

MAKE A HOT PAD FOR THE TABLE • Protect your table from hot casseroles, coffeepots, and serving dishes. Use old computer mouse pads as hot pads. The cloth-topped foam mouse pad is the perfect size to hold most hot containers you bring to the table.

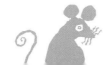

MOUTHWASH

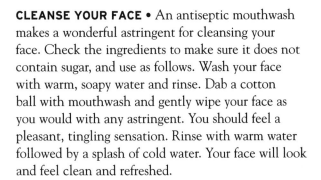

CLEAN A COMPUTER MONITOR SCREEN • Out of glass cleaner? An alcohol-based mouthwash will work as well as, or better than, glass cleaner on your computer monitor or television screen. Apply with a damp, soft cloth and buff dry. Remember to use only on glass screens, not liquid crystal displays. The alcohol can damage the material used in LCDs.

CLEANSE YOUR FACE • An antiseptic mouthwash makes a wonderful astringent for cleansing your face. Check the ingredients to make sure it does not contain sugar, and use as follows. Wash your face with warm, soapy water and rinse. Dab a cotton ball with mouthwash and gently wipe your face as you would with any astringent. You should feel a pleasant, tingling sensation. Rinse with warm water followed by a splash of cold water. Your face will look and feel clean and refreshed.

TREAT ATHLETE'S FOOT • A sugarless antiseptic mouthwash may be all you need to treat mild cases of athlete's foot or toenail fungus. Use a cotton ball soaked in mouthwash to apply to the affected area several times a day. But be prepared; it will sting a bit! Athlete's foot should respond after a few days, but toenail fungus may take up to several months. If you do not see a response by then, make an appointment with a dermatologist or podiatrist.

ADD TO WASHING WATER

Smelly gym socks are often full of bacteria and fungi that may not all come out in the wash—unless you add a cup of alcohol-based, sugarless mouthwash during the regular wash cycle.

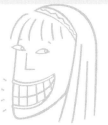

Homemade mouthwash

TIP

❋ *Freshen your breath with your own homemade, alcohol-free mouthwash.*

Place 1 ounce (30 g) whole cloves and/or 3 ounces (85 g) fresh rosemary in a 2-cup (500-ml) jar and add 2 cups (500 ml) boiling water. Cover tightly and steep overnight before straining. If you need mouthwash immediately, dissolve ½ teaspoon (2 ml) baking soda in ½ cup (125 ml) warm water.

CURE UNDERARM ODOR • Regular deodorants mask unpleasant underarm odors with a heavy perfume smell but do little to attack the cause of the problem. To get rid of the bacteria that cause perspiration odor, dampen a cotton ball with a sugarless, alcohol-based mouthwash and swab your armpits. If you've just shaved your armpits, it's best to wait for another day to try this.

DISINFECT A CUT • When you need to clean out a small cut or wound, use an alcohol-based mouthwash to disinfect your skin. Remember that, before it became a mouthwash, it was successfully used as an antiseptic to prevent surgical infections.

GET RID OF DANDRUFF • To treat a bad case of dandruff, wash your hair with your regular shampoo, and rinse with an alcohol-based mouthwash. You can follow with your regular conditioner.

CLEAN YOUR TOILET • If you're out of your regular toilet-bowl cleaner, try pouring ¼ cup (50 ml) alcohol-based mouthwash into the bowl. Let it stand in the water for half an hour, then swish with a toilet brush before flushing. The mouthwash will disinfect germs as it leaves your toilet bowl sparkling clean.

MUSTARD

SOOTHE AN ACHING BACK • Take a bath in yellow mustard to relieve an aching back or arthritis pain. Simply pour a 6–8-ounce (175–250 ml) bottle of prepared mustard into the hot water as the tub fills. Mix well and soak yourself for 15 minutes. If you don't have time for a bath, you can rub some mustard directly on the affected areas. Use only mild yellow mustard and make sure to apply it to a small test area first. Undiluted mustard may irritate your skin.

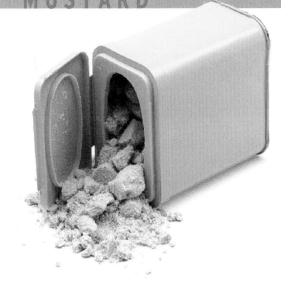

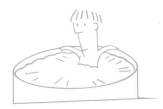

RELAX STIFF MUSCLES • Next time you take a bath in Epsom salt, throw in a few tablespoons of prepared yellow mustard, too. The mustard will enhance the soothing effects of the Epsom salt and also help to relax stiff, sore muscles.

RELIEVE CONGESTION • Relieve congestion with a mustard plaster just like Grandma used to make. Rub your chest with prepared mustard, soak a washcloth in hot water, wring it out, and place it over the mustard.

MAKE A FACIAL MASK • Pat your face with mild yellow mustard for a bracing facial that will soothe and stimulate your skin. Try it on a small test area first to make sure it will not cause irritation.

REMOVE ODOR FROM BOTTLES • If you've got some nice bottles you'd like to keep, but after washing them they still smell like whatever came in them, mustard is a surefire way to kill the smell. After washing, just squirt a bit of mustard into the bottle, fill with warm water, and shake it up. Rinse well and the smell will be gone.

DID YOU KNOW?

Ancient Romans brought mustard back from Egypt and used the seeds to flavor unfermented grape juice, called must. This is believed to be how the mustard plant got its name. The Romans also made a paste from the ground seeds for medicinal purposes and may have used it as a condiment. But the mustard we use today was first prepared in Dijon, France, in the thirteenth century. Dijon-style mustard is made from darker seeds than yellow mustard.

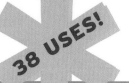

NAIL POLISH

38 USES!

around the house

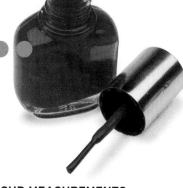

MAKE BUTTONS GLOW IN THE DARK • It happens all the time—the lights are dimmed, you grab the remote control to increase the TV volume and you hit the wrong button and change the channel instead. To put an end to those problems, dab glow-in-the-dark nail polish onto frequently used remote buttons. You can also use phosphorescent polish to mark keys and keyholes and other hard-to-spot items.

MARK YOUR THERMOSTAT SETTING • If you have a dial-type thermostat on your heater and you wake up with a chill and don't have your glasses handy, it's easy to adjust the thermostat if you have already preset it to your preferred temperature and made a thin mark with colored nail polish from the dial into the outside ring.

MARK TEMPERATURE SETTINGS ON SHOWER KNOBS • Don't waste precious shower time fiddling with the water temperature. With the shower on, select your ideal settings, turn off the flow to the shower, and make a small mark with bright nail polish on the stationary lip of both the hot and cold knob indicating the handle position that's best.

MARK LEVELS INSIDE A BUCKET • When you're mixing something in a big bucket, it's usually too heavy for you to be able to lift the bucket to check the quantity. Besides, the bucket you use for mixing might not have the measurements clearly marked on it at all. Make sure you know you're using the right amounts by marking levels at a pint (500 ml), quart, (1 L), half-gallon (2 L), and gallon (4 L) with lines of nail polish. Use a polish color that stands out against the color of your bucket.

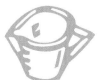

MAKE CUP MEASUREMENTS LEGIBLE • You'll be able to find your measuring cup markings faster, especially if you like to measure 'on the fly' while cooking, if you use a highly visible color of nail polish to trace over the basic measurement levels. This also works well for late-night bottle feedings, when you need to see how much Junior has tanked up. And you won't have to squint to find the correct dosage on little plastic medicine cups if you first mark them with a thin line of dark polish.

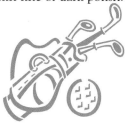

LABEL YOUR SPORTS GEAR • If you share a lot of interests with your golf partner, including the same brand of golf balls, make it clear who got on the green first, by putting a dot of bright nail polish on your golf balls. This also works well with batting gloves and other items that don't have enough room to fit your name on them.

LABEL POISON CONTAINERS • If everyone in your home has easy access to all the cupboards, prevent someone from grabbing dangerous items in haste. Use dark red or other easily visible nail polish color to label the poisons. Draw an unmistakable X on the label as well as on the lid or spout.

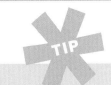

Using nail polish

Bottles of nail polish don't come with instructions, so here are some pointers:

● To keep nail polish fresh and easy to use, store it in the refrigerator. Keep your collection of bottles together in a little square plastic container.

● Shaking a nail polish bottle to mix the color can cause bubbles to form. Gently roll the bottle between your palms instead.

● Wipe the inside threads of your nail polish bottle and cap with a cotton swab dipped in polish remover before closing the bottle. It will open more easily.

SEAL AN ENVELOPE • Brush some nail polish along the underside of the flap, seal it, and it won't open easily. Or try brushing your initial (or any design) in nail polish over the sealed flap tip, as a modern type of sealing wax that doesn't need to be melted first.

SMUDGE-PROOF DRUG LABELS • Preserve the important information on all of your prescription medicine and other important medicine labels with a coat of clear polish, and they won't be smudged as you grab them after getting your glass of water.

WATERPROOF ADDRESS LABELS • When you're sending a parcel on a rainy day, a little clear polish brushed over the address information will make sure your package goes to the right place.

PREVENT RINGS FROM METAL CONTAINERS • If your guests are going to peek into your medicine cabinet, you don't want them to see rust rings on your shelves. Brush nail polish around the bottom of shaving cream cans and other metal containers to avoid those unsightly stains.

MAKE A GLEAMING PAPERWEIGHT

To create paperweights that look like gemstones, or interesting rocks for the base of your potted cactus, try this. Find some palm-sized, smooth clean rocks. Put about 1/2 inch (1 cm) water into a pie pan. Add a drop of clear nail polish on the water and polish will spread over the water's surface. Holding a rock with your fingertips, slowly roll it in the water to coat it with polish. Set the rock on newspaper to dry.

PREVENT RUSTY TOILET SEAT SCREWS • If you're installing a new toilet seat, keep those screws from quickly rusting. Paint them with a coat or two of clear nail polish. It will also help prevent seat wobble by keeping the screws in place.

PAINT SHAKER HOLES TO RESTRICT SALT • If your favorite saltshaker dispenses a little too much salt, paint a few of the holes shut with nail polish. It's a good idea if you're watching your salt intake.

TARNISH-PROOF COSTUME JEWELRY • Inexpensive costume jewelry can add sparkle and color to any outfit, but not if it tarnishes and the tarnish rubs off the jewelry and onto your skin. To keep your fake jewelry and your skin sparkling clean, brush clear nail polish on the back of each piece and allow it to dry before wearing.

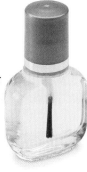

more NAIL POLISH over →

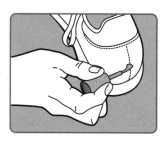

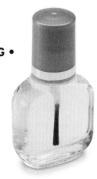

SEAL OUT SCUFFS ON SHOES • On leather shoes, it's the back and toes that really take the brunt of the wear and tear that leaves scratches on the surface. Next time you buy a new pair of shoes—especially ones for a kid or an active adult—give these areas the extra measure of protection they need. Paint a bit of clear nail polish on the outside of the back seam and over the toes. Rub the polish in a little to feather out the shine of the polish. After it dries, you'll be a step ahead of those perennial shoe problems: "driver's heel" and "jump-rope toe."

KEEP LACES FROM UNRAVELING • Neaten the appearance of frayed shoelaces and extend their life by dipping the ends in clear nail polish and twisting the raveled ends together. Repair laces in the evening so that the polish can dry overnight.

PROTECT YOUR BELT BUCKLE'S SHINE • Cover new or just-shined belt buckles with a coat of clear nail polish. You'll prevent oxidation of the metal buckle and guarantee a gleaming first impression.

GET RID OF A WART • Warts are unattractive, embarrassing, and infectious. In order to get rid of warts and prevent spreading the virus to others, cover them with nail polish. The wart should be gone or greatly diminished within a week.

in the sewing room

PROTECT PEARL BUTTONS • Delicate pearl buttons will keep their brand-new sparkle with a protective coat of clear nail polish. It will keep costume pearl buttons from peeling as well.

PREVENT LOSS OF BUTTONS • Keep that brand-new shirt in good shape by putting a drop of clear nail polish on the thread in the buttons. It prevents the thread from fraying, so taking this precaution in advance could save you some embarrassment later on. Put a dab on recently repaired buttons as well.

MAKE NEEDLE THREADING EASIER • Do you fumble with your needle and thread, licking and re-licking the frayed thread end until it's too floppy to go through the eye? Try dragging the cut thread end through the application brush of nail polish once or twice, then roll the thread end between your thumb and forefinger. It will dry in a second, and your thread end stays stiff enough to thread in a flash. Your sewing box is a great place for a nail polish color you no longer use.

PREVENT FRAYED FABRIC FROM UNRAVELING • Do you have wisps peeking out from the bottom of your skirt? Is the nylon lining of your jacket fraying at the cuffs? You can tame those fraying strays by brushing them in place with some clear nail polish.

KEEP RIBBONS FROM FRAYING • The gift is perfect, so make sure the wrapping is just as nice. Brush the cut ends of ribbon with a little clear nail polish to stop them from unraveling. This is also the perfect solution for a little girl's hair ribbons on special occasions. At least one part of her will stay together all day!

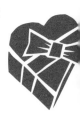

STOP RUNS IN PANTYHOSE • Runs in pantyhose are a real pain. Happily, you can stop them for good and prolong the life of fragile pantyhose with a dab of clear nail polish. Simply apply polish to each end of a run (no need to remove the pantyhose), and let it dry. This invisible fix stops runs and lasts through many hand washings.

making repairs

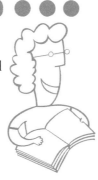

MEND A FINGERNAIL • When you split a nail, but don't have a nail repair kit handy, just grab an unused tea bag instead. Cut the bag open, dump the tea, cut a piece of the bag into the shape of your nail and cover it with clear nail polish. Press it onto your nail and apply colored nail polish. You'll be good to go until the break grows out.

STOP A WINDSHIELD CRACK FROM SPREADING • If you've developed a small crack in your windshield, stop it cold with some clear polish. Working in the shade, brush the crack on both sides of the glass with polish to fill it well. Move the car into the sun so the windshield can dry. You will eventually need to repair your windshield, but this will give you time to shop around for the best deal.

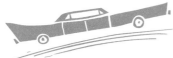

FILL SMALL NICKS ON FLOORS AND GLASS • If some children have been playing hockey on your hardwood floors, fill in those little nicks by dabbing them with some clear nail polish. It will dry shiny, so sand the spot gently with some 600-grit sandpaper. A thick coat of clear nail polish also helps to soften the sharp edge of a nicked mirror or glass pane.

RESET LOOSE JEWELRY STONES • If a piece of jewelry has lost a stone or two, you don't have to put it in the 'play dress-up' box yet. The stone can be reset using a little drop of clear nail polish as the 'glue'. It dries quickly and the repair will be invisible.

REPAIR LACQUERED ITEMS • If you chip a favorite lacquered vase or other lacquered item, try mixing colors of nail polish to match the piece, then paint over the chipped area to make it less noticeable. **WARNING: You may lower the value of an antique by doing this, so only use this method if you're repairing an inexpensive item.**

TEMPORARILY REPAIR GLASSES

You sat on your glasses and one lens has a small crack, but you can't get to the optometrist right away? Seal the crack on both sides with a thin coat of clear nail polish. That will it hold together until you can see your way to the eye doc.

PLUG A HOLE IN YOUR COOLER • A small hole inside your cooler doesn't make it ready for the trash can just yet. Seal the hole with two coats of nail polish to hold in ice and other liquid substances.

FILL WASHING MACHINE NICKS • It's a mystery how they got there, but your washing machine tub has one or two nicks near the holes, and now you're concerned about snags in your clothes or even rust spots. Seal those nicks with some nail polish, feathering the edges so there is no lip.

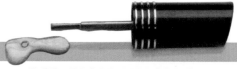

DID YOU KNOW?

Nail polish is certainly not a recent concept. As early as 3000 B.C., ancient Chinese nobility are believed to have colored their long nails with polishes, made from gum arabic, beeswax, gelatin, and pigments. The nobility wore shades of gold, silver, red, or black, while lesser classes were restricted to pastel shades. Colored nails were also popular with ancient Egyptians, who often dyed their nails with henna or stained them with berries. Polish wasn't just for women. In Egypt and Rome, military commanders painted their nails red before going into battle.

more NAIL POLISH over →

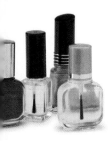

KEEP CHIPPED CAR PAINT FROM RUSTING • If your car's paint has small dings and chips, you can keep them from rusting or enlarging by dabbing clear nail polish on the damaged areas.

SMOOTH WOODEN HANGERS • If you've noticed a few splinters or nicks in your wooden hangers, no need to toss them out. Brush some nail polish over the rough edges to smooth the surface again and keep your coat linings safe.

TIGHTEN LOOSE SCREWS • You may not be rough with your drawers and cupboards, but you may well find yourself tightening certain knob screws once too often. Keep them in place by brushing a little clear polish on the screw threads, insert the screws, and allow to dry before using again. This is also a great solution if you've been keeping a Phillips screwdriver in the kitchen for loose pot handles. You can also use clear nail polish to keep nuts on machine screws or bolts from coming loose, and if you need to take the nuts off, a twist with a wrench will break the seal.

DID YOU KNOW?

Unless you work in a laboratory, you probably don't know that clear nail polish is the respected method used in mounting microscopic slides. Officially referred to as NPM (nail-polish mountant), it is the preferred and inexpensive substance used around a cover glass to seal it onto a slide, thus protecting the specimen from air and moisture.

MEND HOLES IN WINDOW SCREENS • It's not unusual to find that a small hole has been poked in a window or door screen. If the hole is no more than about ¼ inch (6 mm) in diameter, you can block out the insects and keep the hole from getting bigger by dabbing on a bit of clear nail polish.

FIX TORN WINDOW BLINDS • If there's a small tear visible in your window blind, you don't have to start looking for a replacement just yet. Try sealing it with a light dab of clear nail polish.

NAIL POLISH REMOVER

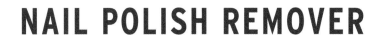

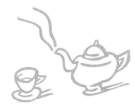

REMOVE STAINS FROM CHINA • If your bone china has assorted stains from years of use, spruce it up by rubbing soiled areas with nail polish remover. Clean spots with a cotton swab and wash dishes as usual.

ELIMINATE INK STAINS • If the ink stains on your skin won't come off with soap and water, they are probably not water soluble. Try using nail polish remover instead. Take a cotton ball and wipe the affected areas with the solution. Once the ink stains are gone, wash your skin with soap and water. Nail polish remover can also eliminate ink stains on the drum of your clothes dryer.

RUB PAINT OFF WINDOWS • Working in a well-ventilated area, dab on nail polish remover in small sections of the pane. Let the solution remain on the painted areas for a few minutes before rubbing it off with a cloth. Once finished, take a damp cloth and go over the areas again.

NAIL POLISH REMOVER

SCIENCE **WORKS!**

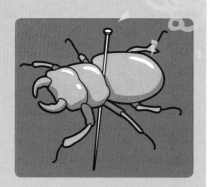

Some children love to study insects, and just like the pros, your budding entomologist can kill and preserve insects, using nail polish remover.

Use a nail polish remover that contains the solvent acetone. (Check the label or sniff it for a banana-like odor.) To preserve the insects, soak some cotton balls with the polish remover and place them in a glass or plastic jar along with several tissues and the selected insects. A wide-mouthed jam jar works well. The tissues prevent the insects from damaging their wings. Seal the jar tightly with a lid and the specimens will quickly dehydrate. Use a straight pin stuck through the insect's body to mount it on corkboard or corrugated cardboard.

CAUTION: Frequent use of nail polish remover containing acetone—check the label—can cause dry skin and brittle nails. All nail polish removers are flammable and potentially hazardous if inhaled for a long time. Use them in a well-ventilated area away from flames and work carefully. They can damage synthetic fabrics, wood finishes, and plastics.

REMOVE STICKERS FROM GLASS • Scraping price stickers from glass objects can be messy, and it often leaves behind a gummy adhesive that attracts dirt and is sticky to the touch. Remove the stickers and clean up the residual glue by wiping the area with acetone-based nail polish remover. The same method can be used for removing stickers and sticky residue from metal surfaces.

DISSOLVE MELTED PLASTIC • Ever get too close to a hot metal toaster with a plastic bag of bread or bagels? The resulting mess can be a real cleaning challenge. But don't let a little melted plastic ruin a perfectly good appliance. Eliminate the sticky mess with nail polisher remover. Firstly, unplug the toaster and wait for it to cool. Then pour a little nail polish remover on a soft cloth and gently rub over the damaged areas. Once the melted plastic is removed, wipe with a damp cloth and dry with a paper towel. Your toaster is now ready for the next round of toast. The same solution works for melted plastic on curling irons.

UNHINGE SUPERGLUE

Superglue will stick tenaciously to anything, including your skin. And trying to peel it off your fingers can actually cause skin damage. Instead, soak a cotton ball with acetone-based nail polish remover and hold it on the skin until the glue dissolves.

CLEAN VINYL SHOES • Patent leather shoes may not reflect up, but they do show off scuff marks, as will white or other light-colored vinyl shoes. To remove the marks, rub them lightly but briskly with a soft cloth or paper towel dipped in nail polish remover. Afterwards, remove any residue with a damp cloth.

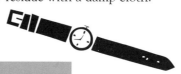

KEEP WATCHES CLEAN • Tired of looking at your watch and seeing unsightly scratches when you check the time? Get rid of them with nail polish remover. If the face of your watch is made from unbreakable plastic, rub the remover over the scratches until they diminish or disappear.

more NAIL POLISH REMOVER over →

CLEAN COMPUTER KEYBOARDS • You can keep computer keyboards clean with nail polish remover and an old toothbrush. Simply moisten the brush with remover and lightly rub the keys.

DILUTE CORRECTION FLUID • To take the goop out of correction fluid or old nail polish, dilute it with nail polish remover. Pour just a few drops into the bottle and shake. Add a little more polish remover to the solution, if needed, to attain the desired consistency.

PREP BRASS FOR RE-LACQUERING • Old or damaged lacquer coatings on brass can be safely removed with nail polish remover. Take a soft cloth and pour a small amount of remover on it, then rub the brass object until the old lacquer has been lifted. Your brass item is now ready to be polished or professionally re-lacquered.

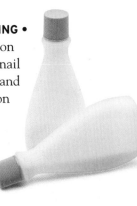

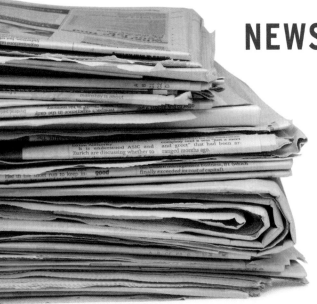

NEWSPAPER

ENCASE YOUR GLASSWARE FOR MOVING

Are you relocating or packing items for long-term storage? Use several sheets of soaking-wet newspapers to wrap up your glass dishes, bowls, drinking glasses, and other fragile items, then let them thoroughly dry before packing. The newspaper will harden and form a protective cast around the glass that will dramatically improve its chances of surviving the move without breaking.

STORE SWEATERS AND BLANKETS • Don't treat moths to a fine meal of your homemade or pricey woolen sweaters and blankets. When putting them into storage, wrap your woolens in a few sheets of newspaper (be sure to tape up the corners). It will keep away the moths and keep out dust and dirt.

CLEAN AND POLISH YOUR WINDOWS • If you're like most people, you probably use a lot of paper towels for drying off your freshly washed windows. Did you know that crumpled-up newspaper dries and polishes windows even better than paper towels? And it's a lot cheaper, too.

DEODORIZE LUGGAGE AND CONTAINERS • Do you have a plastic container or wooden box with a persistent, unpleasant odor? Stuff in a few sheets of crumpled newspaper and seal it closed for three or four days. You can also use this technique to deodorize trunks and suitcases, using more newspaper, of course.

DRY WET SHOES • If your shoes get soaking wet, stuff them with dry, balled-up newspaper to prevent any long-term damage. Place the shoes on their sides at room temperature so the moisture can be absorbed. For severe sogginess, replace the stuffing a few times.

MAKE AN IMPROMPTU IRONING BOARD

If you usually pack a travel iron—just in case you end up in a motel that doesn't provide irons and ironing boards—it's a cinch to make your own on-the-road ironing board. Simply fill a pillowcase with a short stack of newspapers, keeping it as level as possible. Place it on a countertop or the floor and get pressing.

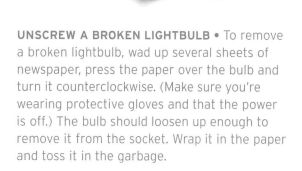

CREATE AN EMERGENCY SPLINT • If someone you're with takes a nasty fall—and you think there may be a bone injury to an arm or leg—it's important to immobilize the limb to prevent pain and additional damage.

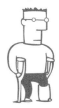

Fashion a makeshift splint by folding up several sheets of newspaper until stiff and attach it beneath the limb using a few pieces of adhesive tape. You may need to overlap a couple of folded sheets to make a splint long enough for a leg injury.

REMOVE OVEN RESIDUE • They may call it a self-cleaning oven, but when it's finished cleaning, you always have to contend with mopping off that ashlike residue. Don't waste a roll of paper towels on the flaky stuff. Clean it up with a few sheets of moistened, crumpled newspaper.

PICK UP BROKEN GLASS SHARDS • Everyone breaks a big glass bowl at least once in a lifetime. A safe way to get up the small shards of glass that remain after you remove the large pieces is to blot the area with wet newspapers. The tiny fragments will stick to the paper, which makes for easy disposal. Just carefully drop the newspaper in your garbage can.

UNSCREW A BROKEN LIGHTBULB • To remove a broken lightbulb, wad up several sheets of newspaper, press the paper over the bulb and turn it counterclockwise. (Make sure you're wearing protective gloves and that the power is off.) The bulb should loosen up enough to remove it from the socket. Wrap it in the paper and toss it in the garbage.

DID YOU KNOW?

America's first newspaper was called *Publick Occurrences, Both Foreign and Domestick.* It was a folded three-panel sheet of paper printed in Boston on September 25, 1690 by Richard Pierce and Benjamin Harris. Unfortunately, British colonial authorities closed it after its first and only issue and quickly issued a decree banning "unlicensed" publications. Ironically, the only known copy isn't found in the United States. It's in the Public Records Office in London.

more NEWSPAPER over →

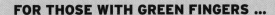

FOR THOSE WITH GREEN FINGERS ...

SLOW-RIPEN TOMATOES IN LATE FALL • Is there an early frost predicted and you still have a bunch of tomatoes on the vine? Relax. Pick your tomatoes and wrap each one in a couple of sheets of newspaper. Store them in airtight containers in a dark cupboard or closet at room temperature. Check each one every three to four days. They will all eventually ripen to perfection.

USE AS MULCH • Newspaper makes terrific mulch for veggies and flowers. It's excellent at retaining moisture and does an equally fine job of fighting off and suffocating weeds. Just lay down several sheets of newspaper and cover the paper with about 3 inches (8 cm) of wood mulch so that it doesn't blow away.

CAUTION: Avoid using glossy stock and colored newspaper for mulching or composting. Colored inks may contain lead or harmful dyes that can leach into the ground. To check your newspaper, contact your local paper and ask about the inks they use; many papers now use only safe vegetable-based inks.

ADD TO COMPOST • Adding moderate amounts of wet, shredded newspaper–black ink only–to a compost heap is a good and relatively safe way to reduce odor and give worms a tasty treat.

KILL EARWIGS • If your garden is under siege by earwigs–those creepy-looking insects with the sharp pincers on their hindquarters–get rid of them by making your own environmentally friendly traps. Tightly roll up a wet newspaper and put a rubber band around it to keep it from unravelling. Place it in the area you've seen the insects and leave it overnight. By morning, it will be standing room only for the insects. Place the newspaper in a plastic grocery bag, tie a knot at the top of the bag, and toss it into the garbage. Repeat until your traps are free of earwigs.

WINTERIZE OUTDOOR FAUCETS • If you live in a cold area and don't have frost-free outdoor spigots, it's a good idea to insulate your outdoor faucets. To prevent damage from ice and cold temperatures, make sure you shut off the valve to each faucet and drain any excess water. Insulate each faucet by wrapping it with a few sheets of newspaper covered with a plastic bag (keep the bag in place by wrapping it with duct tape or a few rubber bands).

PROTECT WINDOWS WHEN PAINTING

Don't bother buying thick masking or carpenter tape when painting around the windows of your home. Simply wet several long strips of newspaper and place them on the glass along the wood you're painting. The newspaper will easily adhere to the surface and keep the paint from the glass or frames, and it is much easier to remove than masking tape.

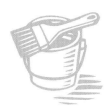

ROLL YOUR OWN FIREPLACE LOGS • Cold winter on the way? Bolster your supply of fireplace logs by making a few of your own out of old newspapers. Just lay out a bunch of sheets end to end, roll them up as tightly as you can, tie up the ends with string or wire, and wet them in a solution of slightly soapy water. Although it will take a while, let them dry thoroughly, standing on end, before using. However, do not use newspaper logs in a wood-burning stove unless the manufacturer specifies that it is OK.

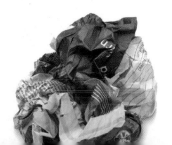

PUT TRACTION UNDER YOUR WHEELS • Unless your vehicle has four-wheel drive, it's always a good idea to keep a small stack of newspapers in the trunk of your car during the winter months to prevent getting stranded on a patch of slushy mud. Placing a dozen or two sheets of newspaper under each rear wheel will often provide just the traction you need to get your car back on the road.

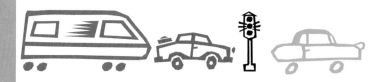

NONSKID TAPE

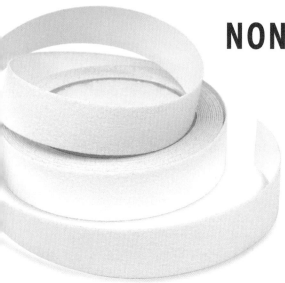

KEEP APPLIANCES IN PLACE • Affixing small pieces of nonskid tape to the bottom of telephones, electric can openers, computer speakers, and similar items will help keep them from sliding off counters or desktops.

ADD TRACTION TO BOOTS • Some rubber boots may be great at keeping out moisture, but don't prevent you from slipping on ice, snow, or slush-covered surfaces. But you can usually improve the traction of waterproof footwear by gluing a few strips of flat nonskid tape on the toe, middle, and heel sections.

GET A GRIP ON TOOLS

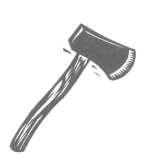

Wrapping the handles of tools such as hammers, axes, and wrenches with flat nonskid tape will not only give you a better and more comfortable grip on them, but it might even prevent wooden handles from getting damaged. Spiral the weather stripping around the handle, overlapping it half a width.

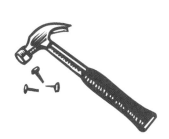

OATMEAL

TREAT CHICKEN POX OR POISON IVY RASH •
Take the itch out of chicken pox or poison ivy rash
with a relaxing, warm oatmeal bath. Simply grind
1 cup (250 g) rolled oats to a fine powder in a
blender, pour it into a piece of cheesecloth, the foot
section of a clean nylon stocking, or the leg of old
pantyhose. Knot the material and tie it around the
faucet of your bathtub, suspending it under the
running water. Fill the tub with lukewarm water and
soak in it for about 30 minutes. For additional relief,
apply the oatmeal pouch directly to the rash.

ADD LUXURY TO A REGULAR BATH • You don't
have to have itchy skin to make a luxurious bath
mix with oatmeal. It beats buying expensive bath
oils. All you need is 1 cup (250 g) rolled oats
and your favorite scented oil, such as rose or
lavender. Grind the oats in a blender, put it in a
cheesecloth bag, add a few drops of the scented
oil and suspend the bag under the running water
as you fill your bathtub. You'll not only find it
sweetly soothing, you can also use the oat-filled
bag as a wascloth to exfoliate your skin.

MAKE A FACIAL MASK • If you're looking for a
quick pick-me-up that will leave you feeling and
looking better, give yourself an oatmeal facial.
Combine ½ cup (125 ml) hot—not boiling—
water and 1/3 cup (75 g) rolled oats. After the water
and oats have settled for 2 or 3 minutes, mix in
2 tablespoons (30 ml) plain yogurt, 2 tablespoons
(30 ml) honey, and a small egg white. Apply a thin
layer of the mixture to your face and let it sit for 10
to 15 minutes. Rinse with warm water. Be sure you
place a strainer in your sink to avoid clogging
the drain with the granules.

DID YOU KNOW?

Thirty minutes. Five minutes. One minute! Oatmeal
cooking times depend on how the oats were milled.
After the inedible hull is removed, the oat is called
a groat. If the groats are just cut into about four
pieces, the oatmeal takes up to 30 minutes to cook.
If the groats are steamed and rolled but not cut
(traditional rolled oats), it takes about 5 minutes. If
they are steamed, rolled, and cut (quick-cooking oats),
the cooking time drops to a minute or so. Steaming,
rolling, and cooking breaks down the fiber, so if you
want a lot of fiber, use 30-minute oats and cook them
until the oatmeal is chewy, not mushy.

MAKE A DRY SHAMPOO • If you occasionally need
to skip washing your hair, keep this dry shampoo on
hand in an airtight container specifically for those
times. Put 1 cup (250 g) rolled oats in the blender
and grind it into a fine powder. Add 1 cup (250 g)
baking soda and mix well. Rub a bit of the mixture
into your hair. Give it a minute or two to soak up
the oils, then brush or shake it out of your hair
(preferably over a towel or bag to avoid getting
it everywhere). This dry shampoo mixture is also
ideal for cleaning the hair of people who are unable
to get into a shower or bathtub due to medical
reasons. Plus, it's equally effective for deodorizing
unpleasant smelling dog hair.

OLIVE OIL

REMOVE PAINT FROM HAIR • It's not that difficult to get almost as much paint in your hair as you do on the walls during a big paint job. Luckily, you can easily remove that undesirable tint by moistening a cotton ball with some olive oil and gently rubbing it into your hair. The same approach is also effective for removing mascara —just be sure to wipe your eyes with a tissue when you're done.

MAKE YOUR OWN FURNITURE POLISH • Restore the lost luster of your wooden furniture by whipping up some serious homemade furniture polish that's just as good as any commercial stuff. Combine 2 parts olive oil and 1 part lemon juice or white vinegar in a clean, recycled spray bottle, shake it up, and spritz it on. Leave the mixture on for a minute or two, then wipe it off with a clean towel or paper towel. If you're in a hurry, apply the olive oil straight from the bottle on a paper towel. Wipe off the excess with another paper towel or an absorbent cloth.

USE AS HAIR CONDITIONER • Is your hair as dry and brittle as a loofah? Put the moisture back into it by heating ½ cup (125 ml) olive oil (don't boil it) and liberally applying it to your hair. Cover your hair with a plastic grocery bag, and wrap it in a towel. Let it set for around 45 minutes, then shampoo and thoroughly rinse.

CLEAN YOUR GREASY HANDS • To remove car grease or paint from your hands, pour 1 teaspoon (5 ml) olive oil and 1 teaspoon (5 ml) salt or sugar into your palms. Vigorously rub the mixture into your hands and between your fingers for several minutes, and wash it off with soap and water. Your hands will be clean and softer as well.

Buying olive oil

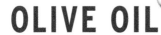

* Expensive extra virgin olive oil is made from olives crushed soon after harvest and processed without the application of excessive heat.

It's great for culinary uses where the taste of the oil is important. But for everyday cooking and non-food applications, lower grades of olive oil— light, extra light, or just plain olive oil—work just as well and save you money.

CLEAR UP ACNE • The notion of applying oil to your face to treat acne does sound a bit wacky. Still, many people swear this works. Make a paste by mixing 4 tablespoons (60 g) salt with 3 tablespoons (45 ml) olive oil. Pour the mixture on your hands and fingers and work it around your face. Leave it on for a minute or two and rinse it off with warm, soapy water. Apply daily for one week and cut back to two or three times weekly. You should see improvement in your condition. The principle is that the salt cleanses the pores by exfoliation, while the olive oil restores the skin's natural moisture.

SUBSTITUTE FOR SHAVING CREAM • If you run out of shaving cream, don't use soap—it could be rough on your skin. Olive oil, on the other hand, is a great substitute for shaving cream. It not only makes it easier for the blade to glide over the face and legs, but it moisturizes the skin as well.

RECONDITION AN OLD BASEBALL GLOVE • If your beloved, aging baseball glove is showing signs of wear and tear—cracking and hardening of the leather—you can give it a second lease on life with an occasional olive oil rubdown. Just work the oil into the dry areas of your glove with a soft cloth, let it set for 30 minutes, then wipe off any excess. Your game may not improve, but at least it won't be your glove's fault. Some people prefer to use bath oil to recondition their baseball glove (see page 77).

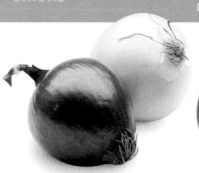
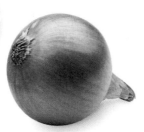

ONIONS

ELIMINATE NEW PAINT SMELL

Your bedroom's new shade of paint looks great, but the smell is keeping you up all night. What to do? Place several freshly cut slices of onion in a dish with a bit of water. It will absorb the smell within a few hours.

REMOVE RUST FROM KNIVES • Forget about using steel wool or harsh chemicals—how's this for an easy way to get the rust off your kitchen or utility knives? Plunge your rusty knife into a large onion three or four times (if it's very rusty, it may require a few extra stabs). The only tears you shed will be ones of joy over your rust-free blade.

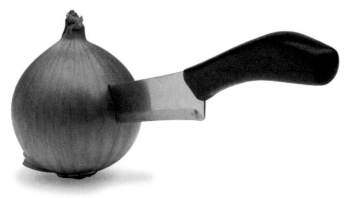

DID YOU KNOW?

How can you keep your eyes from watering when cutting onions? Suggestions range from wearing protective goggles while chopping, to placing a fan behind you to blow away the onion's tear-producing vapors, to rubbing your hands with vinegar before you start slicing. However, the most effective trick is to chill the onions in the freezer for about 30 minutes prior to slicing them. You should also try cutting off the top portion and peeling off the outer layers, but leave the root end intact while you're slicing, because it has the highest concentrations of the sulphur compounds that cause your eyes to water.

CORRECT PET 'MISTAKES' • If Rover or Kitty is still not respecting your property—whether it be by chewing, tearing, or soiling—you may be able to get the message across by leaving several onion slices where the damage has been done. Neither cats nor dogs are particularly fond of the smell of onion, so they'll avoid returning to the scene of their crimes.

SOOTHE A BEE STING • If you have a nasty encounter with a bee at a barbecue, grab one of the onion slices intended for your burger and place it over the area where you got stung. It will ease the soreness. (If you are severely allergic to bee or other insect stings, seek medical attention immediately.)

USE AS SMELLING SALTS • If you happen to be at a party or in a restaurant with someone who feels faint—and smelling salts are not on hand—reach for a freshly cut onion instead. The strong odor is likely to bring them around.

USE AS A NATURAL PESTICIDE • Make an effective insect repellent for your garden. In a blender, puree 4 onions, 2 cloves of garlic, 2 tablespoons (30 ml) cayenne pepper, and 1 quart (1 L) water. Set this aside. Now dilute 2 tablespoons (30 ml) soap flakes in 2 gallons (8 L) water. Pour in the contents of the blender, shake well, and you have a potent, earth-friendly solution to spray on your plants.

MAKE MOSQUITO REPELLENT • Some people find that increasing their intake of onions or garlic in the summer—or rubbing a slice of onion over their exposed skin—is a good way to keep away mosquitoes and other biting insects.

ORANGES

USE FOR KINDLING • Dried orange and lemon peels are a far superior choice for use as kindling than newspaper. Not only do they smell better and produce less creosote than newspaper, but the flammable oils found inside the peels enable them to burn much longer than paper.

MAKE A POMANDER • Pomanders have been used for centuries to fill small spaces with a delightful fragrance as well as to combat moths. They are also incredibly easy to make. Take a bunch of cloves and stick them into an orange, covering the whole surface. Now suspend your pomander using a piece of string, wool, or monofilament fishing line inside a closet or cupboard, and it will keep the space smelling fresh for years.

SIMMER FOR STOVETOP POTPOURRI • Fill your abode with a refreshing citrus scent by simmering several orange and/or lemon peels in 1–2 cups (250–500 ml) water in an aluminium saucepan for a few hours, adding water as needed. This process freshens up the pot as well as the air in your home.

KEEP CATS OFF YOUR LAWN • Are the neighbor's cats still mistaking your lawn for their litter box? Gently point them elsewhere by making a mixture of orange peels and coffee grounds and distributing it around the cats' favorite spots. If they don't take the hint, lay down a second batch and try moistening it with a bit of water.

APPLY AS A MOSQUITO REPELLENT • If you're not crazy about the idea of rubbing onions all over yourself to keep away mosquitoes (*see page 210*), you may be happy to know that you can often get similar results by rubbing fresh orange or lemon peels over your exposed skin. It's said that mosquitoes and gnats are totally repulsed by either scent.

SHOW ANTS THE DOOR • Get rid of the ants in your garden, on your patio, and along the foundation of your home. In a blender, make a smooth puree of a few orange peels in 1 cup (250 ml) warm water. Slowly pour the solution over and into anthills to send the little pests packing. Repeat if they return.

OVEN CLEANER

PUT THE STYLE BACK IN YOUR CURLING IRONS • Before using curling irons that have caked-on gel or hair product stuck to them, spray on a light coating of oven cleaner. Let it sit for an hour, wipe it off with a damp rag, and dry with a clean cloth. Make very sure that you don't use the tongs until they are thoroughly dry.

WIPE AWAY A BATHTUB RING • Get rid of stubborn stains or a ring around your white porcelain bathtub by spraying it with oven cleaner. Let it sit for a few hours and give it a thorough rinsing.
WARNING: Do not apply oven cleaner to colored porcelain tubs; it could cause fading. And be careful not to get the oven cleaner on your shower curtain, as it can ruin both plastic and fabric.

more OVEN CLEANER over →

211

CLEAN GRIMY TILE GROUT LINES • Ready for an all-out attack on grout grunge? First, make sure you have plenty of ventilation: It's a good idea to use your exhaust fan to suck air out of a small bathroom. Then put on your rubber gloves and spray oven cleaner into the grout lines. Wipe the cleaner off with a sponge within 5 seconds. Rinse thoroughly with water to reveal sparkling grout lines.

CLEAN OVENPROOF GLASS COOKWARE • If you've tried everything to scrub baked-on stains from your Pyrex or CorningWare, try this. Put on rubber gloves and cover the cookware with oven cleaner. Place the cookware in a heavy-duty garbage bag, close it tightly with twist ties, and leave it overnight. Open the bag outdoors, keeping your face away from the dangerous fumes. Use rubber gloves to remove and wash the cookware.

CLEAN A CAST-IRON FRYING PAN

If you need to clean and re-season an encrusted secondhand cast-iron skillet you found at a garage sale, start by giving it a good spraying with oven cleaner and placing it in a sealed plastic bag overnight. (This keeps the cleaner working by preventing it from drying.) The next day, remove the pot and scrub it with a stiff wire brush. Wash it thoroughly with soap and water, rinse well, and immediately dry it with a couple of clean, dry cloths. This technique eliminates built-up gunk and grease, but not rust. For that, you'll need to use vinegar. Don't leave it on too long, though. Prolonged exposure to vinegar can damage cast-iron cookware.

CAUTION: Most oven cleaners contain highly caustic lye, which can burn your skin and damage your eyes. Always wear long rubber gloves and protective eyewear when using oven cleaner. The mist from oven-cleaner spray can irritate nasal membranes. Ingestion can cause corrosive burns to the mouth, throat, and stomach that require immediate medical attention. Store oven cleaner well out of children's reach.

REMOVE STAINS FROM CONCRETE • Get those unsightly grease, oil, and transmission fluid stains off your concrete driveway or garage floor by spraying them with oven cleaner. Let it settle for 5 to 10 minutes, scrub with a stiff brush, and rinse it off with your garden hose at its highest pressure. Severe stains may require a second application.

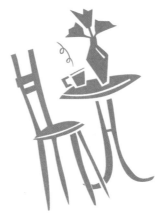

STRIP PAINT OR VARNISH • For an easy way to remove paint or varnish from wooden or metal furniture, try using a can of oven cleaner; it costs less than commercial paint strippers and is easier to apply (if you spray rather than brush it on). After applying, scrub off the old paint with a wire brush. Neutralize the stripped surface by coating it with vinegar, and wash it off with clean water. Allow the wood or metal to thoroughly dry before repainting. Don't use oven cleaner to strip antiques or expensive furnishings; it can darken the wood or discolor the metal.

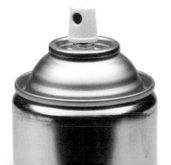

OVEN MITTS

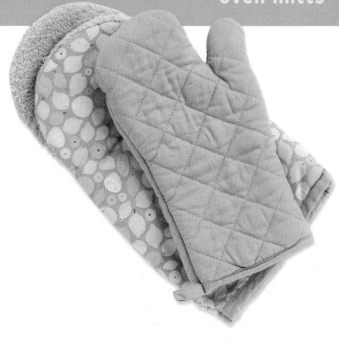

USE AS A BEVERAGE COSY OR EGG WARMER • Keep that mug of java or tea from getting cold when you're called away by placing an oven mitt over it. The mitt's insulation will keep it warm until you get back. You can also use an oven mitt to keep boiled eggs warm for up to half an hour. Conversely, an oven mitt will help keep a cold drink colder longer.

USE FOR DUSTING AND POLISHING • Although oven mitts are typically confined to kitchen duty, they're actually great for dusting and polishing around your house. Use one side of the mitt to apply wax or polish to your furniture and the other side to buff it up. It's a great way to use clean, old mitts or all those extra ones you've collected.

PROTECT YOUR HANDS WHEN PRUNING • Oven mitts are too awkward to use for weeding or planting seedlings, but they can come in handy when pruning trees, hedges, and bushes—particularly thorny ones, such as holly, bougainvillea, and rosebushes.

REMOVE HOT ENGINE PARTS • Keeping an oven mitt in your car's glove compartment or trunk can make life a lot easier when you are confronted with a hot radiator cap or any other too-hot-to-handle parts during a roadside emergency.

CHANGE A HOT LIGHTBULB • When the lightbulb on your reading lamp blows out, don't scorch your fingers when replacing it. Once you've removed the lampshade, put on an oven mitt, remove the dead bulb from the socket, and toss it into the garbage can. That way, you won't still be blowing on your fingertips when screwing in the new bulb.

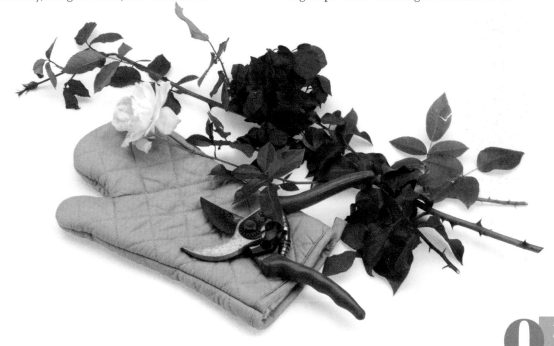

P PAINTBRUSHES

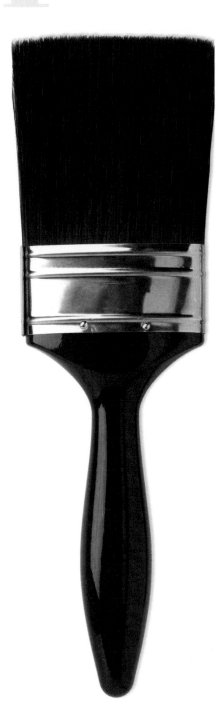

BRUSH OFF SAND • Keep a clean, dry paintbrush in your car specifically for those return trips from the beach. Use it to remove sand from beach chairs, towels, toys, the kids, and even yourself before you open the car door or trunk. You'll wind up with a lot less to vacuum the next time you clean your vehicle.

DUST DELICATE ITEMS • A feather duster or dust rag is fine for cleaning shelves and such, but neither one is much good when you need to get into the tiny cracks and crevices of chandeliers, wicker furniture, baskets, and knickknacks. That's when a small, natural-bristle paintbrush is indispensable. The soft bristles are perfect for cleaning out areas that are otherwise impossible to reach. It's also great for dusting delicate items such as porcelain or carved wooden figurines.

CLEAN OUT A TOASTER • Toasters are notoriously difficult to clean, so much so that many forgo the task entirely. Armed with an unused narrow paintbrush, you can easily clean out the crumb tray and any particles trapped in the slots. Always make sure the toaster is unplugged before attempting any cleaning.

COVER UP SEEDS WHEN SOWING • Sow your seeds with a little TLC. When planting seeds in rows, use large a paintbrush to gently brush them over with soil. This lets you distribute the exact amount of soil needed and prevents overpacking.

CLEAN YOUR WINDOW SCREENS • Are your window screens screaming for a good cleaning? Use a large, clean paintbrush to give them a good dusting. Shake off the brush, dip it into a small dish of kerosene and 'paint' both sides of your screens. Dry off the mesh with a clean cloth.

KEYBOARD CLEANING • Removing debris from your computer's keyboard is essential, but cleaning in those cracks and crevices is a challenge. Keep a small, unused fine-bristle paintbrush at your desk and you can clean the keyboard when the impulse strikes. It's also great for getting rid of the gunk that collects in the hinges of a laptop.

APPLY STAIN REMOVER TO CLOTHES

Let's face it, pouring detergent or stain remover onto a soiled garment is often a hit-or-miss proposition. And when you miss, it usually involves grabbing paper towels to soak up a spill. Make life little a easier by using a small paintbrush to apply liquid stain remover to dirty shirt collars and cuffs. It's neater and a lot more accurate.

GREASE IS THE WORD • You don't need fancy cooking spray to coat loaf pans or muffin tins when baking. Just use a clean paintbrush to evenly apply grease, butter, or oil to your pans. With a paintbrush, you can thoroughly cover the sides and really get into those corners. No more cake sticking to the bottom.

ADD TEXTURES TO FROSTING • Use a spatula or knife to spread frosting on a cake but to take it to the next level, try a paintbrush. To add texture, try different sizes and bristle types (coarse to fine) and create swirls and peaks, too. DIY sites with videos on the web can show you how it's done.

BRUSH ON THE SAUCE • A small synthetic-bristle paintbrush can be invaluable in the kitchen. You can use it to brush on pie glaze, marinades, and sauces while baking or roasting. It's also great for painting on barbecue sauce when grilling burgers and steaks outdoors. Best of all, a paintbrush is easier to clean than most conventional pastry brushes.

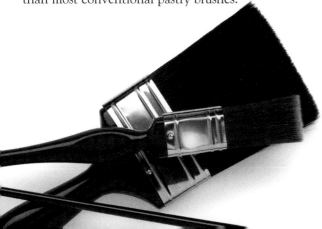

Buying and cleaning paintbrushes

Natural-bristle brushes work best with alkyd/oil-based paint. But use a synthetic-bristle brush with acrylic paint because the water in the paint can ruin natural bristles.

Before cleaning any brush, wipe off any excess paint on newspaper. Clean a brush used with oil-based paint in mineral spirits (turpentine) until you get out all the paint, and then shake it out. To clean out acrylic paint, wash the brush thoroughly with soapy water, rinse clean, and then shake it out. Many acrylic paints contain acrylics that won't wash out completely with soap and water. In this case, finish cleaning up with mineral spirits.

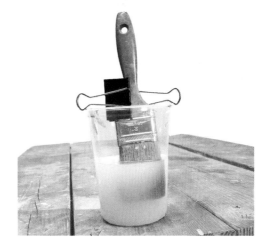

SOAK PAINTBRUSHES WITHOUT BENDING THE BRISTLES •
You're done painting for the day and just want to soak the brush overnight. If you stick it in a jar, the bristles wil touch the bottom and ruin your brush. Here's a simple fix: Attach a large binder clip around the handle (see above) and spread the arms out to span your container so the bristles don't touch bottom. When you're ready to paint, clean off your brush and go.

33 USES!

PANTYHOSE
around the house

• • •

FIND SMALL OBJECTS • Have you ever spent hours on your hands and knees searching through a carpet for a lost gemstone, contact lens, or some other tiny, precious item? If not, count yourself among the lucky few. Should you ever be faced with this situation, try this. Cut a leg off an old pair of pantyhose—make sure the toe section is intact—and pull it up over the nozzle of your vacuum cleaner hose. (If you want additional security, you can even cut off the other leg and slip that over as well.) Secure the hose in place with a tightly wound rubber band. Turn on the vacuum, move the nozzle over the carpet and you'll soon find your lost valuable attached to the pantyhose filter.

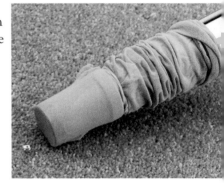

VACUUM YOUR FISH TANK

If you have a wet-and-dry vacuum, you can change the water in your fish tank without disturbing the gravel and tank accessories. (You'll still have to relocate the fish, of course.) Just pull the foot of old nylon pantyhose over the end of the vacuum's nozzle, secure it with a rubber band, and you are ready to suck out the water.

BUFF YOUR SHOES • Bring out the shine in your freshly polished shoes by buffing them with a medium-length strip of pantyhose. It works so well, you may retire that chamois cloth for good.

WRAP UP WRAPPING PAPER • Keep your used rolls of wrapping paper from tearing and unravelling by storing them in tubes made by cutting the leg sections off old pairs of pantyhose. (Don't forget to leave the foot section intact.) Or, if you have a bunch of used rolls, you can simply put one in each leg of a pair of pantyhose and hang them over a hanger in your closet.

KEEP YOUR HAIRBRUSH CLEAN • If you dread the prospect of cleaning out your hairbrush, here's a way to make the job much easier. Cut a 2-inch (5-cm) strip from the leg section of a pair of old pantyhose and stretch it over and around the bristles of your new (or newly cleaned) hairbrush. If necessary, use a bobby pin or a comb to push the hose down over the bristles. The next time your brush needs cleaning, simply lift up and remove the pantyhose layer— along with all the dead hair, lint, and dust on top— and replace it with a fresh strip.

REMOVE NAIL POLISH • If you can't find the cotton balls you've been looking for, just moisten strips of recycled pantyhose with nail polish remover to take off your old nail polish. Cut the hose material into 3-inch (7.5-cm) squares and store a stack of them in an old bandage container or makeup case.

KEEP SPRAY BOTTLES CLOG-FREE • If you recycle your spray bottles to use with homemade cleaners or furniture polishes, you can prevent any potential clogs by covering the open end of the tube—the part that goes inside the bottle—with a small, square-cut piece of pantyhose held in place with a small rubber band. This works especially well for filtering garden sprays that are mixed from concentrates.

SUBSTITUTE FOR STUFFING • Is your kid's teddy bear or doll losing its stuffing? Get out a needle and thread and prepare the patient for an emergency 'stuffing transplant'. Replace the lost filler with narrow strips of clean, worn-out pantyhose (ball them up, if possible). Stitch the hole up well and a complete recovery is guaranteed. This works well with throw pillows and seat cushions, too.

ORGANIZE YOUR SUITCASE • As any seasoned traveler knows, you can squeeze more of your belongings into any piece of luggage by rolling up your clothes. To keep your bulkier rolls from unwrapping, cover them in flexible nylon tubes. Simply cut the legs off a pair of old pantyhose, snip off the foot sections and stretch the stockings over your rolled-up garments. Happy travels!

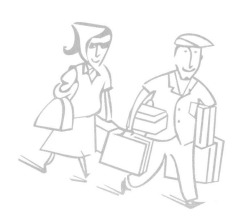

TAKE A CITRUS BATH • Make your own scented bath oil by drying and grinding up orange and/or lemon peels and pouring them into the foot section of recycled pantyhose. Put a knot about 1 inch (2.5 cm) above the peels and leave another 6 inches (15 cm) or so of hose above that before cutting off the remainder. Tie the stocking to the bathtub faucet with the peels suspended below the running water. As well as giving your bath a fresh citrus fragrance, you can use the pantyhose to exfoliate your skin.

HOLD MOTHBALLS OR POTPOURRI • Looking for an easy way to store mothballs in your closet or to make sachets of potpourri to keep in your dresser drawers? Pour either ingredient into the toe section of your recycled pantyhose. Knot off the contents, then cut off the remaining hose. If you plan to hang up the mothballs, leave several inches of material before cutting.

more PANTYHOSE over →

MAKE A PONYTAIL SCRUNCHY • Why buy a scrunchy to make a ponytail when you can easily make one for nothing? Cut a horizontal strip about 3 inches (7.5 cm) wide across a pantyhose leg. Wrap it around your ponytail and you've got a scrunchy!

USE TO HANG-DRY SWEATERS • Avoid getting clothespin marks on your freshly washed sweater by putting an old pair of pantyhose through the neck of the sweater and running the legs out through the arms. Then hang the sweater to dry on your clothesline by clipping the clothespins onto the pantyhose instead of the wool.

BUNDLE BLANKETS FOR STORAGE • For an effortless and foolproof way to keep blankets and quilts securely bundled before they go into temporary storage, wrap them up in large "rubber bands" made from the waistbands of your used pantyhose. You can reuse the bands year after year if needed.

TIE UP BOXES, NEWSPAPERS, MAGAZINES • If you run out of string or you need something stronger for a large stack of glossy magazines, tie up your bundles of boxes, newspapers, and other types of recyclable paper goods using an old pair of pantyhose. Cut off the legs and waistband, and you'll be able to tie up almost anything securely.

in the kitchen

STORE ONIONS IN CUTOFF BUNDLES • Get the maximum shelf life out of your onions by hanging them in nylon holders that provide the good air circulation needed to keep them fresh.

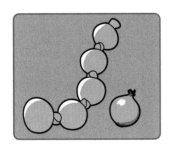

Place the onions one at a time into the leg of a clean pair of pantyhose. Work the first one down to the foot section, then tie a knot above it and add the next one. Repeat until done. Cut off the remaining hose and hang in a cool, dry area of your kitchen. To remove an onion, snip off a knot, starting from the bottom, and the onion will slip out.

MAKE A POT OR DISH SCRUBBER • Make a do-it-yourself scrubbing pad by crumpling up a pair of clean, old pantyhose moistened with a bit of warm water and a couple of drops of dishwashing liquid added. You can also make terrific scrubbers for dishes —as well as walls and other nonporous surfaces— by cutting off the foot or toe section, fitting it over a sponge and knotting off the end.

MAKE A FLOUR DUSTER • Looking for a simple way to dust baking dishes and surfaces with exactly the right amount of flour? Just cut the foot section off a clean, old pantyhose leg, fill it with flour, tie a knot in it and keep it in your flour jar. Give your new flour dispenser a few gentle shakes whenever you need to dust flour onto a baking pan or prepare a surface for rolling out dough for breads or pastries.

KEEP A ROLLING PIN FROM STICKING

Getting dough to the perfect consistency is an art form in itself. Although you can add water to dough that's too dry, it often results in a gluey consistency that winds up sticking to your rolling pin. Avoid the hassle of scraping your rolling pin clean by covering it with a piece of pantyhose. It will hold enough flour to keep even the wettest dough from sticking to the pin.

SECURE GARBAGE BAGS • How many times have you opened your kitchen garbage can only to discover that the liner has slipped down, and that someone in your house has covered it over with fresh garbage anyway? You can prevent such 'accidents' by firmly securing the garbage bag or liner to your garbage can with the elastic waistband from a recycled pair of pantyhose; tie a knot in the band to keep it tight. You can also use this method to keep garbage bags from slipping off the edge of your outdoor trash cans.

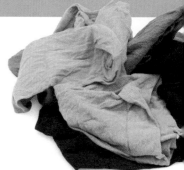

DID YOU KNOW?

You have probably heard that you can temporarily replace a broken fan belt with pantyhose in an emergency. Well, don't believe it—it won't work! Pulleys in most vehicles require flat belts, not the rounded shape pantyhose would present. Even on a V-belt pulley, they fly off as soon as the engine starts. A much better idea is to replace the belts before they get in bad condition.

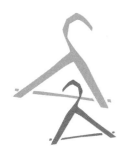

DUST UNDER THE FRIDGE • Having trouble catching all that dust residing underneath and alongside your refrigerator? Round it up by balling up a pair of old pantyhose and attaching it with a rubber band to a coat hanger or broomstick. The dust and dirt will cling to the nylon, which can easily be washed off before being called back into dusting duty.

in the garden

STAKE DELICATE PLANTS • Give your young plants and trees the support they need. Use strips of pantyhose to attach them to your garden stakes. The nylon's flexibility will stretch as the seedlings or saplings fill out and mature—unlike string or wool, which can actually damage plant stalks if you tie it too tightly.

STORE FLOWER BULBS IN WINTER • Pantyhose legs make terrific sacks for storing your flower bulbs over winter, since they let air freely circulate around the bulbs to prevent rotting. Simply cut a leg off a pair of pantyhose and place your bulbs inside, knot off the end and place ID tags on each sack using a strip of masking tape. Hang them up in a cool, dry place and they'll be ready for planting in the spring.

PREVENT SOIL EROSION IN HOUSEPLANTS • When moving a houseplant to a larger or more appropriate-sized container, put a piece of pantyhose at the bottom of the new pot. It will act as a liner that lets the excess water flow out without draining the soil along with it.

SUPPORT MELONS • Keep small melons, such as cantaloupes and honeydews, off the ground—and free of pests and diseases—by making protective sleeves for them from your old pantyhose. Cut the legs off the pantyhose. As your young melons start to develop, slide each one into the foot section and tie the leg to a stake to suspend the melon above the ground. The nylon holders will stretch as the melons mature, while keeping them from touching the damp soil, where they would be susceptible to rot or invasion by hungry insects and other garden pests.

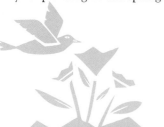

more PANTYHOSE over →

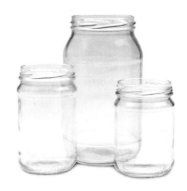

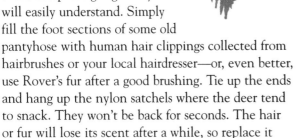

KEEP DEER OUT OF YOUR GARDEN • If you've been catching Bambi and friends nibbling on your crops, put up a 'No Trespassing' sign they will easily understand. Simply fill the foot sections of some old pantyhose with human hair clippings collected from hairbrushes or your local hairdresser—or, even better, use Rover's fur after a good brushing. Tie up the ends and hang up the nylon satchels where the deer tend to snack. They won't be back for seconds. The hair or fur will lose its scent after a while, so replace it every four or five days as needed.

CLEAN UP AFTER GARDENING • Here are two recycling tips in one: Save your leftover slivers of soap and place them in the foot section of an old pair of pantyhose. Knot it off and hang it next to an outdoor faucet. Use the soap-filled hose to quickly wash off your hands after gardening and other outdoor work without worrying about getting dirt on the door handles or bathroom fixtures indoors.

COVER A KIDS' INSECT JAR

What child doesn't like to catch fireflies–and hopefully release them–on a warm summer night? When making an insect jar for your child, don't bother using a hammer and nail to punch holes in the jar's metal lid (in fact, save the lids for other projects). It's much easier to just cut a 6-inch (15-cm) square from an old pair of pantyhose and attach to the jar with a rubber band. A nylon cover lets plenty of air into the jar, and makes it easier to get the insects in and out.

for the do-it-yourselfer ● ● ●

APPLY STAIN TO WOOD CREVICES • Getting wood stain or varnish into the tight corners and crevices of an unfinished bookcase or table that you just bought can be maddening. A brush often just won't fit into them and give them an even coating. But there's really nothing to it once you know the secret. Just cut a strip from an old pair of pantyhose, fold it over a few times and use a rubber band to fix it to the tip of a wooden popsicle stick. Dip your homemade applicator into the stain or varnish and you'll have no trouble getting into those hard-to-reach spots.

PATCH A HOLE IN A SCREEN • Don't invite insects in for a bite. Use a small square of pantyhose to temporarily patch holes in window screens. You can secure each patch by simply applying some rubber cement around the holes before pressing the patch in place. When you're ready to fix the holes with a piece of screening, peel off the nylon and the glue. If you want the patches to last a bit longer, sew them onto the window screen.

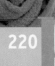

TEST A SANDED SURFACE FOR SNAGS • Think you did a pretty good job sanding down a woodworking project? Put it to the pantyhose test. Wrap a long piece of pantyhose around the palm of your hand and rub it over the wood. If the pantyhose snags on any spots, sand them until you're able to freely move the nylon over the surface without any catches.

CLEAN YOUR POOL • Want a more effective way to skim the debris off the surface of your pool water? Cut a leg off a pair of pantyhose and fit it over your pool's skimmer basket. It will catch a lot of tiny dirt particles and hairs that would otherwise make their way into—and possibly clog—your pool's filter unit.

MAKE A PAINT STRAINER • Strain your paint like the pros, by using a pantyhose filter to remove lumps of paint from an old can of paint. First, cut a leg off a pair of old pantyhose, clip the foot off the leg, and make a cut along the leg's length so that you have a flat piece of nylon. Cut the leg into 12-inch (30-cm) sections to make the filters. Stretch the nylon over a clean bucket or other receptacle and hold it in place with a rubber band or perhaps even the waistband from the pantyhose. Now slowly pour the paint into the bucket.

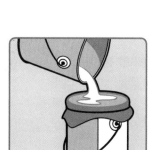

PAPER BAGS
around the house

26 USES!

DUST OFF YOUR MOPS • Dust mops make it a breeze to get the dust bunnies and pet hair around your home, but how do you get the stuff off the mop? Place a large paper bag over the mop head and use a piece of string or a rubber band to keep it from slipping off. Now give it several good shakes (a few gentle bumps wouldn't hurt either). Lay the mop on its side for a few minutes to let the dust in the bag settle. Then carefully remove the bag for easy disposal of your dusty dirt.

more PAPER BAGS over →

paper bags

PAPER BAGS

paper bags

paper bags

paper bags

PAPER BAGS

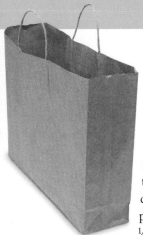

CLEAN ARTIFICIAL FLOWERS • Authentic silk flowers are actually pretty rare these days. Most are now made of nylon or some other man-made material. Whether they're silk or something else, you can easily freshen them up by placing them in a paper bag with ¼ cup (50 g) salt. Give the bag a few gentle shakes and your flowers will emerge as clean as the day you purchased them.

CARRY YOUR LAUNDRY • If your laundry basket is overflowing or the plastic handle suddenly gives out, you can always use a sturdy paper shopping bag to pick up the slack. A bag with handles will probably make the job easier, but any large bag will do in a pinch. Just make sure your laundry is completely dry before using the bag on the return trip. Otherwise, your freshly cleaned clothes could wind up under your feet.

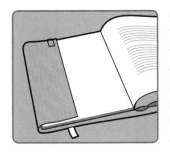

COVER YOUR KIDS' TEXTBOOKS • Helping your children make book covers for their textbooks isn't only fun, it's also a subtle way to teach kids to respect public property. And few materials rival a paper bag when it comes to making a rugged book cover. Firstly, cut the bag along its seams to make it a flat, wide rectangle, then place the book in the center. Then fold in the top and bottom edges so the bag is only slightly wider than the book's height. Next, fold over the sides to form sleeves over the book covers. Cut off the excess, leaving a few inches on either side to slide over the front and back covers. Put a piece of masking tape on the top and bottom of each sleeve (over the paper, not the book) to keep it on tightly and you're done. Lastly, let your child put his or her personal design on each cover.

CREATE A TABLE DECORATION • Use a small designer shopping bag with handles to make an attractive centerpiece for your dining room table or mantelpiece. Fill a small cup with some water and place it in the middle of the bag. Place a few freshly cut flowers in the glass and it's done.

MAKE YOUR OWN WRAPPING PAPER • When you need to wrap a present in a hurry, don't rush out to buy wrapping paper. Just cut a large paper bag along the seams until it's a flat rectangle. Position it so that any printing is facing up at you, put your gift on top, and fold, cut, and tape the paper around your gift. If you wish, personalize your homemade wrapping paper by decorating it with markers, paint, or stickers.

REUSE AS GIFT BAGS

What to do with those small gift bags with handles favored by most boutiques? Why not use them to hold your own gifts? They're ideal for items such as bath supplies, jewelry, perfume, and even

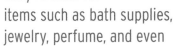

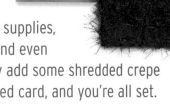

most books. Simply add some shredded crepe paper, a personalized card, and you're all set.

RECYCLE AS TOWEL OR TISSUE DISPENSERS • Add a simple but elegant touch to your guest bathrooms by using small "boutique bags" as paper towel or tissue dispensers. You can even embellish them with your own personal touches, such as ribbons or stickers that match your decor.

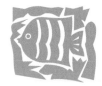

RESHAPE KNITS AFTER WASHING • Put the shape back into your woolen sweater or mittens by tracing the contours of the item on a paper bag before you wash it. Then use your outline to stretch the item back to its original shape after washing it.

STORE LINEN SETS • Have you ever emptied the contents of your linen closet looking for the flat sheet to match the fitted one you just pulled out? You can easily spare yourself some grief by using medium-sized paper bags to store your complete linen sets. Not only will your shelves be better organized, but you can also keep your linens smelling fresh by placing a used fabric softener sheet in each bag.

USE AS A PRESSING CLOTH • If your ironing board's cover appears to have seen its last steam iron, don't worry. You can easily make a temporary pressing cloth by splitting open one or two paper bags. Dampen the bags and lay them over your ironing board to get those last few shirts or skirts pressed in time for the work week.

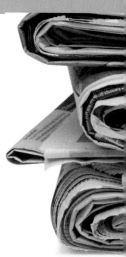

DID YOU KNOW?

Are paper shopping bags really better for the environment than their plastic counterparts? Not according to the Environmental Protection Agency. Paper bags generate 70 percent more air pollutants and 50 times more water pollutants than plastic bags. What's more, it takes four times as much energy to make a paper bag as it does to manufacture a plastic bag and 91 percent *more energy* to recycle paper than plastic. On the other hand, paper bags come from a renewable resource (trees), while most plastic bags are made from nonrenewable resources (polyethylene). So what's the answer? Take your own reuseable cloth shopping bags with you when you go to the supermarket!

BAG YOUR RECYCLED NEWSPAPERS

Double up on your recycling efforts by using large paper bags to hold your newspapers for collection. It not only spares you the time and effort needed to tie up the bundles with string, but it also makes it easier to sort out your magazines, newspapers, and glossy pages.

PACK YOUR BAGS • Getting ready to leave on a family holiday? Don't forget to pack a few large paper shopping bags–the kind with handles–in your luggage. They're guaranteed to come in handy for bringing home the souvenirs you pick up, or your soiled laundry, or beach towels.

in the kitchen

MAKE CLEANUPS EASIER • Cut open one or two paper bags and spread them out over your countertop when peeling vegetables, husking corn, shelling peas, or doing any other messy job. When you're done, simply fold up the paper and toss it into the compost heap for fast and easy clean-up.

KEEP BREAD FRESH • If you live in a high-humidity area, your bread will stay fresher if it's stored inside a paper bag rather than those plastic ones that they are sold in. Paper's ability to "breathe" will keep the bread's crust crisp while allowing the center of the loaf to stay soft and moist.

more PAPER BAGS over →

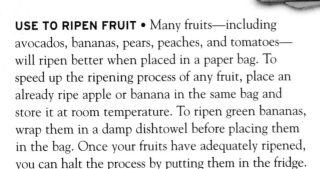

USE TO RIPEN FRUIT • Many fruits—including avocados, bananas, pears, peaches, and tomatoes—will ripen better when placed in a paper bag. To speed up the ripening process of any fruit, place an already ripe apple or banana in the same bag and store it at room temperature. To ripen green bananas, wrap them in a damp dishtowel before placing them in the bag. Once your fruits have adequately ripened, you can halt the process by putting them in the fridge.

STORE MUSHROOMS • Remove your store-bought mushrooms from their mesh packaging and place them in a paper bag inside your refrigerator to keep them fresh for up to five days.

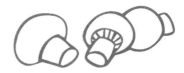

in the garden

STORE GERANIUMS IN WINTER • If you live in an area of snow or heavy frost, you can help your geraniums survive the winter. First, remove the plants from their pots or carefully dig them up from your flower bed, shake off as much soil as possible, and place each plant in its own paper bag. Cover each bag with a second paper bag turned upside down and store them in a cool, dry place. When spring arrives, cut off all but 1 inch (2.5 cm) of stem and repot. Place them in a sunny spot, water regularly, and watch your plants 'spring' back to life.

FEED YOUR PLANTS • Bonemeal is an excellent source of nutrients for all the plants in your garden. You can easily make your own by drying your leftover chicken bones in a microwave (depending on the quantity, cook them for 1 to 4 minutes on *High*). Then place the dried bones in a sturdy paper bag and grind them up using a mallet, hammer, or rolling pin. When done, distribute the powder around your plants and watch them thrive.

ADD TO COMPOST • Brown paper bags are a great addition to any garden compost heap. Not only do they contain less ink and pigment than newsprint, but they will also attract more earthworms to your pile. In fact, the only thing the worms like better than paper bags is cardboard. It's best to shred and wet the bags before adding to your pile. Also, make sure you mix them in well to prevent them from blowing away after they dry.

Kids' Stuff

Make a life-sized body poster of your child. Start by cutting up 4-6 paper bags so they lie completely flat (any print should be facing downwards). Arrange them into one big square on the floor and tape the undersides together. Then have your child lie down in the middle and use a crayon to trace the outline of his or her entire body. Give him or her crayons or watercolor paints to fill in the face, clothing and other details. When your child is finished, hang it up in his or her room as an unique and fun wall decoration.

DRY YOUR HERBS • To dry fresh herbs, first wash each plant under cold water and dry thoroughly with paper towels. Make sure the plants are completely dry before you proceed, to reduce the risk of them getting moldy. Take five or six plants, remove the lower leaves, and place them upside down inside a large paper bag. Gather the end of the bag around the stems and tie it up. Punch a few holes in the bag for ventilation and store it in a warm, dry area for at least two weeks. Once the plants have dried, inspect them carefully for any signs of mold. If you find any, toss out the whole bunch. You can grind them up, once you've removed the stems, with a rolling pin or a full soft-drink bottle, or keep them whole to retain the flavor longer. Store your dried herbs in airtight containers and away from sunlight.

MOVE SNOW OFF YOUR WINDSHIELD • If you're tired of having to constantly scrape ice and snow off your car's windshield during the winter months, keep some paper bags on hand. When there's snow in the forecast, go out to your car and turn on the wipers. Shut off the engine with the wipers positioned near the middle of your windshield. Now, split open a couple of paper bags and use your car's wipers to hold them in place. After the last snowflake falls, pull off the paper to instantly clear your windshield. To prevent damaging your car's wipers, don't turn on the ignition until you've removed the snow and paper from the windshield.

MAKE A FIRE STARTER • Looking for an easy way to get a fire going in your fireplace? Simply fill a paper bag with some balled-up newspaper and perhaps some bits of candle wax. Stick the bag under your logs, light it, then sit back and enjoy your roaring fire.

BUILD A BAG KITE • Make a simple bag kite for your children to play with by folding over the top of a paper bag to keep it open. Glue on pieces of party streamers under the fold. Reinforce the kite by gluing in some strips of balsa wood or a few thin twigs along the length of the bag. Poke a couple of holes above the opened end and attach two pieces of string or wool. Put a piece of masking or transparent tape over the holes to prevent them from tearing, and tie the ends onto a roll of kite string. It should take off when the kids start running.

SPRAY-PAINT SMALL ITEMS • You don't have to make a mess every time you need to spray-paint a small item. Just place the object to be painted inside a large paper shopping bag and spray away. The bag will contain the excess spray. Once the item has dried, simply remove it and toss away the bag.

PAPER CLIPS

USE AS HOOKS FOR HANGING • Paper clips make great impromptu hooks. Making a hanging ceramic plaque? Insert a large, sturdy paper clip on the back before the clay hardens.

USE AS A ZIPPER PULL • Don't throw away your jacket or personal organizer just because the zipper-pull broke. Untwist a small paper clip enough to slip it through the hole. Twist it closed and zip! For a more decorative look, thread beads over the paper clip or glue on sequins.

OPEN SHRINK-WRAPPED COMPACT DISCS

Opening shrink-wrap, especially on CDs, can be a test of skill and patience! To save your fingernails and teeth from destruction, just twist out the end of a paper clip and slice the wrap. To prevent scratches, slip the clip under the folded section of wrap and lift up.

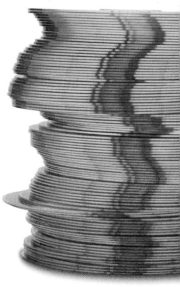

more PAPER CLIPS over →

HOLD THE END OF TRANSPARENT TAPE • If you've got a roll of transparent tape without a dispenser, don't drive yourself nuts trying to locate and lift the end of the tape. Simply stick a paper clip under the end the next time you use the roll.

MAKE A BOOKMARK • Paper clips make great bookmarks because they don't fall out. A piece of ribbon or colorful string attached to the clip will make it even easier to use and find.

PIT CHERRIES • Need a seedless cherry for a recipe? Don't like to pit the cherry while you're eating it? Clip it to pit it! Over a bowl or sink, unfold a clean paper clip at the center and, depending on the size of the cherry, insert either the clip's large or small end through the top. Loosen the pit and pull. To pit cherries but leave stems intact, insert the clip in the bottom. Cherry juice stains, so watch your clothing.

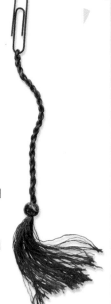

EXTEND A CEILING-FAN CHAIN • Put away the stepladder and put an end to your ballet routine while trying to reach a broken or too-short ceiling fan chain, if your ceiling fan operates with one. To extend the chain, just fasten a chain of paper clips to its end.

SCIENCE **WORKS!**

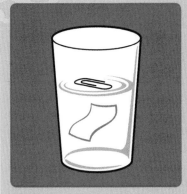

Want to amaze your friends? Challenge them to make a paper clip float on water.

Give them a cup of water and a paper clip. When they fail, show them how to do it. Tear off a piece of paper towel—larger than the clip—and place it on top of the water. Put the paper clip on top of the paper towel and wait a few seconds. The towel will sink, leaving the clip floating. It's magic! Actually, it's the surface tension of the water that allows the clip to float. As the paper towel sinks, it lowers the paper clip onto the water without breaking the surface tension.

PAPER PLATES

PROTECT STORED DISHES
Prevent stored dishes from clattering and breaking, especially when you are moving, by inserting a paper plate between each dish when packing.

MAKE INDEX CARDS • It's inevitable—at the eleventh hour your child tells you they need index cards to deliver a presentation. If you don't have any, use paper plates and a ruler. Measure out a 3 x 5-inch (8 x 13-cm) or 4 x 6-inch (10 x 15-cm) card on the plate and cut. Use the first card as a template for the rest.

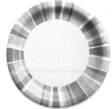

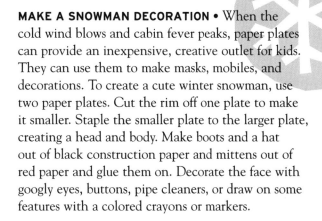

MAKE A PAINT CAN DRIP CATCHER • Painters more often than not scrape the paintbrush on the side of the can to remove excess paint. To prevent drips from falling on the floor, place a paper plate under the can.

MAKE FRISBEE FLASH CARDS • Drilling your kids with flash cards can be a drag, but here's a way to make it fun. Write the numbers, letters, words, or shapes you are teaching on paper plates and let the kids toss them like Frisbees across the room when they get a correct answer.

MAKE A SNOWMAN DECORATION • When the cold wind blows and cabin fever peaks, paper plates can provide an inexpensive, creative outlet for kids. They can use them to make masks, mobiles, and decorations. To create a cute winter snowman, use two paper plates. Cut the rim off one plate to make it smaller. Staple the smaller plate to the larger plate, creating a head and body. Make boots and a hat out of black construction paper and mittens out of red paper and glue them on. Decorate the face with googly eyes, buttons, pipe cleaners, or draw on some features with a colored crayons or markers.

PAPER TOWELS

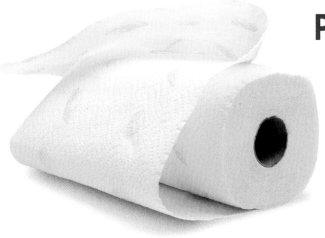

COOK BACON WITHOUT THE MESS • Here's a sure-fire way to cook bacon in a microwave oven. Layer two paper towels on the bottom of your microwave. Lay slices of bacon side by side on the paper towels. Cover with two more paper towels. Run your microwave on *High* at 1-minute intervals, checking for crispness. It should take 3 to 4 minutes to cook. There's no pan to clean and the towels absorb the grease. Toss them in the garbage can for easy cleanup.

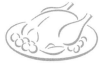

CLEAN SILK FROM FRESH CORN • If you hate picking the silk off a freshly husked ear of corn, a paper towel can help. Dampen one and run it across the ear. The towel picks up the silk and the corn is ready for the boiling pot or the grill.

KEEP PRODUCE FRESH FOR LONGER • Don't you hate it when you open the vegetable crisper in the fridge and find last week's moldy carrots mixed with the now-yellow lettuce? Make your produce last long enough so you can eat it. Line your vegetable crisper with paper towels. They absorb the moisture that causes your fruits and vegetables to rot. It also makes cleaning up the crisper easier.

REMOVE THE FAT FROM STOCK • When a pot of chicken stock has been bubbling for hours, but you don't want to skim off the fat, use a paper towel to absorb it instead. Place another pot in the sink, put a colander (or a sieve) in the new pot and put a paper towel in the colander. Now pour the stock through the paper towel into the waiting pot. You'll find that the fat stays in the paper towel, while the cleaner stock streams through. Make sure you wear oven mitts or use potholders to avoid burning your hands with the boiling-hot liquid.

more PAPER TOWELS over →

paper towels
PAPER TOWELS
paper towels
paper towels
PAPER TOWELS
paper towels

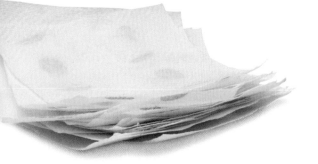

KEEP FROZEN BREAD FROM GETTING SOGGY • If you like to buy bread in bulk, this tip will help you freeze and thaw your bread better. Place a paper towel in each bag of bread to be frozen. When you're ready to eat that frozen loaf, the paper towel absorbs the moisture as the bread thaws.

CLEAN A CAN OPENER

Have you ever noticed that strange gunk that collects on the cutting wheel of your can opener? You don't want that in your food. Clean your can opener by 'opening' a paper towel. Close the wheel on the edge of a paper towel, close the handles, and turn the crank. The paper towel will clean off the gunk as the wheel cuts through it.

KEEP CAST-IRON POTS RUST-FREE • Stop rust from invading your prized collection of cast-iron pots. After they've been cleaned, place a paper towel in each to absorb any moisture. Store lids separately from the pots, separated by a lining of paper towels. This way there won't be any ugly surprises when you reach for the pot again.

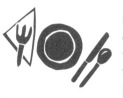

MAKE A PLACEMAT FOR KIDS • Whenever you're having children over to visit, it's a distinct possibility that there will be a big mess to clean up after mealtime. Use paper towels to make cleaning up quick and easy by using a paper towel as a placemat. It will catch spills during the meal and save the trouble of washing fabric placemats.

CLEAN A SEWING MACHINE • If you're worried about getting grease from your sewing machine on the fabric you're sewing, just thread the sewing machine and stitch several lines on a paper towel first. That should take care of any residual grease so you'll be ready to resume your sewing projects.

SCIENCE **WORKS!**

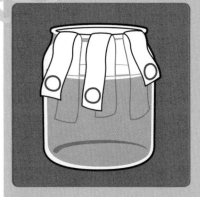

Learn how all other colors are actually mixes of the primary colors of red, blue, and yellow.

Cut a paper towel into strips. With a marker, draw a rectangle or large circle on one end of each strip. Try different shades of orange, green, purple, or brown. Black is good, too. Place the other end of the strip into a glass jar filled with water, leaving the colored end dry and draped over the side of the jar. As the water from the jar slowly (about 20 minutes) moves down the towel and into the color blot, you'll see the colors separate. This also demonstrates capillary attraction—the force that allows the porous paper to soak up the water and carry it over the side of the jar.

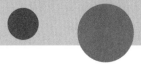

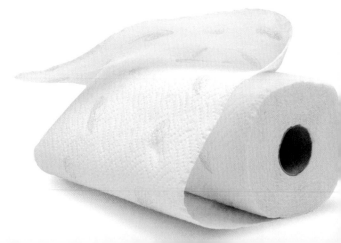

TEST VIABILITY OF OLD SEEDS • If you've got a collection of seed packets hanging around and you just found a packet of watermelon seeds dated two years ago, should you bother to plant them or has their shelf life expired and they're best off planted in the garbage can? To find out for certain, dampen two paper towels and lay down a few seeds. Cover with two more dampened paper towels. Over the next two weeks, keep the towels damp and keep checking on the seeds. If most of the seeds sprout, you can plant the rest of the batch in the garden.

MAKE A BEAUTIFUL KIDS' BUTTERFLY • Use colored markers to draw a bold design on a paper towel. Then lightly spray water on the towel. It should be damp so that the colors start to run, but don't saturate the paper. When the towel is dry, fold it in half, open it up and gather it together using the fold line as your guide. Loop a pipe cleaner around the center to make the body of the butterfly and twist it closed. To make antennae, fold another pipe cleaner into a V shape and slip it under the first one at the top of the butterfly.

PEANUT BUTTER

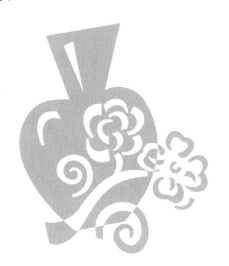

GET CHEWING GUM OUT OF HAIR • If you happen to find that a piece of chewing gum you gave to your child not 10 minutes ago is now a wadded mess in their hair, don't panic. Apply some peanut butter to the wad and rub the gum until it comes out. Your child's hair may smell like peanut butter until you shampoo it, but it's better than having to cut the gum out.

REMOVE PRICE-TAG ADHESIVE • After you've removed the price tag from something you've just purchased, you're often left with that annoying gummy glue on the glass. Remove it easily by rubbing peanut butter on it.

BAIT A MOUSETRAP

When the mice are scurrying around at night, it's time to get tough. Lay traps, but bait them with peanut butter. They can't resist, and it's nearly impossible for them to swipe without tripping the trap. You'll be rid of them in no time.

ELIMINATE STINKY FISH SMELL • If you're trying to eat more fish for health reasons, but hate the smell that hangs around the kitchen after you've cooked it, try this trick. Put a dollop of peanut butter in the frying pan with the frying fish. The peanut butter absorbs the odor instead of your furnishings.

PLUG AN ICE-CREAM CONE • Ice-cream cones are fun to eat but a bit messy, too. Here's a delectable solution. Plug up the bottom of an ice-cream cone with a bit of peanut butter. Now, when munching through a scoop of double chocolate fudge, you'll be protected from leaks. And there's a peanutty surprise at the end of the treat.

PENCIL ERASERS

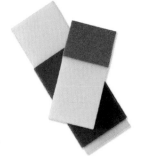

SHINE YOUR COINS • If you've got a rather grimy looking coin collection, but you'd like to see it with more luster, try using a pencil eraser to shine up the coins. Don't do this with rare and valuable coins—you can erase their value along with their surface patina.

STORE PINS OR DRILL BITS • A box is not the most handy place to keep sewing pins. What if the box spills? What if you have a hard time grabbing just one when you're laying out pattern pieces? Here's the solution. Stick pins in a eraser. They won't fall out and it's easy to grab the ones you need. This is also a good tip if you're storing several small drill bits.

CLEAN OFF CRAYON MARKS • If a toddler has gone wild with the crayons and drawn on your walls, not on paper, and you've tried everything to get it off, try using a pencil eraser. You'll be erasing the crayon marks to get the wall back to a clean slate.

REMOVE SCUFF MARKS ON VINYL FLOORS • New black shoes have a bad track record for leaving black streak marks on vinyl flooring. However, a pencil eraser will take them off in no time. Give the kids a eraser each and get them to do it!

CLEAN RESIDUE FROM STICK-ON LABELS • That gray, gummy substance on the new picture frame you just purchased is a sight to behold and not coming off with plain soap and water. Rub the residue with a eraser and watch the stuff just peel away.

CLEAN YOUR PIANO KEYS • Whether it's a baby grand piano that fills the corner of the living room, a more conventional upright, or just a fold-away electronic keyboard, cleaning the keys of dust and fingerprints can be a nightmare project. And when you clean it, it's hard to reach some spots to remove dirt. The sides of black keys are especially difficult to clean. Find a pencil eraser that fits between the ivories and the black keys and you'll have cured the problem. This works well whether you have a piano with real ivory keys or the more common plastic ones.

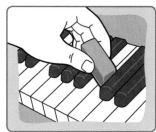

CUSHION PICTURE FRAMES • Don't you hate it when a heavy mirror or picture frame is slightly crooked? If you're tired of worrying about the black marks and scrapes the frame is making on the wall, just glue erasers to the bottom corners of the frame. The pictures will now hang straighter and not leave a mark.

PENCILS

EASE A NEW KEY INTO A LOCK • If you have a new house key made, but it doesn't seem to fit into your front door lock, rub a pencil over the teeth of the key. The graphite powder should help the key slide easily into the lock.

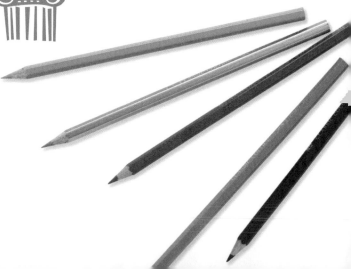

SCIENCE **WORKS!**

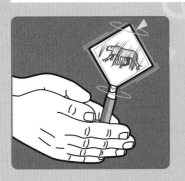

Are your eyes deceiving you?

Cut a small piece of paper, about 2 inches (5 cm) square. Turn the square so it's a diamond. On one side, draw an animal or a person. On the other side, draw a setting for the animal or a hat and hair for a person. Try a zebra and grasslands or a boy with a hat. Next, tape the bottom point of the diamond onto the point of a pencil. Then, holding the pencil so the picture is upright, twirl the pencil rapidly between your hands. You should see both images from the two sides of the paper at the same time.

USE AS A HAIR ACCESSORY • Take a pencil to school to help with your ... hair. A pencil can help give lift to curly hair if you don't have a wide comb. Two pencils crossed in an X can stabilize and decorate a bun, plus provide you with a new writing tool if you lose yours during the day.

DECORATE A PICTURE FRAME • Dress up the frame for this year's class picture with pencils. Glue two sharpened pencils lengthwise to the frame. Sharpen down two other pencils to fit the width of the frame.

REPEL MOTHS WITH PENCIL SHAVINGS • If you're tired of finding your woolen sweaters filled with moth holes after you've stored them for the season, this may help. Empty the wood shavings from a pencil sharpener into little cloth sacks to use as sachets in your closet. The wood shavings will make those pesky moths skedaddle.

STAKE A SMALL PLANT • If you've got a small plant that needs some support, but don't know if it needs watering, a pencil can help with both problems. It's the perfect-sized stake for a small plant, tied with piece of old pantyhose or a cloth strip. Or stick a pencil in the pot of a houseplant to see if the soil needs watering.

LUBRICATE A STICKY ZIPPER • When a zipper gets sticky or the zipper teeth constantly get caught, pick up a pencil and run the lead tip along the teeth of the zipper to unstick them. It works like a charm.

PEPPER

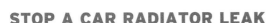

STOP A CAR RADIATOR LEAK

A heat wave has hit your town, and your old, leaking car radiator isn't too happy about it. If it's overheating because of a small leak, pepper can help. Before you bring your car to a mechanic for a more thorough repair, pour a handful of pepper into your radiator. It will temporarily plug the leaks until you can get some professional help.

USE AS A DECONGESTANT • Is your nose stopped up? Are your ears plugged? Do you have a cold? Forget over-the-counter medications. Nothing gets things flowing faster than cayenne pepper. Sprinkle it on your food and rush to grab some tissues.

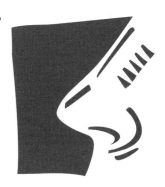

more PEPPER over →

231

KEEP COLORS BRIGHT • That new cherry-red shirt you just purchased is fantastic, but just think how faded the color will look after the shirt has been washed a few times. Add 1 teaspoon (5 ml) of pepper to the wash. Pepper keeps bright colors bright and prevents them from running, too.

GET INSECTS OFF PLANTS • There's nothing more frustrating than a swarm of insects nibbling at your fledgling garden. Just when things are starting to pop up, the insects are there, chewing away. Mix black pepper with flour and sprinkle around your plants.

DETER DEER FROM YOUR GARDEN • If you live in an wooded area with lots of deer, you may soon learn that they will find their way into your garden for a snack. They'll find another place to dine if you spray your bushes with a cayenne-and-water mixture.

DID YOU KNOW?

The black pepper on your table actually starts out as a red berry on a bush. When the pea-sized berry is placed in boiling water for 10 minutes, it shrinks and turns black, becoming the familiar peppercorn that we use to fill our pepper grinders. Of course, some of us skip that step and buy pepper already ground. Either way, black pepper is an ancient spice and the most common one in the world.

KILL AN ANT COLONY • If you find the ants' home colony a little too close to yours and it is causing them to relocate to your kitchen, cayenne pepper can help get rid of it. Pour the pepper down the ant hole and say goodbye to ants.

KEEP ANTS OUT OF THE KITCHEN

Two or three of your annual summer visitors have invaded your kitchen. Those ants are looking for sugar, so give them some pepper instead. Cayenne pepper sprinkled in spots where you see ants, such as the back of countertops or along the baseboards, will send out a clear message to them: "No sugar ahead."

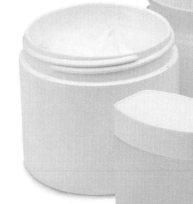

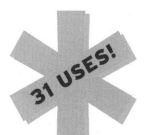
31 USES!

PETROLEUM JELLY
for personal grooming

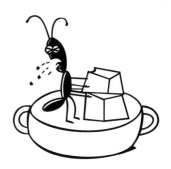

MOISTURIZE YOUR LIPS AND MORE • If you don't want to pay a lot for expensive lip balm, makeup remover, or a facial moisturizer, your answer is a jar of petroleum jelly. It can soothe lips, take off foundation, eye shadow, mascara, and more. It will even act as a light moisturizer for your face.

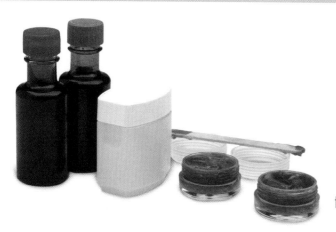

EMERGENCY MAKEUP

Oh no! You've run out of your favorite eye shadow. What do you do now? It's easy! Make your own. Add a bit of food coloring to petroleum jelly and apply as usual. This is a quick way to make some temporary blush, lipstick, or eye shadow.

LENGTHEN THE LIFE OF PERFUME • You've picked out a great scent to wear on your night out, but it's got to last. Worry not; dab a bit of petroleum jelly on your pulse points, then spray on the perfume. Now you can go out knowing your perfume won't turn in early.

SMOOTH WILD EYEBROW HAIRS • If you have runaway eyebrows—the ones where the hairs won't lie flat but curl up instead, control the wildness with some petroleum jelly. Rub a dab into your brows. They'll calm down and behave.

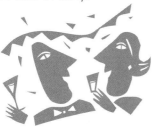

REMOVE A STUCK RING • If you have a ring stuck on your finger, trying to get it off can take a lot of tug and pull, not to mention pain. Apply some petroleum jelly around your finger and it will glide right off.

SOFTEN CHAPPED HANDS • If you're constantly applying hand lotion to your tired, chapped hands, but then taking it off again so you can get more work done, try this tip. Apply a liberal amount of petroleum jelly to your hands just before you go to bed. By morning, they'll be soft and smooth.

NO MORE MESSY MANICURES • During home manicures, keeping nail polish off your cuticles can be tricky. Petroleum jelly can help your manicures look more professional. Dab some along the base of your nails and the sides. If polish seeps off the nail during the manicure, all you do is wipe off the petroleum jelly and the sloppy nail polish is gone.

JELLY BABIES!

HELP PREVENT DIAPER RASH • No Mommy wants to hear a baby experiencing the pain of diaper rash. Help is just a few moments away. Petroleum jelly sets up a protective coating on the skin so the rash can heal. No more pain.

NO MORE SHAMPOO TEARS • Thinking of buying special no-tears shampoo for your child? Forget about it. If you have some petroleum jelly, you have the solution. Rub a fair amount into your baby's eyebrows. It acts as a protective shield against shampoo running down into their eyes.

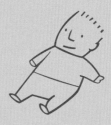

more PETROLEUM JELLY over →

STOP HAIR DYE RUNS • There's nothing more embarrassing than a home hair color job gone awry. Imagine finishing applying that new auburn shade to your tresses when you notice that you've dyed your hairline and part of your forehead, too. Next time, run a bit of petroleum jelly across your hairline. If dye seeps off your hair, the petroleum jelly will catch it.

HEAL WINDBURNED SKIN • You've just been on a fabulous drive through the countryside with the top down, but the drive has left you with an unpleasant souvenir: windburn. Grab a jar of petroleum jelly and apply it liberally to your face or wherever you've been chapped. You'll find that the jelly helps to relieve the pain.

around the house

SMOOTHER CLOSING SHOWER CURTAINS • Stop the water from squirting out onto the bathroom floor by getting that shower curtain into place quickly. Lubricate the curtain rod with petroleum jelly and you'll whip that curtain across the shower in no time.

TAKE OUT LIPSTICK STAINS • You set the table at that lovely dinner party with your favorite cloth napkins, but your friends left their mark all over them. Now dotted with lipstick stains, those napkins may be headed for the trash. But try this first. Before you wash them, blot petroleum jelly on the stain. Launder as usual and with a little luck, you can kiss those stains goodbye.

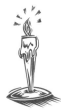

REMOVE WAX FROM CANDLESTICKS • Long red tapers used for a candlelit dinner are a beautiful sight until you see the candle wax drippings left in the candleholders. Before a dinner party, apply petroleum jelly to the insides of your candleholders before you put the candles in. That way, the wax will pop out for easy cleaning.

REMOVE CHEWING GUM FROM WOOD • If you discover chewing gum stuck under the dining room table or behind the headboard of your child's bed, don't freak out. Just squeeze some petroleum jelly on the offending wad, rub it in until the gum starts to disintegrate, and you can remove the gum.

FIT VACUUM PARTS TOGETHER SMOOTHLY • It's nice that your vacuum cleaner comes with so many accessories and extensions, but it's frustrating when the parts get stuck together and you have to yank them apart. Apply a bit of petroleum jelly to the rims of the tubes and the parts will easily slide together and apart.

SHINE PATENT-LEATHER SHOES • You've got a great pair of patent-leather shoes and a dynamite bag to match. The luster will stay longer if you polish both of them with petroleum jelly.

DID YOU KNOW?

Although there are many generic versions of petroleum jelly, the only real major brand is Vaseline. The online American Package Museum included a jar of Vaseline in its collection of classic packaging designs that also include Alka-Seltzer and Bayer Aspirin. Why did the site include Vaseline? "Vaseline is a well-established brand with a 145-year-old history," says Ian House, who created the site. "It also seems to enjoy popularity as a cultural icon for humorous reasons. Nobody knows quite what to do with it ... but nobody can live without it!"

RESTORE LEATHER JACKETS • You don't need fancy leather moisturizer to take care of your favorite leather jacket. Petroleum jelly does the job just as well. Apply, rub it in, wipe off the excess and you're ready to go.

KEEP ANTS AWAY FROM PET FOOD BOWLS • Pet food bowls are often invaded by ants. Since your pet would prefer to eat without them, help her out with this idea. Ring her food bowl with petroleum jelly. The ants will no longer be tempted by the food if they have to cross a mountain of petroleum jelly.

KEEP A BOTTLE LID FROM STICKING • If you're having a hard time unscrewing that bottle of glue or nail polish, remember this tip for when you finally do get it open. Rub a little petroleum jelly along the rim of the bottle. Next time, the top won't stick.

SOOTHE SORE PET PAWS • Sometimes your cat's or dog's paw pads can get cracked and dry. Give them a little tender loving care by squirting a little bit of petroleum jelly on the affected pads to stop pain and further cracking. They'll love you for it.

GREASE A BASEBALL GLOVE

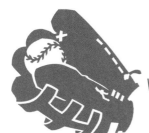

Got a new baseball glove, but it's as stiff as a board? Soften it up with petroleum jelly. Apply liberal amounts. Work it into the glove, and tie it up with a baseball inside. Do this in the winter and by springtime, you'll be ready to take the field.

for the do-it-yourselfer

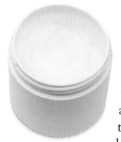

MASK DOORKNOBS WHEN PAINTING • When you're about to undertake painting the family room, you don't really want to fiddle with removing all the metal fixtures, including the doorknobs. Petroleum jelly rubbed on the metal will prevent paint from sticking. When you're done with painting, just wipe off the jelly and the unwanted paint is gone.

STOP BATTERY TERMINAL CORROSION • It's no coincidence that your car battery always dies on the coldest winter day. Low temperatures increase electrical resistance and thicken engine oil, making the battery work harder. Corrosion on the battery terminals also increases resistance and might just be the last straw that makes the battery give up. Before winter starts, disconnect the terminals and clean them with a wire brush. Reconnect them and smear with petroleum jelly. The jelly will prevent corrosion and help keep the battery cranking all winter long.

PROTECT STORED CHROME • If you're getting ready to store the kids' bikes for the winter or stow that stroller until your next baby comes along, stop before you stash. Take some petroleum jelly and apply it to the chrome parts of the equipment. When it's time to take those items out of storage, they'll be rust-free. The same method works for machinery stored in your garage.

more PETROLEUM JELLY over →

KEEP OUTDOOR LIGHT BULBS FROM STICKING • Have you ever unscrewed a light bulb and found yourself holding the glass while the metal base remains in the socket? It won't happen again if you remember to apply petroleum jelly to the base of the bulb before screwing it into the fixture. This is an especially good idea for light bulbs that are used outdoors.

SEAL A PLUMBER'S PLUNGER • Before you reach for that plunger to unclog the bathroom toilet, find some petroleum jelly. Apply it along the rim of the plunger and it will help create a tighter seal.

LUBRICATE CABINETS AND WINDOWS • If you can't stand hearing your medicine cabinet door creak on its runners, or that window you have to force open every time you want a breeze in the house, do something about it. With a small paintbrush, apply petroleum jelly to the window sash channel and cabinet door runners and they will slide easily.

STOP SQUEAKING DOOR HINGES • It's so annoying when a squeaky door makes an ill-timed noise when you're trying to keep quiet. Put petroleum jelly on the hinge pins of the door. It'll get rid of the squeaks.

REMOVE WATERMARKS ON WOOD • If your most recent party left lots of watermark rings on your wooden furniture, make them disappear by applying petroleum jelly and letting it sit overnight. In the morning, wipe the watermarks away with the jelly.

KEEP SQUIRRELS AWAY FROM A BIRD FEEDER • Feed the birds, not the squirrels. Keep them off the pole of your bird feeder by greasing it with petroleum jelly. They'll slide right off, so the birds can eat in peace.

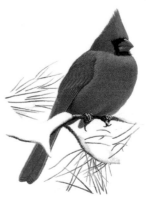

PILLOWCASES

DUST CEILING FAN BLADES • Have you ever seen clumps of dust careening off your ceiling fan when you turn it on for the first time in weeks? Grab an old pillowcase and place it over one of the ceiling fan blades. Slowly pull off the pillowcase. The blades get dusted and the collected dust stays in the pillowcase, instead of parachuting to the floor.

CLEAR OUT COBWEBS • There's a cobweb way up high in the corner of your dining room. Before you take a broom to it, cover the broom with an old pillowcase. Now you can wipe away the cobweb without scratching the wall paint or leaving a dirty mark. It's also easier to remove the cobweb from the pillowcase than to pull it out of broom bristles.

COVER A BABY'S CHANGING TABLE

Have you priced those expensive changing table covers lately? Instead, pick up a few of the cheapest white pillowcases you can find and use those to cover the changing table pad. When one is soiled, just slip it off and replace with a clean one.

Kids' Stuff

Kids love to personalize their bedrooms. You can help kids as young as 4 or 5 do just that by making a pillowcase into a wall hanging. Let the child choose a pillowcase color then slit a hole about an inch (2 cm) long in each side seam. Use fabric paints to create a design or scene or let the child rubber-stamp a picture on the pillowcase. Stick a dowel through the seam openings. Cut a length of wool about 30 inches (75 cm) long and tie one end of the wool to each end of the dowel. Hang the wall hanging up in the artist's room.

MAKE A SET OF LINEN NAPKINS • Who needs formal linen napkins that need pressing every time you use them? Cheap pillowcases are available in a wide array of colors and designs. Pick a color or design you like and start cutting. If you're really ambitious, sew a ½-inch (1-cm) hem on each edge. You'll have a new set of colorful napkins for a fraction of the cost of regular cloth napkins.

PREPARE TRAVEL PILLOWS • Road trips can be a lot of fun, but a bit dirty, too. Your children may want to bring their own pillows along, but they'll stain them with candy, food, and pens. Take their favorite pillows and layer several pillowcases on each pillow. When the outside one gets dirty, remove it for a fresh start.

USE FOR WRAPPING PAPER • Trying to wrap a basketball or an odd-shaped piece of art is tricky. Instead of regular wrapping paper, place the gift in a colored pillowcase and tie it closed with a ribbon.

KEEP MATCHING SHEETS TOGETHER • Rummaging around to find bedsheets is a common problem when friends come over to stay the night. Your recently arrived overnight guests want to go to bed, but it's not made, and you'd like to avoid giving them sheets that don't match, or that look as though they are ready to recycle as rags. Next time, file away your linens. Place newly laundered and folded sheets in their matching pillowcase before putting them in the linen closet.

MACHINE-WASH YOUR DELICATES • To prevent sweaters and pantyhose from being pulled out of shape when they twist around in the washing machine, first toss them into a pillowcase and close the opening, set the machine for delicates and add soap.

PILLOWCASE PROTECTION

STORE YOUR SWEATERS • Stored in plastic, winter sweaters can get quite musty. But stored just in a closet, they're prey to moths. The solution can be found among your linens. Put them in a pillowcase for seasonal storage. They will stay free from dust but the pillowcase fabric will allow them to breathe.

PROTECT CLOTHING HANGING IN A CLOSET • You've just laundered a favorite dress shirt or skirt and you know you won't be wearing it again for a while. To protect the garment, cut a hole in the top of an old pillowcase and slip it over the hanger and clothing.

STASH YOUR LEATHER ACCESSORIES • You reach up to pull a leather purse or suede shoes down from a shelf. Of course, the item is dusty and now you have to clean it. Save yourself the time and hassle next time by storing infrequently used items in a pillowcase. They'll be clean and ready to use when the occasion arises.

more PILLOWCASES over →

MACHINE-WASH STUFFED ANIMALS •

Children's stuffed toys may be cute but they get mighty dusty. When it's time for a bath, place them in a pillowcase and throw it in the washing machine. The pillowcase will ensure they get a gentle but thorough wash. If any parts fall off the stuffed animals, they'll be caught in the pillowcase so you can reattach them after their wash.

USE AS A TRAVELING LAUNDRY BAG •

When you travel, you always want to keep your dirty laundry separate from your clean clothes. Stick a pillowcase in your suitcase and toss it in the dirty laundry as it accumulates. When you get home, just empty the pillowcase into the washing machine and throw in the pillowcase as well.

WASH LOTS OF LETTUCE IN THE WASHING MACHINE

Expecting a large crowd for an outdoor lunch? Do you have 20 heads of lettuce to wash? Here's your solution: Place one pillowcase inside another, pull apart the lettuce heads and fill the inside case with lettuce leaves. Close both pillowcases with string or a rubber band and throw the whole package in the washing machine with another large item, such as a towel, to balance it. Now run the spin cycle for a few seconds. Your leaves come out dried. Works better than a salad spinner.

PIPE CLEANERS

DECORATE A PONYTAIL •

Need a fresh look for your hair? Tired of using plain old ribbons? Once you have your hair in a ponytail, twist a pipe cleaner around the hair band. Twist a couple together for an even brighter effect.

SAFETY PIN HOLDER •

Safety pins come in so many sizes, it's hard to keep them together and organized. Thread safety pins onto a pipe cleaner, through the bottom loop of each pin, for easy access.

USE AS AN EMERGENCY SHOELACE •

Your shoelace broke and you're about to go out on the court to play that grudge match in basketball. A pipe cleaner is a good temporary tie-up. Just thread it in your sneaker as you would a shoelace and twist it up at the top.

CLEAN GAS BURNERS •

Have you noticed that your stovetop burners are not firing on all their jets? Do you see an interrupted circle of blue when you turn a burner on? Poke a pipe cleaner through the little vents. This cleans the burner and allows it to work more efficiently. This works for safety valves on pressure cookers, too.

MAKE NAPKIN RINGS •

Colorful pipe cleaners are an easy and fast resource for making napkin rings. Just twist around the napkin and place on the table. If you want to get adventurous, use two—one for the napkin ring, and the other pipe cleaner attached to it, shaped into a heart, shamrock, flower, curlicue, or something else.

USE AS A TWIST TIE • If you have a smelly bag of kitchen garbage to go out, and you discover you're out of twist ties, just grab a pipe cleaner instead.

USE AS A TRAVEL TOY • If you're worried about having a bored, wiggly child on your hands during your next long car or plane ride, throw a bunch of pipe cleaners into your bag. Whip them out when the 'Are we there yet?' questions start coming your way. Colorful pipe cleaners can be bent and shaped into fun figures, animals, flowers, or whatever. They even make fun temporary bracelets and necklaces.

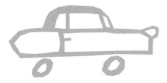

USE AS A MINI-SCRUBBER • Pipe cleaners are great for cleaning in tight spaces. Use one to remove dirt from the wheel of a can opener or to clean the bobbin case in a sewing machine.

DID YOU KNOW?

According to reliable sources, pipe cleaners were invented in the late nineteenth century in New York by J. Harry Stedman. Although pipe smoking has declined dramatically since then, pipe cleaners have flourished, having been co-opted by the arts-and-crafts community. Technically, the pipe cleaners used in children's arts and crafts activities are called chenille sticks. These stems come in various colors and widths and are fuzzier and softer than the real pipe cleaners that pipe smokers use.

DECORATE A GIFT • To give a special touch to a birthday or Christmas present, shape a pipe cleaner into a bow or a heart. Poke one end through a hole in the card and affix it to the package with a dab of glue.

49 USES!

PLASTIC BAGS
around the house

LINE A CRACKED FLOWER VASE • A beautiful heirloom flower vase is a sight to behold when it's filled with posies, but problems arise when an older vase leaks from large cracks. To fix this problem, line the vase with a plastic bag before you fill it with water and add the flowers, giving fresh life to a treasured heirloom.

BULK UP CURTAIN VALANCES • You've picked out snazzy new curtain balloon valances for your bedroom. The problem is the manufacturer has only sent you enough stuffing to make the valances look a bit better than limp. Recycle some plastic bags by stuffing them in the valances for a resilient pouf.

more PLASTIC BAGS over →

STUFF CRAFTS OR PILLOWS • There are a number of ways to stuff a craft project: with beans, rice, fabric filler, plastic beads, pantyhose, and so on. But have you ever tried stuffing a craft item or throw pillow with plastic bags? There are plenty on hand, so you don't have to worry about running out and you're recycling at the same time.

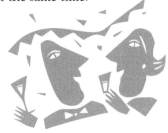

MAKE PARTY DECORATIONS • Here is an easy way to create streamers for a party using plastic bags. Cut each bag into strips starting from the open end and stopping short of the bottom. Then attach the bag bottom to the ceiling with tape.

DRAIN BATH TOYS • Don't let Rubber Ducky and all of the rest of your child's bath toys get moldy and create a potential hazard in the bathtub. Instead, after bathtime is over, gather them up in a plastic bag that has been punctured a few times. Hang the bag by its handles on one of the faucets to let the water drain out. This way the toys are collected in one place, ready for the next bath playtime.

KEEP KIDS' MATTRESSES DRY • There's no need to buy an expensive mattress guard if bed-wetting is a problem. Instead, line the mattress with plastic garbage bags. Big bags are also useful to protect toilet-training toddlers' car seats or upholstery for children coming home from the swimming pool.

DID YOU KNOW?

You still hear the question "Paper or plastic?" at the supermarket checkout. Plastic bags have been around for nearly 50 years but didn't get wide use at supermarkets until 1977. Within two decades, plastic had replaced paper as the most common grocery bag. Today, supermarkets have started recycling programs for plastic bags and are now encouraging the use of alternatives in the form of reusable cloth bags.

MAKE A LAUNDRY POCKET PICKIN'S BAG • You may think that the laundry's all done, until you open the dryer to find a tissue left in someone's pocket has shredded and is now plastered all over the dryer drum, not to mention the clothes in there. Hang a plastic bag near where you sort laundry and before you start the wash, go through all pockets and dump any contents in the bag for later sorting.

TREAT CHAPPED HANDS • If your hands are cracked and scaly, try this solution. Rub a thick layer of petroleum jelly on your hands then place them in a plastic bag. The jelly and your body's warmth will help make your hands supple in about 15 minutes.

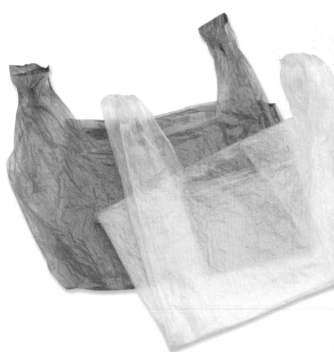

for storing stuff

STORE EXTRA BABY WIPES • If you picked up a jumbo box of baby wipes at a great price, you'll have enough wipes to last for several months, as long as they don't dry out before you can use them. To protect your good investment, keep the opened box of wipes in a plastic bag sealed with a twist tie.

COLLECT CLOTHES FOR A THRIFT SHOP • If you're constantly setting aside clothes to give to charity, then find them back in your closet or drawers, try this solution. Hang a large garbage bag in your closet.

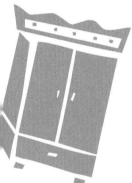

That way, the next time you find something you want to give, you just toss it in the bag. Once it's full, you can take it to the local donation center. Don't forget to hang a new bag in the closet.

COVER CLOTHES FOR STORAGE • If you've got a seersucker suit you'd like to save until it's fashionable again, grab a large, unused garbage bag and slit a hole in the top and push the hanger through for an instant dustcover.

STORE YOUR SKIRTS • If you find you have an overstuffed closet but plenty of room to spare in your chest of drawers, conduct a clothes transfer. Roll up your skirts and place them each in a plastic bag, to help them stay wrinkle-free.

for keeping things clean

PROTECT HAND WHEN CLEANING A TOILET • When cleaning your toilets with a long-handled brush or a shorter tool, first wrap your hand in an old plastic bag. You'll be able to do the scrubbing without your hand getting dirty in the process.

Storing plastic bags

✳ *If all your reuseable shopping bags spill out of the third drawer down in the kitchen, here are other ways to store them.*

● Squeeze the air out and stuff them inside an empty tissue box for easy retrieval.

● Poke a bunch of them down into a cardboard tube, such as a paper towel or mailing tube or even a section of a carpet tube.

● Fill a clean, empty gallon (4 L) plastic jug. Cut a 4-inch (10-cm) hole in the bottom. Stuff it with plastic bags and hang it by its handle on a hook. Pull the bags out of the spout.

● Make a bag 'sock'. Fold a dishtowel lengthwise with the wrong sides facing out. Stitch the long edges together. Sew ½-inch (1-cm) casings around the top and bottom openings and thread elastic through them, securing the ends. Turn the sock right side out, sew a loop of ribbon or string on the back to hang it up, stuff bags into the top opening, and pull them out from the bottom one.

KEEP PURSES IN SHAPE • When storing handbags and purses, fill them with clean, empty plastic bags to help the bags retain their original shape.

PREVENT STEEL WOOL FROM RUSTING • Steel wool pads have a habit of sitting useless in their own pool of rust at the edge of the sink. Next time, when you're not using a pad, toss it into a plastic bag where it won't rust so you'll be able to use it again.

more PLASTIC BAGS over →

MAKE BIBS FOR KIDS • The grandkids just popped in, and they're hungry. But you don't have any bibs to protect their clothes while they eat. Make some by tying a plastic bag loosely around the kids' necks so their clothes stay free of stains. You can make quick aprons this way, too.

CREATE A HIGH-CHAIR DROP CLOTH • Baby stores are quite happy to sell you an expensive drop cloth to place under your child's high chair, but why spend the money on a sheet of plastic when you have all those large garbage bags that can do the job? Split the seams of a bag and place it under the high chair to catch all the drips and dribbles. When it gets filthy, take it outside and shake, or just toss it.

LINE THE LITTER BOX • Nobody likes to change the cat's litter box. Make the job quick and easy by lining it with an open plastic bag before pouring in the litter. Use two bags if you think one is flimsy. When it's time to change the litter, just remove the bags, tie them up, and throw them into the garbage.

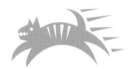

NEEDLE-FREE CHRISTMAS TREE REMOVAL • O Christmas tree, O Christmas tree, how lovely are thy branches! Until those needles start dropping, that is. When it's time to take down your Christmas tree, place a large garbage bag over the top of the tree and pull down. If it doesn't fit in one bag, use another from the bottom and pull up. You can quickly remove the tree without needles trailing behind you.

KEEP POLISH OFF YOUR HAND • If you've got a pair of scruffy white sandals that you'd like to freshen up, but you figure you're going to get more polish on your hands than your shoes, just wrap your hand in a plastic bag before inserting it into the sandal to start polishing. When polish runs off the sandal straps, your hand is protected. Leave the bag in the sandal until the polish is dry.

SCIENCE **WORKS!**

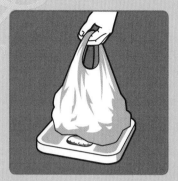

It is said that a plastic bag can carry about 20 pounds (9 kg) of groceries before you need to double-bag. Find out how much a bag can hold without its handles breaking.

For this experiment, you will need a kitchen scale, a plastic bag, and a bunch of rocks. Place the bag on the scale. Fill it with rocks until the scale reads 10 pounds (4.5 kg). Lift the bag. Does it hold? Add more rocks in 2 pound (1 kg) increments, testing the bag's strength after each addition. When the handles tear, you'll know the bag's actual strength.

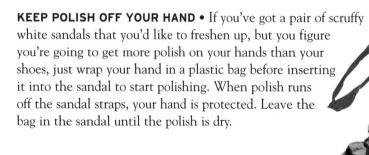

in the kitchen   ● ● ●

COVER A COOKBOOK

You're trying a new recipe from a borrowed cookbook that you don't want to get splattered during cooking. Cover the book with a clear plastic bag. You'll be able to read the directions and the book will stay clean.

BAG THE PHONE • Picture this: You're in the middle of making your famous chocolate chip cookies. You're up to your elbows in cookie dough and the phone rings. Now what? Wrap your hands in a plastic bag and answer the phone. You won't have to miss a call or clean the phone afterwards.

SCRAPE DISHES • Your extended family of 25 has just finished their Sunday dinner. Time to clean the dishes. Here's an easy way to get rid of the table scraps. Line a bowl with a plastic bag and scrape scraps into it. Once it's full, just gather up the handles and toss. Place the bowl in a prominent place in your kitchen so everyone can scrape their own dishes when bringing them to the sink.

CRUSH GRAHAM CRACKERS • Don't spend money on a a box of graham cracker crumbs. It's much cheaper and easier to crush them yourself. Just crumble several plain, graham crackers into a plastic bag. Lay the bag on the kitchen counter and go over it several times with a rolling pin. In no time, you'll have all the crumbs you need, plus the remainder of a box of graham crackers to snack on as well.

REPLACE A MIXING BOWL • If you're cooking for a crowd and are short on mixing bowls, try using a plastic bag instead. Place all the dry ingredients to be mixed in the bag, gather it up and gently shake. If the ingredients are wet, use your hands to mix.

SPIN DRY SALAD GREENS • The kids will enjoy helping you with this one. Wash lettuce and shake out as much water as you can in the sink. Then place the greens in a plastic grocery bag that has been lined with a paper towel. Grab the handles and spin the bag in large circles in the air. After several whirls, you'll have dry lettuce.

RIPEN FRUIT
Some of the fruit from that case of peaches you just bought at the local farmers' market are as hard as rocks. Place the fruit with a few already ripe pieces or some ripe bananas in a plastic bag. The ripe fruit will help soften the others through the release of their natural gas. But don't leave them for more than a day or two or you'll have purple, moldy peaches.

more PLASTIC BAGS over →

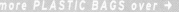

in the garden

PROTECT PLANTS FROM FROST • When frost threatens your small plants, grab a bunch of plastic bags to protect them. Just cut a hole in the bottom of each bag. Slip one over each plant and anchor it inside using small rocks. Pull the bags over the plants, roll them closed, and secure them with clothespins or paper clips. You can open up the bags again when the weather turns warm.

START POINSETTIA BUDS FOR XMAS • Christmas poinsettia usually look their best by the time the holidays arrive. You can speed up Mother Nature by placing the poinsettia in a large, dark garbage bag for several weeks to wake up the plant's buds.

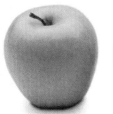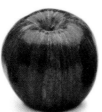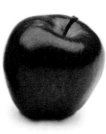

PROTECT FRUIT ON THE TREE • Are there some apples in your orchard you want to protect or some plums that need a bit more time on the tree? Slip the fruit into clear plastic bags while still on the trees. You'll keep out insect pests while the fruit continues to ripen.

PROTECT YOUR SHOES FROM MUD • If, after a hard rainfall you need to get out in the garden to do your regular weeding, but you're worried about getting mud all over your shoes, cover them in plastic bags. The mud gets on the bag, not on the shoes, and your feet remain dry so you can stay out in the garden.

DID YOU KNOW?

Worried about the growing number of plastic bags filling landfills, countries across the globe have started putting restrictions on the seemingly indispensable item. Bangladesh has banned plastic bags, blaming them for clogging drainage pipes and causing a flood. Some Australian towns also have banned plastic bags, and there's a national movement pushing stores to halve their use of bags (estimated at around 7 billion annually) within a few years. If you want to use a plastic bag in Ireland, you'll be charged about 19 cents a bag. In Taiwan, it's 34 cents a bag.

CLEAN A BARBECUE EASILY • That neighborhood barbecue was fun, but your grill is a sorry mess now. Take the racks off and place them in a garbage bag. Spray oven cleaner on the grill and close up the bag. The next day, open the 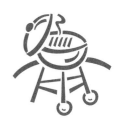 bag, making sure to keep your face away from the fumes. All that burned-on gunk should wipe right off.

COVER GARAGE-SALE SIGNS

If you've gone to the trouble of advertising an upcoming garage sale with signs but worry that rain may hurt your publicity campaign even before the early birds show up, protect the signs by covering them with pieces cut from clear plastic bags. Passersby can still see the lettering, which will be protected from being smeared by the rain.

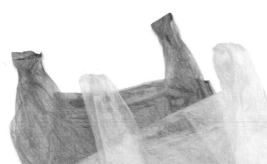

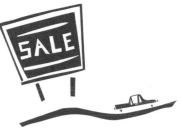

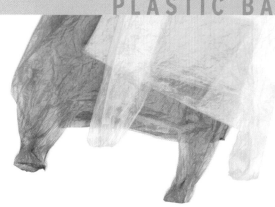

STORE OUTDOOR EQUIPMENT MANUALS • Your weed-wacker's spindle just gave out and you have to replace it. But how? Stash all your outdoor equipment's warranties and owner's manuals in a plastic bag and hang it in your garage. You'll know exactly where to look for help.

PROTECT YOUR CAR MIRRORS • If you live in a cold area and snow is forecast for the next day, save yourself time and get a step ahead by covering your car's side mirrors with plastic bags before the storm. When you're cleaning off the car the next morning, just remove the bag. No ice to scrape off.

MAKE A JUMP ROPE • If 'I'm bored!' is what the kids cry as you're trying to finish your work in the garden, here's a simple solution. Make a jump rope by twisting up several plastic bags and tying them together end to end. Talk about cheap fun!

on the go

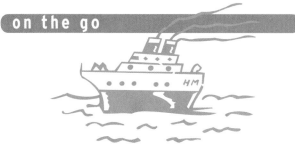

PACK YOUR SHOES • If your next cruise vacation requires a variety of shoes for different occasions, but you worry that packing them in the suitcase will get everything else dirty. Just wrap each pair in its own plastic bag. It will keep dirt off the clothes and you can clearly see that you've packed complete pairs.

PROTECT YOUR HANDS WHEN PUMPING GAS • When you stop at the gas station for a fill-up before meeting friends for lunch, the last thing you want is to greet them with hands that smell of gasoline. Keep a stash of plastic bags in your car and use one to cover your hands while you pump.

MAKE AN INSTANT PONCHO • Leave a large garbage bag in your car and the next time it rains unexpectedly, cut some arm slits in it and another one for your head. Slip on your impromptu poncho and you'll be sure to stay dry.

STASH YOUR WET UMBRELLA • When you're out in the rain and running to your next appointment, who wants to deal with a soggy umbrella dripping all over your clothes and car? One of those plastic bags that newspapers are delivered in is the perfect size to cover your umbrella the next time it rains. Just fold the umbrella up and slip it into the bag.

SCOOT IN THE SNOW • If there's a 6-inch (15-cm) snowfall and your children are hoping to take advantage of it right now, grab some garbage bags, tie one around each of their waists and let them slide down the hills on their fanny.

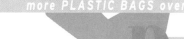
more PLASTIC BAGS over →

for the do-it-yourselfer

COVER CEILING FANS • You're painting the sunroom ceiling, and you don't want to remove the ceiling fan for the process. Cover the blades with plastic bags to protect them from paint splatters. Use masking tape to keep the bags shut.

STORE PAINTBRUSHES • You're halfway through painting the living room when it's time to break for lunch. No need to clean the paintbrush. Just stick it in a plastic bag and it will remain wet and ready to use when you return. Going to finish next weekend, you say? Stick the bag-covered brush in the freezer. Defrost next week and you are ready to go.

CONTAIN PAINT OVERSPRAY • If you've got a few small items to spray paint, use a plastic bag to control the overspray. Just place one item at a time in the bag, spray paint and remove to a spread-out newspaper to dry. When you're finished, toss the bag into the garbage for an easy cleanup.

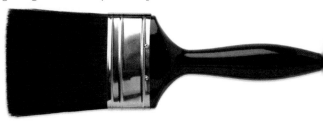

26 USES! PLASTIC BOTTLES

around the house

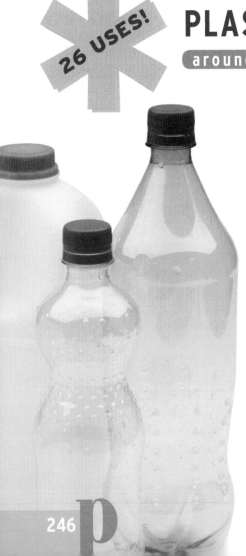

MAKE A FOOT WARMER • Walking around on cold winter days can leave you with cold and tired tootsies. But you don't need to shell out your hard-earned money on a heating pad or a hot water bottle to ease your discomfort. Just fill up a 64-ounce (2 L) soft drink bottle with hot water, sit down, and roll it back and forth under your feet.

USE AS A BOOT TREE • Want to keep your boot tops from getting wrinkled or folded over when you put them in storage? Insert a clean, empty 32-ounce (1 L) soft drink bottle into each boot. For added tautness, put a few old socks on the bottles or wrap them in towels.

MAKE A BAG OR STRING DISPENSER • An empty 64-ounce (2 L) soft drink bottle makes the perfect container for storing and dispensing plastic grocery bags. Just cut off the bottom and top ends of the bottle and mount it with screws upside down inside a kitchen cabinet or cupboard. Put washers under the screw heads to keep them from pulling

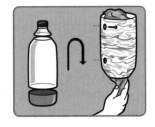

through the plastic. Fill it with your recycled bags (squeeze the air out first) and pull them out as needed. Make a string dispenser the same way, using a 32-ounce (1 L) bottle and let the cord come out the bottom.

RECYCLE AS A CHEW TOY • If your dog has been chewing on your slippers instead of fetching them, she needs new chew toys. Just give her an empty plastic 32-ounce (1 L) soft drink bottle to chew on. Maybe it's the crunchy sound they make, but dogs love them! Just make sure you remove the label and bottle cap (as well as the loose plastic ring under it). Replace it before it gets too chewed up—broken pieces of plastic are choking hazards.

PLACE IN THE TOILET TANK

Unless your house was built relatively recently, chances are you have an older toilet that uses a lot of water each flush. To save water and a bit of money on your water bills, fill an empty 32-ounce (1 L) soft drink bottle with water. Remove any labels and put it in the toilet tank to cut the amount of water in each flush.

CUT OUT A TOY CARRYALL • If you're fed up with Lego or erector-set pieces underfoot, make a simple carryall to store them in by cutting a large hole in the side of a clean plastic bottle with a handle. Cut the hole opposite the handle so you or your child can easily carry the container back to the playroom after putting the pieces away. For an easy way to store craft materials, crayons, or small toys, cut the containers in half and use the bottom part to stash your stuff.

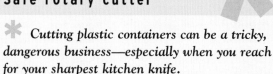

Safe rotary cutter

Cutting plastic containers can be a tricky, dangerous business—especially when you reach for your sharpest kitchen knife.

But you can greatly minimize the risk by visiting your local fabric or craft shop and picking up a rolling cutter knife (this is not the same device used to slice pizza, by the way). The device shown in the picture below with the hint 'Make a scoop or boat bailer', usually sells for less than $20. Be careful, though. These knives use blades that are razor sharp, but they make life much easier when it's time to cut into a hard plastic container.

STORE YOUR SUGAR • The next time you bring home a 2-pound (1 kg) bag of sugar from the store, try pouring it into a clean, dry, large plastic bottle with a handle. The sugar is less likely to harden and the handle makes pouring much easier.

FASHION A FUNNEL • To make a handy, durable funnel, cut a cleaned milk, bleach, or liquid detergent container with a handle in half across its midsection. Use the top portion (with the spout and handle) as a funnel for easy pouring of paints, rice, coins, and anything else suitable.

away from home

• • •

MAKE A SCOOP OR BOAT BAILER • Cut a clean, plastic half-gallon (2 L) milk bottle with a handle diagonally from the bottom so that you have the top three-quarters of the bottle intact. You now have a handy scoop that can be used for everything—from removing leaves and other debris from your gutters, to cleaning out a cat litter box, to scooping up poo after your dog. Use it to scoop dog food from the bag, spread sand on slippery paths in winter, or bail water out of your boat. You might want to keep the cap on for this last application.

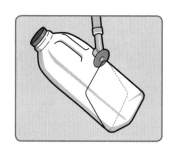

more PLASTIC BOTTLES over →

KEEP THE COOLER COLD • Don't let your cooler lose its cool while you're on the road. Fill a few clean plastic bottles with water or juice and keep them in the freezer for use when transporting food in your cooler. This is not only good for keeping food cold: You can actually drink the water or juice as it melts. It's also not a bad idea to keep a few frozen bottles in your freezer if you have extra space; a full freezer actually uses less energy and can save money on your electricity bill. Leave room for the water to expand as it freezes.

FOR ROAD EMERGENCIES IN WINTER • Don't get stuck in your car the next time a surprise winter storm hits. If you live in a cold area, keep a couple of large, clean plastic bottles, with handles, filled with sand or cat litter in the trunk of your car. You'll be prepared to sprinkle the material on the road surface to add traction under your wheels when you need to get moving on a slippery road. The handle makes it easier to pour out the sand or litter.

in the garden

FEED THE BIRDS • Why spend money on a plastic bird feeder when you probably have one in your recycling bin? Take a clean half-gallon (2 L) juice or milk bottle and carve a large hole on its side to remove the handle. You could even drill a small hole under the large one to insert a sturdy twig or dowel for a perch. Then poke a hole in the middle of the cap and suspend it from a tree with a piece of strong string or monofilament fishing line. Fill it up to the opening with birdseed and enjoy the show.

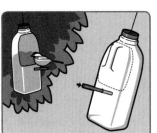

CREATE A DRIP IRRIGATOR FOR PLANTS • During dry spells, a good way to get water to the roots of your plants is to place several drip irrigators around your garden. You can make them from large, clean juice or detergent bottles. Cut a large hole in the bottom of a bottle, then drill 2–5 tiny, 1/16-inch (about 2 mm) holes in or around the cap. Bury the capped bottle upside down about three-quarters submerged beneath the soil near the plants you need to water. Fill through the hole on top and refill as needed.

MAKE A WATERING CAN • If you don't have a watering can, make one from a large, clean juice, milk, or bleach bottle with a handle. Drill about a dozen 1/16-inch (about 2 mm) holes just below the spout of the bottle on the side opposite the handle. Or carefully make punch holes with a skewer. Fill it with water, screw the cap on, and start sprinkling.

MARK YOUR PLANTS • Want an easy way to make identification badges for all the vegetables, herbs, and flowers in your garden? Cut vertical strips from a couple of large, clear water bottles. Make the strips the same width as your seed packets but double their length. Fold each strip over an empty packet to protect it from the elements, and staple it to a strong popsicle stick or chopstick.

SECURE GARDEN NETTING • If you find yourself having to constantly re-stake the loose netting or plastic lining over your garden bed, just place large, water-filled, plastic bottles around the corners to keep the material in place.

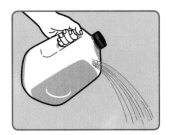

USE A CARRY-ON GARBAGE CAN OR HARVEST BASKET •
Here's a tip for weekend gardeners. Cut a large hole opposite the handle of a half-gallon (2 L) container and loop the handle through a belt or rope on your waist. Use it to collect debris, such as rocks, weeds, and broken stems, that you encounter as you mow the lawn or stroll through your garden. Use the same design to make an portable basket for harvesting berries, cherries, and other small fruits or vegetables.

SPACE SEEDS IN THE GARDEN •
Want an easy way to perfectly space seeds in your garden? Use an empty soft drink bottle as your guide. Find the distance that the seed company recommends between seeds and cut off the tapered top of the bottle so its diameter equals that distance. When you start planting, firmly press your bottle, cut edge down, into the soil and place a seed in the center of the circle it makes. Then line up the bottle so that its edge touches the curve of the first impression and press down again. Plant a seed in the center and repeat until you've filled your rows.

ISOLATE WEEDS WHEN SPRAYING HERBICIDES •
When using herbicides to kill weeds in your garden, you have to be careful not to also spray and kill surrounding plants. To isolate the weed you want to kill, cut a half-gallon (2 L) soft drink bottle in half and place the top half over the weed you want to spray. Then direct your pump's spraying wand through the regular opening in the top of the bottle and blast away. After the spray settles down, pick up the bottle and move on to your next target. Always wear goggles and gloves when spraying chemicals in the garden.

SET UP A BACKYARD SPRINKLER •
If local water restrictions permit, when temperatures soar outdoors, keep your kids cool with a homemade backyard sprinkler. Just cut three 1¼-inch (3 cm) vertical slits in one side of a clean half-gallon (2 L) soft drink bottle. Or make the slits at different angles so the water will squirt in different directions. Attach the nozzle of the hose to the bottle top with a few strips of duct tape (make sure it's fastened on tight), turn on the faucet, and let the fun begin!

BUILD AN INSECT TRAP

Do wasps swarm around you every time you set foot in the garden? Use an empty half-gallon (2 L) soft drink bottle to make an environmentally friendly trap for them. First, dissolve ½ cup (125 g) sugar in ½ cup (125 ml) water in the bottle. Then add 1 cup (250 ml) apple cider vinegar and a banana peel (squish it to fit it through). Screw on the cap and give the mixture a good shake before filling the bottle halfway with cold water. Cut or drill a ¾-inch (2 cm) hole near the top of the bottle and hang it from a tree branch where insects seem especially active. When the trap is full, toss it into the garbage and replace it with a new one.

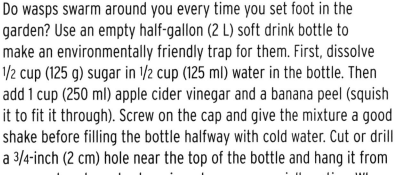

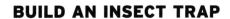

more PLASTIC BOTTLES over →

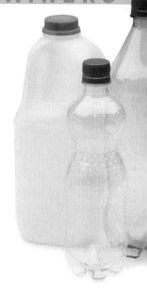

for the do-it-yourselfer

BUILD A PAINT BUCKET • Tired of splattering paint all over as you work? Make a neat paint dispenser by cutting a large hole opposite the handle of a large, clean bottle. Pour in the paint so it's a few inches below the edge of the hole and use the edge to remove any excess paint from your brush before you lift the brush. You can also cut bottles in half and use the bottom halves as disposable paint buckets when several people work on the same job.

STORE YOUR PAINTS • Why keep leftover house paints in rusted or dented cans when you can keep them clean and fresh in plastic bottles? Use a funnel to pour the paint into a clean, dry, milk or water bottle, and add a few marbles (they help mix the paint when you shake the container before your next paint job). Label each container with a piece of masking tape, noting the paint manufacturer, color name, and the date it was opened.

USE AS WORKSHOP ORGANIZERS • Are you always searching for the right nail to use for a particular job, or for a clothespin, picture hook or small fastener? Bring some organization to your workshop with a few half-gallon (2 L) bottles. Cut out a section near the top of each bottle on the side opposite the handle. Use the containers to store and sort all the small items that seem to 'slip through the cracks' of your workbench. The handle makes it easy to carry a bottle to where you're working.

USE AS A LEVEL SUBSTITUTE • How can you make sure that the shelf you're about to put up is straight if you don't have a spirit level on hand? Easy. Fill a 32-ounce (1 L) soft drink bottle about three-quarters full with water. Replace the cap and lay the bottle on its side. When the water is level, so is the shelf.

MAKE A WEIGHT FOR ANCHORING OR LIFTING

Fill a large, clean, dry bottle with a handle with sand and cap it. You now have an anchor that is great for holding down a paint tarp, securing a shaky patio umbrella, or steadying a table for repair. The handle makes it easy to move or attach a rope. Or use a pair of sand-filled bottles as exercise weights, varying the amount of sand to meet your lifting capacity.

PLASTIC CONTAINERS

TRAP PLANT-EATING SLUGS • Sock it to those slugs eating your just-planted vegetable plants, by digging a hole the size of a plastic container near the plant. Place the container, flush with the ground, in the hole. Fill the container with beer or salted water and place cut potatoes around the rim to attract the slugs. The slugs will crawl in and die.

WIPE OUT DANGEROUS WASPS • When wasps get a little too close for comfort, threatening to bring your child's outing to the park to a screeching halt, simply take a plastic container and fill it with water that's sweetened with sugar and cut a hole in the lid. Wasps will be attracted to the water, crawl inside, and get trapped inside the container.

KEEP ANTS AWAY FROM YOUR PICNIC TABLE • You watch helplessly as the ants march up the picnic table leg, onto the tabletop, and into your meal. Here's a foolproof way to stop them in their tracks. Place a plastic container on the bottom of each picnic table leg. Fill with water. The ants won't be able to crawl past.

ORGANIZE YOUR SEWING AREA • You're sitting down at your sewing area to start your Christmas craft projects. But instead of sewing, you're hunting for that extra bobbin or the right colored thread. Plastic containers can help you bring order to your sewing materials. Fill some with thread spools, others with tools such as seam rippers and measuring tapes. Another container can be filled with pins.

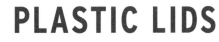

USE AS A PORTABLE DOG DISH • The next time you go out in the woods with your dog, pack a portion of his food and some treats in a plastic container while you pack another container with a snack for yourself. An empty container also makes a great water bowl on the go.

PLASTIC LIDS

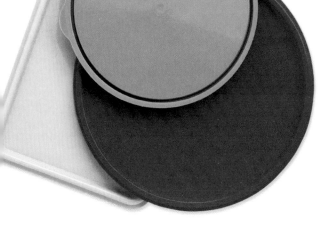

KEEP THE FRIDGE CLEAN • Drippy bottles and containers with leaks can create a mess on your refrigerator shelves. Create coasters from plastic lids to keep things clean. Place the lids under food containers to stop any potential leaks. If they get dirty, throw them in the dishwasher, while your fridge shelves stay free of a sticky mess.

USE AS COASTERS FOR HOUSEPLANTS • Plastic lids are the perfect water catcher for small houseplants. One under each plant will help keep water marks off your wooden furniture.

more PLASTIC LIDS over →

STOP A SINK OR TUB

If your drain plug has disappeared, but you need to stop the water in the sink or bathtub, here's a temporary solution. Place a plastic lid over the drain. The vacuum created keeps the water from slip-sliding away.

USE AS KIDS' COASTERS • Entertaining a crowd of kids and want to make sure your tabletops survive? Or at least give them a fighting chance! Give kids plastic lids to use as coasters. Write their names on the coasters so they won't get their drinks mixed up.

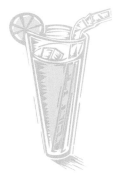

SCRAPE NONSTICK PANS • We all know that stuff often sticks to so-called nonstick pans. And, of course, using steel wool to get it off is a no-no. Try scraping off the gunk with a plastic lid.

SEPARATE FROZEN HAMBURGER PATTIES • If you're planning a big barbecue and you want to get organized in advance, season the meat as desired and shape it into patties. Place each patty on a plastic lid, stack them up, place in a plastic bag, and freeze. When the grill is fired up, you'll have no trouble separating your preformed hamburger patties.

PREVENT PAINTBRUSH
DRIPS • Worried about getting messy paint drips all over yourself while you're touching up the ceiling? Try this trick. Cut a slot in the middle of a plastic lid. The kind of plastic lid that comes on coffee cans is the perfect

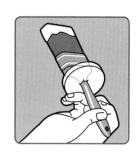

size for most paintbrushes. Insert the handle of your paintbrush through the lid so that the lid is on the narrow part of the handle just above your hand. The lid will catch any paint drips. Even with this shield, always be careful not to put too much paint on your brush when you're painting overhead.

CLOSE A BAG • Out of twist ties? Need to get that smelly garbage bag out of the house? Grab a plastic lid, cut a slit in it, gather the top of the bag and thread it through. The bag's now completely sealed and ready for disposal.

PLASTIC TABLECLOTHS

COLLECT LEAVES

Save all that bending at leaf-raking time. Don't pick the leaves up to put them in a wheelbarrow to transport them to the compost or leaf pile. Just rake the leaves onto an old plastic tablecloth, gather up the four corners and drag the tablecloth to the compost or leaf pile.

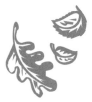

MAKE A SHOWER CURTAIN • A colorful plastic tablecloth can make a great-looking shower curtain to match your bathroom decor. Punch holes about 6 inches (15 cm) apart and ½ inch (1.25 cm) from one edge of a hemmed tablecloth. Insert shower curtain rings or loop strings through the holes and loosely tie to the curtain rod.

MAKE A HIGH-CHAIR DROP CLOTH • Bombs away! It's par for the course for a baby to get more food on the floor than in his or her mouth. Catch the debris and protect your floor by spreading a plastic tablecloth under the high chair.

PLASTIC WRAP

KEEP ICE CREAM SMOOTH • Ever notice how ice crystals form on ice cream in the freezer once the container has been opened? The ice cream will stay smooth and free of those annoying, yucky crystals if you rewrap the container completely in plastic wrap before you return it to the freezer.

KEEP THE FRIDGE TOP FOREVER CLEAN • Make the next time you clean the top of your refrigerator the last time. After you've got it all clean and shiny, cover the top with overlapping sheets of plastic wrap. Next time it's due for a cleaning, all you need do is remove the old sheets, toss them in the garbage, and replace with new layers of wrap.

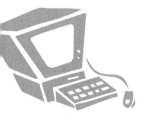

PROTECT YOUR COMPUTER KEYBOARD • When you're on vacation and away from that computer keyboard for a couple of weeks, cover the keyboard with plastic wrap. During long periods of inactivity, dust and grime start to settle in between the keys.

REPAIR A KITE • Flying kites with the kids is a lot of fun, but it can also be frustrating when the kite gets torn by a tree branch or fence. For a temporary fix that will keep the kite airborne for a while, cover the tear with plastic wrap and fix it to the kite with a few carefully placed strips of transparent tape.

FIRST AID

TREAT A HANGNAIL • Get rid of a hangnail overnight while you sleep. Before going to bed, apply hand cream to the affected area, wrap the fingertip with plastic wrap, and secure it in place with transparent tape. The plastic wrap will confine the moisture and soften the cuticle.

TREAT PSORIASIS • Here is a method often recommended by dermatologists to treat individual psoriasis lesions. After you apply a topical steroid cream, cover the area with a small piece of plastic wrap and use adhesive tape to fix the wrap to your skin. The wrap will enhance the effect of the steroid, seal in moisture, and inhibit proliferation of the rash.

ENHANCE LINIMENT EFFECT • For pain in your knee or other sore spots, rub in some liniment and wrap the area with plastic wrap. The wrap will increase the heating effect of the liniment. Make sure to test on a small area first to make sure your skin does not burn.

more PLASTIC WRAP over →

KEEP STORED PAINT FRESH • Your leftover paint will stay fresher longer if you stretch a sheet of premium plastic wrap over the top of the can before tightly replacing the lid.

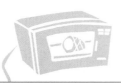

CAUTION: When microwaving foods covered with plastic wrap, always turn back a corner of the wrap or cut a slit in it to let steam escape. Never use plastic wrap when microwaving foods with a high sugar content; they can become extremely hot and melt the wrap.

DID YOU KNOW?

Saran or plastic wrap (polyvinylidene chloride) was accidentally discovered in 1933 by Ralph Wiley, a Dow Chemical Company lab worker. One day, Ralph came across a vial coated with a smelly, clear, green film he couldn't scrub off. He called it eonite, after an indestructible material featured in the 'Little Orphan Annie' comic strip. Dow researchers analyzed the substance and dubbed the greasy film Saran. Soon the armed forces were using it to spray fighter planes, and car manufacturers used it to protect upholstery. Dow later got rid of the green color and unpleasant odor and transformed it into a solid material, which was approved for food packaging after World War II and as a contact food wrap in 1956.

PLUNGERS

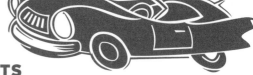

REMOVE CAR DENTS

Before forking over big bucks to have an auto body shop pull a dent out of your car, try wetting a plumber's plunger, pushing it over the dent, and pulling it out sharply. It's always worth a try.

CATCH CHIPS WHEN DRILLING A CEILING • Before you use a star drill to make an overhead hole, remove the handle from a plunger and place the cup over the shank of the drill. The cup will catch falling chunks of plaster, cement, or brick from the ceiling.

USE AS AN OUTDOOR CANDLE HOLDER • Looking for a place to put one of those mosquito-deterring citronella candles? Plant a plunger handle in the ground and put the candle in the rubber cup.

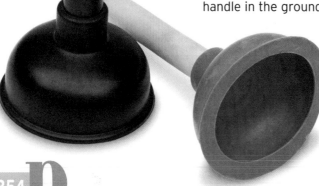

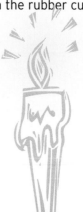

POPSICLE STICKS

EMERGENCY SPLINT FOR A FINGER • If you suspect your child has a broken finger, use a popsicle stick as a temporary splint before going to the hospital. Use adhesive tape to stabilize the finger until it can be set.

FOR FUTURE ARTISTS AND WRITERS • Popsicle sticks are just the thing for spreading finger paint. Or, for a fun way to help young children practice their letters, let them use popsicle sticks to write letters in a pile of shaving cream, whipped cream, or yogurt.

SKEWER KIDS' FOOD

It's more fun to eat food if you get to play with it first, as the parents of many picky eaters know. Popsicle sticks are good to have in your bag of tricks at mealtime. Skewer bites of sausage, pineapple, melon, and more. Or give kids a stick and have them spread their own peanut butter.

Kids' Stuff

Here's a great gift to encourage young readers. Paint a popsicle stick in a bright color. When it's dry, write on one side a reading slogan such as 'I love to read' or 'I'll hold the page'. Now cut a shape, such as a heart, flower, a cat or a dog, out of craft paper. Glue the shape to the top of the stick and you have a homemade bookmark.

KEEP TRACK OF PAINT COLORS • You're searching through cans of leftover paint. Did you paint the living room Whipped Cream or Sand? To avoid this again, dip a popsicle stick in the can, let it dry, then write the name of the paint and where it was used on the stick. You'll know what color to use when it's time to paint again. This can also help an interior decorator pick out fabrics and decorative items.

LABEL YOUR PLANTINGS • Is that parsley, sage, rosemary, or thyme popping up from your garden? Remember what you planted by using popsicle sticks as plant labels. Just write the type of seeds you planted on the stick with indelible marker.

POTATOES

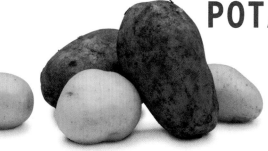

REMOVE STAINS ON HANDS • Your family's favorite carrot soup is simmering on the stove, and you've got the orange hands to show for it. Hard-to-remove stains on hands from peeling carrots or handling pumpkin come right off if you rub your hands with a raw, cut potato.

EXTRACT SALT FOR SOUP • If you go overboard when salting the soup, it's not a problem. Just cut a few potatoes into large chunks. Toss them into the soup pot still on the stove. When they start to soften, in about 10 minutes, remove them and the excess salt they have absorbed. Save them for another use, such as potato salad.

REMOVE A BROKEN LIGHT BULB • You're changing a light bulb in the bedside lamp and it breaks off in your hand. So now the glass is off, but the stem's still inside. Unplug the lamp, cut a potato widthwise and place it over the broken bulb. Twist, and the rest of the light bulb should come out easily.

more POTATOES over →

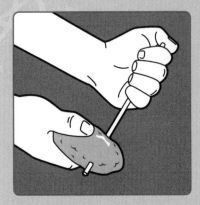

SCIENCE **WORKS!**

Here's a way to demonstrate the power of air pressure.

Grasp a plastic straw in the middle and try to plunge it into a potato. It crumples and bends, unable to penetrate the potato. Now grasp another straw in the middle, but this time, put your finger over the top. The straw will plunge right into the tuber. When the air is trapped inside the straw, it presses against the straw's sides, stiffening the straw enough to plunge into the potato. In fact, the deeper the straw plunges, the less space there is for the air and the stiffer the straw gets.

REMOVE TARNISH ON SILVERWARE • High tea is being served at your house later today, and you're out of silver polish. Grab a bunch of potatoes and boil them up. Remove them from the water and save them for another use. Place your silverware in the remaining water and let it sit for an hour. Then remove the silverware and wash. The tarnish should have disappeared.

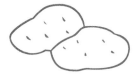

MAKE A HOT OR COLD COMPRESS

Potatoes retain heat and cold well. The next time you need a hot compress, boil a potato, wrap it in a dishtowel and apply to the area. Refrigerate the boiled potato if you need a cold compress.

FOR THOSE WITH GREEN FINGERS ...

LURE WORMS IN HOUSEPLANTS • The worms crawl in and the worms crawl out of the roots of your favorite house plant. The roots are suffering. What to do? Slice raw potato around the base of the plant to act as a lure for the worms. They'll crawl up to eat and you can grab them and toss them into the garden.

FEED NEW GERANIUMS • A raw potato can give a fledgling geranium all the nutrients it could desire. Carve a small hole in a potato. Slip a geranium stem into the hole, then plant the whole thing, potato and all.

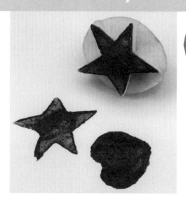

MAKE A DECORATIVE STAMP

Forget those expensive rubber stamps that go for up to $20 or more apiece. A potato can provide the right medium for making your own stamp for decorating greeting cards and envelopes. Cut a potato in half widthwise. Carve a design on one half and start stamping as you would with a wooden stamp.

KEEP SKI GOGGLES CLEAR • You can't keep a good lookout for trees and other skiers through snow goggles that fog up during your downhill descent. Rub raw potato over the goggles before you get on the ski lift and the ride down should be crystal clear.

HOLD A FLOWER ARRANGEMENT IN PLACE • If you have a small flower arrangement that you'd like to stabilize but have none of that green floral foam on hand to stick the flower stems in, try a large baking potato. Cut it in half lengthwise and place it cut side down. Poke holes where you want the flower stems to go and insert the stems.

END PUFFY 'MORNING' EYES • We all hate waking up in the morning and looking at our mug in the mirror. What are those puffy spots on your face? Oh yeah, those are your eyes. A little TLC is what you need. Apply slices of raw, cold potatoes to your eyes to make the puffiness go away.

RESTORE OLD, BEATEN-UP SHOES • Try as you might, your old shoes are just too scuffed to take a shine anymore. They don't have holes, and they are so nice and comfy that you hate to throw them away. Before you give them the brush-off, cut a potato in half and rub those old shoes with the raw potato. After that, polish them; they should come out nice and shiny.

POTS AND PANS

CATCH DRAINING ENGINE OIL • No need to run out and buy an oil-collecting pan. When it is time to change the oil in your car engine, just stick an old 5 quart (5 L) or larger, pot beneath the drain plug.

CREATE AN INSTANT BIRDBATH • You can quickly provide feathered visitors to your backyard with a place to refresh themselves. Just set an old pan on top of a flowerpot and keep it filled with water.

USE AS A LARGE SCOOP • Leave those 40-pound (20 kg) sacks of fertilizer in the garden shed and use a pot to carry what you need to where you need it. A small pot with a handle also makes a terrific boat bailer or dog-food scoop.

MAKE AN EXTRA GRILL • You've got a big barbecue planned, and your grill is not big enough to handle all those burgers and sausages. Improvise an auxiliary grill by building a fire in an old, large pot. Cook on a cake rack placed over the pot. After you are finished, put the pot's cover on to choke the fire and save the charcoal for another barbecue.

p 257

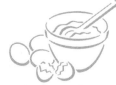

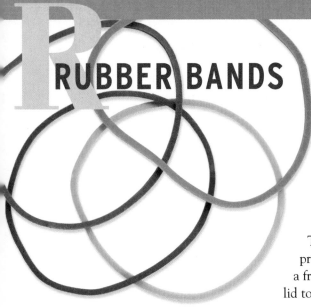

RUBBER BANDS

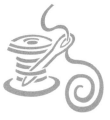

STOP SLIDING SPOONS • When the spoon slips into the mixing bowl again, and you have to fish it out of the messy batter, try another tack next time. After you rinse off the spoon, wrap a rubber band around the top of the handle to catch the spoon and avoid the mess.

SECURE YOUR CASSEROLE DISH LIDS • Don't spill it! That's what you say when you hand somebody your lovingly prepared casserole dish to transport in the car on the way to a friend's house. But you won't have to worry if you secure the lid to the base with a couple of wide rubber bands.

ANCHOR YOUR CUTTING BOARD • Do you find yourself chasing the cutting board around the kitchen counter when you're chopping up vegetables? Give the board some traction by putting a rubber band around each end.

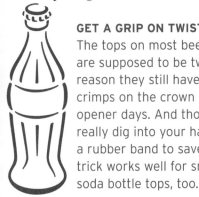

GET A GRIP ON TWIST-OFF TOPS • Ouch! The tops on most beer bottles these days are supposed to be twist-off, but for some reason they still have those sharp little crimps on the crown seal from the bottle opener days. And those little crimps can really dig into your hand. Wrap the top in a rubber band to save the pain. The same trick works well for smooth, tough-to-grip soda bottle tops, too.

GET A GRIP ON DRINKING GLASSES • Does arthritis make it tough for you to grasp a drinking glass securely, especially when it is wet with condensation? Wrap a couple of rubber bands around the glass to make it easier to grip. Works well for kids, too, whose small hands sometimes have a hard time holding a glass.

RESHAPE YOUR BROOM • No need to toss out that broom because the bristles have become splayed with use. Wrap a rubber band around the broom a few inches from the bottom. Leave it for a day or so to get the bristles back in line.

CHILDPROOF KITCHEN AND BATH CUPBOARDS • The grandkids are coming! Time to get out the rubber bands and temporarily childproof the bathroom and kitchen cupboards you don't want them to get into. Just wrap the bands tightly around pairs of handles.

KEEP THREAD FROM TANGLING

Tired of tangled thread in your sewing box? Just wrap a rubber band around the spools to keep the threads from unraveling

MAKE A HOLDER FOR YOUR CAR VISOR • Snap a couple of rubber bands around the sun visors of your car. Now you have a handy spot to slip toll receipts, directions, or your cellphone when it's shut off.

THUMB THROUGH PAPERS WITH EASE • Stop licking your finger. Just wrap a rubber band around your index finger a few times the next time you need to shuffle papers. Not too tight, though—you don't want to cut off circulation to your fingertip.

WIPE OFF YOUR PAINTBRUSH • Every time you dip your paintbrush, you wipe the excess against the side of the can. Before you know it, paint is dripping off the side of the can and the little groove around the rim is so full of paint that it splatters everywhere when you go to hammer the lid back on. Avoiding all this mess is easy. Just wrap a rubber band around the can from top to bottom, going across the middle of the can opening. Now, when you fill your brush, you can just tap it against the rubber band and the excess paint will fall back into the can.

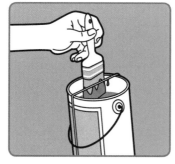

TIGHTEN FURNITURE CASTERS • Furniture leg casters can become loose with wear. To tighten one, wrap a rubber band around the stem and reinsert.

GAUGE YOUR LIQUIDS • Hmm, just how much floor finish is left in that can up on the shelf? Snap a rubber band around the liquid containers in your garage or shed and move them down as you use more. You'll always know how much is left at a glance.

PUMP LESS, SAVE MORE • Are you wasting precious –and expensive–soap, detergent, or lotion? Control portions of products that dispense from a pump, especially for kids who can't get enough. Wrap a rubber band tightly around the neck of the pump dispenser to limit the amount of each "squirt."

KEEP TRACK OF WINE GLASSES • Wrap a different colored rubber band around the stem of each glass the next time you have a dinner party or gathering. No more mixed-up drinks.

CUSHION YOUR REMOTE CONTROL

To protect your fine furniture from scratches and nicks, wrap a wide rubber band around both ends of the television remote control. You'll also be protecting the remote by making it less likely to slide off a table and be damaged

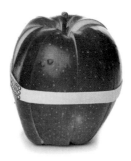

SAVE A SLICED APPLE • Bringing fruit for lunch? If you slice an apple into wedges and put them all back together, a rubber band wrapped around the apple will keep the wedges from turning brown or drying out. Plus, it's much better for the environment than using sandwich bags.

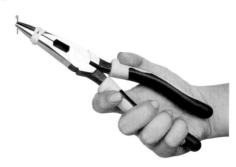

MAKE A SMALL-PARTS CLAMP • Need an extra pair of hands? Wrap a rubber band around the jaws of needle-nose pliers. It keeps the jaws of the pliers clamped together for holding small items. Works especially well for getting nuts into inaccessible spots or for starting small finishing nails.

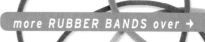

more RUBBER BANDS over →

EXTEND A BUTTON • Having trouble taking a big, deep breath? Maybe that top shirt button is a tad too tight. Stick a small rubber band through the buttonhole, then loop the ends over the button. Put on your tie, relax, and you can breathe easy.

SECURE BED SLATS • Nothing is more annoying than having your mattress fall through the slats in your bed just as you're getting ready for a dreamy night sleep. Here's how to secure those slippery boards. Wrap rubber bands around their ends to make them stay in place.

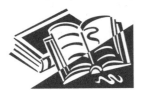

USE AS A BOOKMARK • While paper bookmarks can work well, they often slip out of the book. Before you lose your place in that exciting mystery novel, try wrapping a rubber band from top to bottom around the part of the book you've already read. Your place is now secured, even if you drop the book.

DID YOU KNOW?

The first rubber band was patented in 1845 by Stephen Perry, who owned a manufacturing company in London. A key ingredient in making rubber bands is sulphur. It is added to the rubber and heated—a process known as vulcanization—which makes the rubber strong and stretchy and prevents it from rotting. The process of making rubber bands is surprisingly similar to making a loaf of bread. The dry ingredients are mixed with natural rubber and the resulting friction and chemical reaction heats and partially vulcanizes the rubber. The rubber is cooled and rolled out like bread dough. It's extruded into a long tube, which is heated to finish the vulcanization. Finally, it's rinsed, cooled, and sliced into bands.

RUBBER JAR RINGS

KEEP A RUG FROM SLIPPING • If you have a throw rug that tends to skate across the floor, keep it in place by sewing a rubber jar ring or two on the underside in each corner.

PLAY INDOOR QUOITS • What else can kids do to keep cabin fever at bay on a rainy day? Turn a stool or small table upside down and let get them to try tossing rubber jar rings over the legs.

PROTECT TABLETOPS • Protect your tabletops from scratches and watermarks by placing a rubber jar ring under vases and lamps.

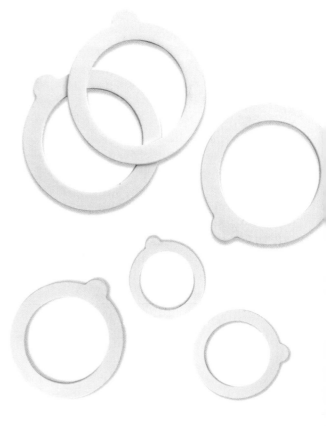

RUBBING ALCOHOL

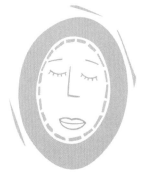

CLEAN VENETIAN BLINDS • Rubbing alcohol does a terrific job of cleaning the slats of venetian blinds. Wrap a flat tool—a spatula or a 6-inch (15-cm) cement trowel—in cloth and secure with a rubber band, dip in some rubbing alcohol, and go to work.

KEEP WINDOWS SPARKLING AND FROST-FREE • Do your windows frost up during winter? Wash them with a solution of ½ cup (125 ml) rubbing alcohol to 1 quart (1 L) water to prevent frost. Polish the windows with newspaper after you wash them to make them shine.

REMOVE INK STAINS • If you get ink on your favorite shirt or dress, try soaking the spot in rubbing alcohol for a few minutes before putting it into the wash.

PREVENT A RING AROUND THE COLLAR • To stop your neck from staining a shirt collar, wipe your neck with rubbing alcohol each morning before you dress.

REMOVE HAIR SPRAY FROM MIRRORS When you are spritzing your head with hair spray, some of it inevitably winds up on the mirror. A quick wipe with rubbing alcohol will whisk away that sticky residue and leave your mirror looking sparkling clean and shiny again.

DISSOLVE WINDSHIELD FROST • If you live in a cold-weather area, rather than scrape, scrape, scraping the frost from your car windows, fill a spray bottle with rubbing alcohol and squirt the car glass. You'll be able to wipe the frost right off after staying inside and enjoying your morning coffee for a little while longer.

CLEAN BATHROOM FIXTURES • Just reach into the medicine cabinet the next time you need to clean chrome bathroom fixtures. Pour some rubbing alcohol straight from the bottle onto a soft, absorbent cloth and the fixtures. No need to rinse—the alcohol just evaporates. It does a great job of making chrome sparkle, plus it will kill any germs in its path.

CAUTION: Don't confuse denatured alcohol with rubbing alcohol. Denatured alcohol is ethanol (drinking alcohol) to which poisonous and foul-tasting chemicals have been added to render it unfit for drinking. Often, the chemicals used in denatured alcohol are not ones you should put on your skin. Rubbing alcohol is made of chemicals that are safe for skin contact—it's usually 70 percent isopropyl alcohol and 30 percent water.

more RUBBING ALCOHOL over →

ERASE PERMANENT MARKERS • If you have the unhappy task of removing permanent marker from your countertop, don't worry, most countertops are made of nonpermeable material such as plastic laminate or granite. Rubbing alcohol will dissolve the marker into a liquid so you can wipe it right off.

REMOVE DOG TICKS • Ticks hate the taste of rubbing alcohol as much as they love the taste of your dog's blood. Before you pull a tick off of Rover, dab the tick with rubbing alcohol to make it loosen its grip. Grab the tick as close to the dog's skin as you can, using tweezers if you have them, and pull it straight out. Wet a cotton ball and dab the spot again to disinfect the wound. This works on people, too.

MAKE A SHAPEABLE ICE PACK • The problem with ice packs is that they won't conform to the shape of an injured body part. To make a slushy, conformable ice pack, mix 2 parts rubbing alcohol with 3 parts water in a ziplock plastic bag. The next time that sore knee acts up, wrap the bag of slush in a cloth and apply it to the area.

STRETCH TIGHT-FITTING NEW SHOES • This doesn't always work, but it's worth a try. If your new leather shoes are pinching your feet, try swabbing the tight spot with a cotton ball soaked in rubbing alcohol. Walk around in the shoes for a few minutes to see if they stretch enough to be comfortable. If not, the next step is to take them back to the shoe store.

GET RID OF FRUIT FLIES

The next time you see fruit flies hovering in the kitchen, get out a fine-misting spray bottle and fill it with rubbing alcohol. Spraying the little flies knocks them out and makes them fall to the floor, where you can sweep them up. The alcohol is less effective than insecticide, but it's a lot safer than spraying poison around your kitchen.

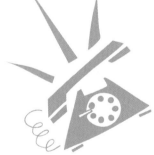

CLEAN YOUR PHONE

Is your phone getting a bit grubby? Wipe it down with rubbing alcohol. It will not only remove the grime, but also disinfect your phone at the same time.

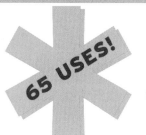

65 USES!

SALT

around the house

KEEP WICKER LOOKING NEW • Wicker furniture can yellow with age and exposure to the sun and elements. To keep your wicker natural-looking, scrub it with a stiff brush dipped in warm salt water. Let the piece dry in the sun. Repeat this process every year or two.

GIVE BROOMS A LONGER LIFE • A new straw broom will last longer if you soak its bristles in a bucket of hot, salty water. After about 20 minutes, remove the broom and let it dry.

EASY FIREPLACE CLEANUP • When you're ready to turn in for the night but the fire is still glowing in the hearth, douse the flames with salt. The fire will burn out more quickly, so you'll wind up with less soot than if you let it smolder. Cleanup is easier, too, because the salt helps the ash and residue gather into easy sweepings.

MAKE BRASS AND COPPER POLISH • When exposure to the elements dulls brass or copper items, there's no need to buy expensive cleaning products. To shine your candlesticks or remove green tarnish from copper pots, make a paste by mixing equal parts salt, flour, and vinegar. Use a soft cloth to rub this over the item, rinse with warm, soapy water, and buff back to its original shine.

REMOVE WINE FROM CARPET • Red wine spilled on a white carpet is the worst. But there's hope. First, while the red wine is still wet, pour some white wine on it to dilute the color. Then clean the spot with a sponge and cold water. Sprinkle the area with salt and wait about 10 minutes. Now vacuum up the whole mess.

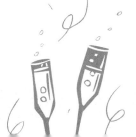

FLOWER POWER

CLEAR FLOWER RESIDUE IN A VASE • Once your beautiful bouquet is gone, the souvenir it leaves behind is not the kind of reminder you want: deposits of minerals on the vase interior. Reach inside the vase, rub the offending ring of deposits with salt, and wash with soapy water. If your hand won't fit inside, fill the vase with a strong solution of salt and water, shake it or brush gently with a bottlebrush, then wash. This should clear away the residue.

CLEAN ARTIFICIAL FLOWERS • You can quickly freshen up artificial flowers—whether they are authentic silk ones or the more common nylon variety—by placing them in a paper bag with 1/4 cup (50 g) of salt. Give the bag a few gentle shakes and your flowers will emerge as clean as the day you bought them.

HOLD ARTIFICIAL FLOWERS IN PLACE • Salt is a great medium for keeping artificial flowers in the arrangement you want. Fill a vase or other container with salt, add a little cold water and arrange your artificial flowers. The salt will solidify and the flowers will stay put.

more SALT over →

CLEAN GREASE STAINS FROM RUGS • If someone in your family is paying more attention to watching football than the greasy food on their plate, and it ends up on your nice white carpet, don't kill them. Just mix up 1 part salt to 4 parts rubbing alcohol and rub it hard on the grease stain, being careful to rub in the direction of the carpet's natural nap.

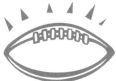

REMOVE WATERMARKS ON WOOD • Watermarks left from glasses on a wood table really stand out. Make them disappear by mixing 1 teaspoon (5 ml) salt with a few drops of water to form a paste. Gently rub the paste on the ring with a soft cloth or sponge and work it over the spot until it's gone. Restore the luster of your wood with furniture polish.

RESTORE A SPONGE • Hand sponges and mop sponges usually get grungy beyond use long before they are really worn out. To restore sponges to a pristine state, soak them overnight in a solution of about ¼ cup (50 g) salt per quart (1 L) water.

RELIEVE STINGS, BITES, AND POISON IVY • Salt works well to lessen the pain of bee stings, insect bites, and poison ivy rash:

■ Stung by a bee? Immediately wet the sting and cover it with salt. It will lessen the pain and reduce the swelling. Of course, if you are allergic to bee stings, seek medical attention immediately.

■ For relief from the itching of mosquito and chigger bites, soak the area in salt water, then apply a coating of lard or vegetable oil.

■ When poison ivy erupts, relieve the itching with a soak in hot salt water. If the case is severe, you might want to immerse yourself in a whole bathtub filled with salt water.

FROST-FREE WINDOWS AND WINDSHIELDS • As you know, if you live in a cold-climate area, salt greatly decreases the temperature at which ice freezes. You can use this fact to keep the windows in your home frost-free by wiping them with a sponge dipped in salt water, then letting them dry. In the winter, keep a small cloth bag of salt in your car. When the windshield and other windows are wet, rub them with the bag. The next time you go out to your car, the windows won't be covered with ice or snow.

DEODORIZE YOUR SNEAKERS

Sneakers and other canvas shoes can get pretty smelly, especially if you wear them without socks in the summer time. Knock down the odor and soak up the moisture by occasionally sprinkling a little salt in your canvas shoes.

MAKE A SCENTED AIR FRESHENER • Buying fragranced air fresheners can get expensive. Here is a wonderful way to make your room smell like a rose any time of the year. Layer rose petals and salt in a pretty jar with a tight-fitting lid. Remove the lid to freshen the room.

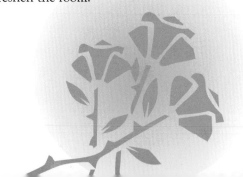

FISHY FACTS

GIVE GOLDFISH A PARASITE-KILLING BATH • The next time you take your goldfish out of its tank to change the water, put the fish in an invigorating saltwater bath for 15 minutes while you clean the tank. Make the bath by mixing 1 teaspoon (5 ml) noniodized salt into 1 quart (1 L) fresh water. (Just like the tank water, you should let faucet water sit overnight first to let chlorine evaporate.) The salt water kills parasites on the fish's scales and helps the fish absorb electrolytes. Don't add salt to the fish's tank, though. Goldfish are freshwater fish and can't spend a lot of time in salt water.

CLEAN YOUR FISH TANK • To remove mineral deposits from hard water in your fish tank, rub the inside of the tank with salt, then rinse the tank well before reintroducing the fish. Use only plain, not iodized, salt.

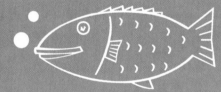

REPEL FLEAS IN PET HABITATS • If your dog enjoys his doghouse, chances are fleas do, too. Keep fleas from infesting your pet's home by washing down the interior walls and floor every few weeks with a solution of salt water.

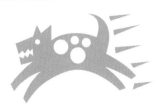

END THE ANT PARADE • If ants are beating a path to your home, intercept them by sprinkling salt across the door frame or directly on their paths. Ants will be discouraged from crossing this barrier.

DID YOU KNOW?

According to the U.S Geologic Survey, in 2012, six salt producers–China, U.S., India, Germany, Australia and Canada–accounted for more than half the world's 259 million metric tons (mmt) of salt produced. China was the leader at 70 mmt, followed by the U.S. (37.2 mmt), India (17 mmt), Germany (11.9 mmt), and Australia and Canada, both with 10.8 mmt.

in the kitchen

REMOVE BAKED-ON FOOD • Yes, you can remove food that has been baked onto cooking pans or serving plates. In fact, it's easy. Baked-on food can be 'lifted' with a pre-treatment of salt. Before washing, sprinkle the stuck-on food with salt. Dampen the area, let it sit until the salt lifts the baked-on food, then wash it away with soapy water.

KEEP OVEN SPILLS FROM HARDENING • The next time food bubbles over in your oven, toss some salt on it while it is still liquid. When the oven cools, you'll be able to wipe up the spill with a cloth. The same technique works for spills on the stovetop. Salt will remove odors, too, and if you'd like to add a pleasant scent, mix a bit of cinnamon in with the salt.

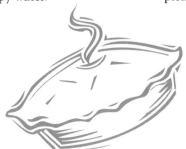

more SALT over →

MAKE GLASSES SPARKLE

CLEAN DISCOLORED GLASS • Did your dishwasher fail to remove those stubborn stains from your glassware? Hand-scrubbing failed, too? Try mixing a handful of salt in a quart (1 L) of vinegar and soak the glassware overnight. Stains should wipe off by morning.

REMOVE LIPSTICK FROM GLASSWARE • Lipstick smudges on glassware can be hard to remove, even in the dishwasher. That's because the emollients designed to help lipstick stay on your lips do a good job sticking to glassware, too. Before washing your stemware, rocks glasses, or water tumblers, rub the edges with salt to erase lipstick stains.

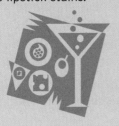

SOAK STAINS OFF ENAMEL PANS • You can run out of elbow grease trying to scrub burned-on stains from enamel pans. Skip the sweat. Soak the pan overnight in salt water, then boil salt water in the pan the next day. The stains should lift right off.

SCRUB OFF BURNED MILK • Burned milk is one of the toughest stains to remove, but salt makes it a lot easier. Wet the burned pan and sprinkle it with salt. Wait about 10 minutes, then scrub the pan. The salt absorbs that burned-milk odor, too.

CLEAN GREASY IRON PANS • Grease can be tough to remove from iron pans, because it is not water-soluble. Take a shortcut by sprinkling salt in the pan before you wash it. The salt will absorb most of the grease. Wipe the pan out and wash as usual.

CLEAN YOUR CAST-IRON WOK • No matter how thoroughly you dry them, cast-iron woks tend to rust when you wash them in water. Instead, when you've finished cooking, but while your wok is still hot, pour in about ¼ cup (50 g) salt and scrub it with a stiff wire brush. Wipe it clean and apply a light coating of sesame or vegetable oil before stowing it. Don't clean a wok with a nonstick coating this way, because it will scratch the coating.

BRIGHTEN UP YOUR CUTTING BOARDS • After you wash cutting boards and breadboards with soap and water, rub them with a damp cloth dipped in salt. The boards will lighten and brighten.

CLEAN THE REFRIGERATOR • We all have to do it sometime. After you've removed all the food and the racks from the fridge, mix up a handful of salt in about a gallon (4 L) of warm water and use it with a sponge to clean the inside of the fridge. The mixture isn't abrasive, so it won't scratch surfaces. And you won't be introducing chemical fumes or odors.

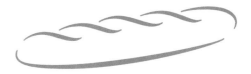

SPEED CLEANUP OF MESSY DOUGH

Here's a way to make short work of the cleanup after you've rolled out dough or kneaded breads. Sprinkle your floury countertop with salt. Now you can neatly wipe everything off with a sponge. No more sticky lumps.

ERASE TEA AND COFFEE STAINS • Tea and coffee leave stains on cups and in pots. You can easily scrub away these unattractive rings by sprinkling salt on a sponge and rubbing in little circles across the ring. If the stain persists, mix white vinegar with salt in equal proportions and rub with a sponge.

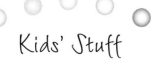

Kids' Stuff

Here's a craft dough easily fashioned into detailed ornaments, miniature foods, and dolls. In a bowl, slowly stir 1 cup (250 g) salt into 1 cup (250 ml) boiling water. After the salt dissolves, stir in 2 cups (500 g) all-purpose white flour. Turn dough out on a work surface and knead until smooth. If the dough sticks, add some flour, a little at a time until it is pliant. It should be easy to shape into balls, tubes, wreaths, and other shapes. Air-dry your creations or bake them in a 200°F (100°C) oven for up to 2 hours (time depends on thickness). Or microwave on *High* for 1 to 2 minutes. Apply paint, then protect and shine with a coat of clear nail polish or varnish.

SHINE YOUR TEAPOT SPOUT • Teapots with seriously stained spouts can be cleaned with salt. Stuff the spout with salt and let it sit overnight or at least several hours. Then run boiling water through the pot, washing away the salt and revealing the old sparkle. If the stain persists, treat the rim with a cotton swab dipped in salt.

CLEAN YOUR COFFEE PERCOLATOR • If your percolated coffee tastes a bit bitter these days, try this. Fill the percolator with water and add ¼ cup (50 g) salt, and percolate as usual. Rinse the percolator and all its parts well and the next pot you make should have the delicious flavor you love.

REVIVE OVERCOOKED COFFEE • If you make a pot of coffee, then get distracted for an hour, the coffee continues to cook in the pot and becomes bitter. Before you throw out such a brew, try adding a pinch of salt to the cup before pouring.

PREVENT GREASE SPLATTERS • How many times have you been burned by splattering grease while cooking bacon when all you wanted was a hearty breakfast? Next time, add a few dashes of salt to the pan before beginning to fry foods that can splatter. You'll cook without pain and you won't have to clean grease off your cooktop.

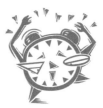

SPEED UP COOKING TIME

In a hurry? Add a pinch or two of salt to the water you are boiling food in. This makes the water boil at a higher temperature so the food you are cooking will require less time on the stove. Keep in mind, though, that salt does not make the water boil faster.

MAKE PERFECT POACHED EGGS •
It's possible to keep the whites intact when you poach eggs—you've had them in a café. No matter how careful you are, the whites always diffuse into the water when you poach eggs at home. Here's the secret. Sprinkle ½ teaspoon (2 ml) salt into the water just before you add your eggs. This helps to 'set' the whites in a neat package. A dash of vinegar also helps, and improves the taste of the eggs, too.

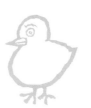

more SALT over →

DID YOU KNOW?

Salt was surely the first food seasoning. Prehistoric people got all the salt they needed from the meat that made up a large portion of their diet. When people began turning to agriculture as a more reliable food source, they discovered that salt—most likely from the sea—gave vegetables that salty taste they craved. As the millennia passed, salt gradually made life more comfortable and certain as people learned to use it to preserve food, cure hides, and heal wounds.

SHELL HARD-BOILED EGGS WITH EASE • Ever wonder whether there's a secret to peeling hard-boiled eggs without breaking the shell into a million tiny pieces? There is, and now it's out of the box! Add 1 teaspoon (5 ml) salt to the water before adding in the eggs to boil.

TEST AN EGG'S FRESHNESS • In doubt about whether your eggs are fresh? Add 2 teaspoons (10 ml) salt to 1 cup (250 ml) water and gently place the egg in the cup. A fresh egg will sink, an old one will float.

PICK UP SPILLED EGGS • If you've ever dropped an uncooked egg, you know what a mess it is to clean up. Cover the spill with salt. It will draw the egg together and you can easily wipe it up with a sponge or paper towel.

SHELL PECANS EASIER

Pecans can be tough nuts to crack. And once you do crack them, it can be tough to dig out the meat. Soak the nuts in salt water for several hours before shelling, and the meat will come cleanly away from the shells.

WASH KALE MORE EASILY • Fresh kale leaves are healthy and versatile, but their curvy, bumpy surface makes it difficult to wash away all the dirt that collects in the crevices. Try this trick: Wash kale leaves in salted water. Dirt is driven out along with salt in the rinse water, so you can cut the rinses down to just one.

KEEP SALAD CRISP • Do you need to prepare leafy salad in advance of a dinner party? Lightly salt the salad immediately after you prepare it and it will remain crisp for several hours.

REVIVE WRINKLED APPLES • Do your apples need a facelift? Soak them in mildly salted water to make the skin smooth again.

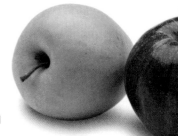

STOP CUT FRUIT FROM BROWNING • If you're preparing for a party by making the fruit salad ahead of time, you'll want to make sure your freshly cut fruit looks appetizing when you serve the dish. To ensure that cut apples and pears retain their color, soak them briefly in a bowl of lightly salted water.

SALT WHIPPING CREAM AND EGGS • The next time you whip cream or beat eggs, add a pinch of salt first. The cream will whip up lighter. The eggs will beat faster and higher, and they'll firm up better when you cook them.

KEEP YOUR MILK FRESH • Add a pinch of salt to a carton of milk to make it stay fresher longer. This works with cream, too.

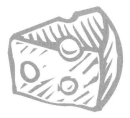

PREVENT MOLD ON CHEESE

Cheese is much too expensive to throw away because it has become moldy. Prevent mold by wrapping cheese in a napkin soaked in salt water before storing it in the refrigerator.

DID YOU KNOW?

The concentration of salt in your body is nearly one-third of the concentration found in seawater. This is why blood, sweat, and tears are so salty. Many scientists believe that humans, as well as all animals, need salt because all life evolved from the oceans. When the first land dwellers crawled out of the sea, they carried the need for salt—and a bit of the supply—with them and passed it on to their descendants.

EXTINGUISH GREASE FIRES • Store a box of salt next to the stove. Should a grease fire erupt, toss the salt on it to extinguish the flames. Never pour water on a grease fire—it will cause the grease to splatter and spread the fire. Salt is the solution when barbecue flames from meat drippings get too high. Sprinkling salt on the coals will quell the flames without causing a lot of smoke and cooling the coals, as water does.

in the laundry

CLEAN YOUR IRON'S METAL SOLEPLATE • It seems to happen on a regular basis. No matter how careful you are while ironing, something melts onto the iron, forming a rough surface that is difficult to remove. Salt crystals are the answer. Turn your iron to *High*, sprinkle table salt on a section of newspaper on your ironing board, run the hot iron over the salt, and you'll iron away the bumps.

MAKE A QUICK PRE-TREATMENT

If you're dining out with friends and notice that a little salad dressing has spotted your slacks, you know it can't be fixed with water, but here's an idea that will stop the stain from ruining your clothing. Cover the spot in salt to absorb the grease. When you get home, wash as usual.

REMOVE PERSPIRATION STAINS • Salt's the secret to getting rid of those stubborn yellow perspiration stains on shirts. Dissolve ¼ cup (50 g) of salt in 1 quart (1 L) of hot water. Just sponge the garment with the solution until the stain disappears.

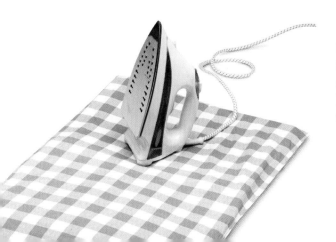

more SALT over →

SET THE COLOR IN NEW TOWELS • The first two or three times you wash new, colored towels, add 1 cup (250 g) salt to the wash. The salt will set the colors so your towels will remain bright much longer.

in the garden

STOP WEEDS IN THEIR TRACKS • Those weeds that pop up in the cracks of your paths can be tough to eradicate. But salt can do the job. Bring a solution of about 1 cup (250 g) salt in 2 cups (500 ml) water to a boil. Pour directly on the weeds to kill them. Another equally effective method is to spread salt directly on the weeds or unwanted grass that come up between patio bricks or blocks. Sprinkle with water or just wait until rain does the job for you.

RID YOUR GARDEN OF SNAILS AND SLUGS • These little fellas are not good for your plants. But there's a simple, chemical-free solution. Take a container of salt into the garden and douse the offenders. They won't survive for long.

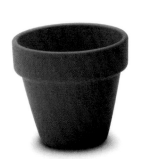

CLEAN FLOWERPOTS WITHOUT WATER • When you need to clean out a flowerpot for reuse, instead of making a muddy mess by washing the pot in water, just sprinkle in a little salt and scrub off the dry dirt with a stiff brush. This method is especially handy if your potting bench is not near a water source.

in the bath

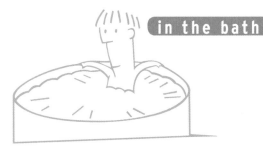

your bathtub and soak as usual. Your skin will be noticeably softer. Buy sea salt for a real treat. It comes in larger chunks and can be found in health food stores or the gourmet section of supermarkets.

A PRE-SHAMPOO DANDRUFF TREATMENT • The abrasiveness of ordinary table salt works well for scrubbing out dandruff before you shampoo. Grab a saltshaker and shake some salt on your dry scalp. Then work it through your hair, giving your scalp a massage. You'll find you've worked out the dry, flaky skin and are ready for a shampoo.

CONDITION YOUR SKIN • Most people have heard of bath salts, but usually this conjures images of scented crystals that bubble up in your tub and may contain coloring and other stuff that leave a dreaded bathtub ring behind. Now strip that picture to its core, and you've got salt. Dissolve 1 cup (250 g) table salt in

GIVE YOURSELF A SALT RUBDOWN • To remove dead skin particles and boost your circulation, try this. Either while still in the tub, or just after stepping out—while your skin is still damp—give yourself a massage with dry salt. Ordinary salt works well; those larger sea salt crystals also do the job.

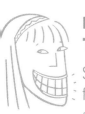

FRESHEN YOUR BREATH THE OLD-FASHIONED WAY

Store-bought mouthwash can contain food coloring, alcohol, and sweeteners, and it isn't cheap. Use this recipe and your breath will be just as sweet. Mix 1 teaspoon (5 ml) salt and 1 teaspoon (5 ml) baking soda into 1/2 cup (125 ml) water. Rinse and gargle.

OPEN HAIR-CLOGGED DRAINS • It's tough to keep hair and shampoo residues from collecting in the bathtub drain and clogging it. Dissolve the mess with 1 cup (250 g) salt, 1 cup (250 g) baking soda, and 1/2 cup (125 ml) white vinegar. Pour the mixture down the drain. After 10 minutes, follow with 2 quarts (2 L) boiling water, and run the hot water until the drain flows freely.

REMOVE SPOTS ON BATHTUB ENAMEL • Yellow spots on enamel bathtubs or sinks can be lessened by mixing up a solution of salt and turpentine in equal parts. Using rubber gloves, rub away the discoloration and rinse thoroughly. Be sure to ventilate the bathroom while you perform this task.

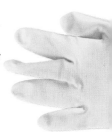

SALTSHAKERS

CUT BACK ON SUGAR • You can cut back on sugar but still keep your sweet tooth happy if you fill a saltshaker with sugar. For sugar-restricted diets, use your sugar shaker as an alternative to dipping into the sugar bowl and sprinkle lightly over food.

USE AS A CINNAMON-SUGAR DISPENSER • Cinnamon toast is a great comfort food, and everyone likes it made a certain way. Mix sugar and cinnamon to your taste in a saltshaker. Once you've found the proportions you like, you can make it easily and consistently every time. Your cinnamon-sugar shaker is also perfect for sprinkling extra flavor on cereal.

USE FOR FLOUR-DUSTING • Baking is sometimes a messy job, so make at least one part of it tidier by putting flour into a large saltshaker. It's perfect for dusting your cake pans or muffin tins. Keep it neat and keep it handy in the cupboard, especially if you have an aggressively helpful junior chef!

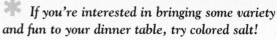

Colored salt

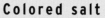 *If you're interested in bringing some variety and fun to your dinner table, try colored salt!*

Put a few tablespoons of salt into a plastic sandwich bag and add a few drops of food coloring. Work it gently with your fingers to mix, then let it to dry in the open bag for about a day. Just cut a hole in the corner of the bag to pour the festive salt into your saltshaker. As a bonus, your colored table or kosher salt makes wonderful homemade glitter!

USE TO APPLY DRY FERTILIZER • If you use dry fertilizer, try putting it in a saltshaker to use when fertilizing seedlings. It gives you lots of application control so you can prevent fertilizer burn on your tender babies.

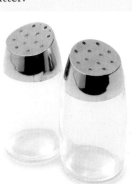

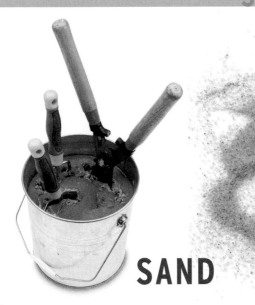

SAND

PROTECT AND STORE GARDEN TOOLS • Your gardening tools are meant to last longer than your perennials, so keep them clean and protected from the elements. Fill a 5-gallon (19-L) bucket with builder's sand (available from masonry supply and home centers) and pour in about 1 quart (1 L) clean motor oil. Plunge shovels and other tools into the sand a few times to clean and lubricate them. To prevent rust, leave the tool blades in the bucket of sand for storage. A coffee can, filled with sand and a little motor oil, will provide the same protection for your pruners and hand trowels.

CLEAN A NARROW-NECK VASE • All vases get gunk and dirty watermarks stuck to their insides, and it isn't always easy to clean off. If the vase neck is too narrow for your hand, put a bit of sand and warm, soapy water into the vase and swish gently. The sand will clean off the residue that you can't reach inside.

HOLD ITEMS WHILE GLUING • Repairing small items, such as broken china, with glue would be easy if you had three hands—one for each piece along with one to apply the glue. Since you only have two hands, try this. Stick the biggest part of the item in a small container of sand to hold it steady. Position the large piece so that when you set the broken piece in place, the piece will balance. Apply glue to both edges and stick on the broken piece. Leave the mended piece there and the sand will hold it steady until the glue dries.

USE FOR TIRE TRACTION • A bag of sand kept in the trunk of your car is good insurance in icy weather against getting stuck or spinning out from a parking spot. Throw in a clean margarine tub as well, to use as a scoop. For rear-wheel-drive vehicles, a bag or two of sand will also give you some extra traction.

SANDPAPER

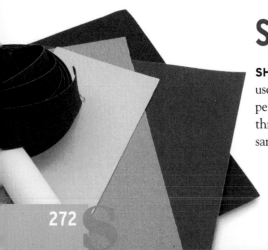

SHARPEN SEWING NEEDLES • Think twice before throwing out a used piece of fine-grit sandpaper. The unused edges or corners are perfect for tucking into your sewing box. Poking your sewing needles through sandpaper a few times, or twisting them inside a folded piece of sandpaper, will make them sharper than new.

Kids' Stuff

You or your little Leonardo can make a beautiful one-of-a-kind T-shirt. Have your child use crayons to draw a bold design on the rough side of a sheet of sandpaper. Lay the T-shirt on your ironing board and slip a sheet of aluminium foil inside, between the front and back of the shirt. Place the sandpaper on the T-shirt, design side down. Using an iron on the warm setting, press the back of the sandpaper in one spot for about 10 seconds, then move on to the next spot until the entire design has been pressed. Let the shirt cool to set the design, launder on a cool setting, and hang to dry.

SHARPEN SCISSORS • Are your scissor cuts less crisp than they used to be? Try cutting through a sheet of fine-grit sandpaper to sharpen the edges and keep cuts clean.

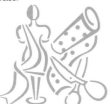

REMOVE FUZZY PILLS ON SWEATERS • If you're fighting a losing battle with pilling on your sweaters, a bit of sandpaper will handle them. Use any grit, and rub lightly in one direction.

REMOVE SCORCHES ON WOOL • Take some medium-grit sandpaper to any small scorch spots on your woolen clothing. The mark left by a careless spark will be less noticeable with some light sanding around the edges.

HOLD PLEATS WHILE IRONING • Keep some fine- or medium-grit sandpaper where you store your iron, for putting under pleats to hold them in place while you iron a nice sharp fold.

ROUGHEN SLIPPERY LEATHER SOLES

New shoes with slippery soles can send you flying, so take a scrap of sandpaper and a little time to sand across the width of the soles and roughen up the slick surface. It's cheaper and easier than taking your new shoes to a repair shop to have rubber soles put on.

REMOVE INK STAINS AND SCUFF MARKS FROM SUEDE • A bit of fine-grit sandpaper and a gentle touch is great for removing or at least minimizing an ink stain or small scuff mark on suede clothing or shoes. Afterwards, bring up the nap with a toothbrush or nailbrush. You just might avoid an expensive trip to the dry cleaners!

DETER SLUGS • Slugs and snails are unwelcome guests that never leave, but you can stop them from getting into your potted plants in the first place. Put used sanding disks to work under the bases of your pots, making sure the sandpaper is wider than the pot base.

REMOVE STUBBORN GROUT STAINS • Sometimes your bathroom abrasive cleaner is just not abrasive enough. Get tough on grout stains with fine-grit sandpaper. Fold the sandpaper and use the folded edge to sand in the grout seam. Be careful not to sand the tile and scratch the finish.

OPEN A STUCK JAR • If you're having a tough time opening a jar, grab a piece of sandpaper and place it grit side down on the lid. The sandpaper should improve your grip enough to do the job.

MAKE AN EMERY BOARD • If you don't have an emery board handy the next time you need to smooth your nails, just raid the sandpaper stash in the garage workshop. Look for a piece marked 120 grit or 150 grit on the back.

sandwich and freezer bags
sandwich and freezer bags
SANDWICH AN

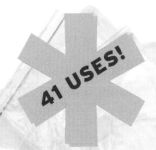

41 USES!

SANDWICH AND FREEZER BAGS

around the house

PROTECT YOUR PICTURES • You just picked up a batch of beautiful photos of your overseas vacation. Before you show them around to your friends and family, encase each in a small, clear sandwich bag. Then enjoy the oohs and aahs without any smudges on your pictures.

FREEZE A WASHCLOTH FOR A COLD PACK • It's hard to predict when someone in your household will suffer a burn, teething pain, or another bump or scrape, so be ready. Freeze a wet washcloth in a sandwich or freezer bag. Pull it out of the freezer the next time someone needs some cold care.

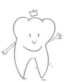

DISPLAY BABY TEETH

When small children lose their first tooth, it's only natural they want to show it off. To make sure they don't lose that precious memento, place the tooth in a small sealable plastic bag. That way, they can easily display it and you won't have to worry about the tooth getting lost.

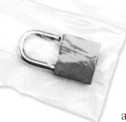

PROTECT YOUR PADLOCKS • When the weather is cold enough to freeze your padlocks on the backyard shed or garage, remember that a sandwich bag can help. Slip one over the lock and you'll avoid frozen tumblers.

MOLD SOAP SCRAPS INTO A NEW BAR • The penny pinchers among us hate to throw out a sliver of soap. Yet they're impossible to use when they get small. Instead, start collecting them all in a resealable plastic bag. When you have several, place the bag in a pan of warm, not boiling, water. Watch the soap pieces melt. When the mixture cools, you'll have a new bar of soap.

MAKE A FABRIC-SOFTENER DISPENSER • Who can ever remember to add the fabric softener to the washing machine at the right time? You won't have to again with this tip. Punch some pinholes in a sealable plastic bag and, holding it over the laundry tub, fill it with fabric softener. Seal the plastic bag and toss it into the laundry. The softener dispenses slowly through the pinholes during the wash and you won't have to remember that extra step.

MAKE BABY WIPES ON THE CHEAP • You could buy outrageously expensive baby wipes at the supermarket or purchase some in bulk and hope they don't dry out before you use them up. Or you can just take the crafty way out. Make your own baby wipes by placing soft paper towels in a sealable plastic bag with 1 tablespoon (15 ml) gentle antibacterial soap, 1 teaspoon (5 ml) baby oil, and 1/3 cup (75 ml) water. Use enough of the mixture to get the wipes damp, not drenched.

DID YOU KNOW?

Of course, we haven't always carried our ham-and-cheese sandwiches to work in plastic bags. Sandwich-sized plastic bags were first introduced in the U.S. in 1957. Seven years later, Mobil Corp. introduced sandwich bags with tuck-in flaps, also known as Baggies. Just in case you are too young to remember, before plastic bags, we wrapped our sandwiches in grease-proof paper or wax paper, like they still do in most delicatessens.

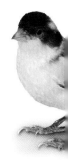

STARCH CRAFT ITEMS • You've just completed that handmade Christmas stocking for your grandchild. But the last fabric ornaments to attach need to be starched. Throw them in a resealable plastic bag that contains a bit of starch. Shake until covered, remove, and allow to dry thoroughly. Save the starch in the bag for your next craft project.

FEED THE BIRDS • Be kind to the birds in your garden during the lean winter months. Mix some birdseed with peanut butter in a resealable bag. Seal the bag and mix the ingredients by kneading the outside of the bag. Then place the glob in a small net bag or spread on a pinecone. Attach it to a tree, and await the grateful flock.

in the kitchen

STORE GRATED CHEESE • Pasta or pizza is always better with a dash of freshly grated Parmesan cheese. But who wants to bother with getting the grater out every time you want that taste? Instead, take a wedge of Parmesan cheese, grate the whole thing at once, and double bag it in two resealable bags to protect the freshness. Or stick the grater in the bag with the cheese wedge and pull it out for a short grate when the pesto gets to the table. That way you won't have to clean the grater after each use.

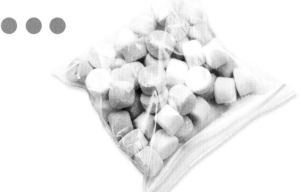

SOFTEN HARD MARSHMALLOWS • If you grab a bag of marshmallows from your kitchen cupboard for toasting around an open fire, and you notice that their once-fluffy form has turned to rock, just warm some water in a saucepan, place the marshmallows in a resealable plastic bag, seal it, and place it in the pan. The warmth will soften them up in no time.

MAKE A PASTRY BAG • Pastry bags can be cumbersome, expensive, and hard to clean. Stop scrounging around the kitchen drawer for the pastry bag tips. Place the food to be piped, be it deviled-egg mix or decorating icing, in a resealable plastic bag. Squish out the air and close the top. Snip off a corner of the bag to the size you want—start small—and you are ready to begin squeezing.

DISPOSE OF COOKING OIL • Don't clog your kitchen drain with used cooking oil, instead, wait for it to cool, then dump it in a resealable plastic bag. Toss the bag into the garbage.

COLOR DOUGH WITHOUT STAINED HANDS • Experienced bakers know what a mess your hands can be after coloring cookie dough. Here's a an idea for keeping them clean. Place your prepared dough in a bag, add the drops of food coloring and squish around until the color is uniform. You can use the dough now or stick it in the freezer, ready to roll out when the next occasion arises.

PREVENT ICE CRYSTALS ON ICE CREAM • It's annoying to open up a container of chocolate-chip ice cream from the freezer to find unappetizing ice crystals on it. Stop this from happening by placing a half-full ice-cream container in a sealable plastic bag and no crystals will form.

more SANDWICH AND FREEZER BAGS over →

sandwich and freezer bags
sandwich and freezer bags
SANDWICH AN

STORE EXTRA ICE CUBES • It's a common experience. You open the freezer to grab some ice cubes from it and find they're all stuck together, sometimes even clogging the ice cube dispenser on the front of the fridge. When the tray fills up, toss the cubes in a resealable freezer bag. They won't stick together and you'll have easy access to the ice.

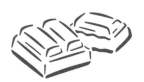

MELT CHOCOLATE WITHOUT A MESS

Melting chocolate in a microwave or double boiler leaves you with a messy bowl or pot to wash. Here's a mess-free method. Warm (don't boil) some water in a pan. Place the chocolate you want to melt in a sealable freezer bag. Seal and place the bag in the pan. In a few minutes, you'll have melted chocolate, ready for baking or decorating. You can even leave the bag sealed and snip off a bottom corner to pipe the chocolate onto a cake. When you're done, toss the bag in the garbage can.

KEEP SODA FROM GOING FLAT • If you have to go out for a meeting and you don't want to take the soda you've just opened with you, leave the opened bottle or can contained in a large resealable plastic bag. That should help keep the fizz in until you get back.

Kids' Stuff

Dyed dry pasta in different shapes and sizes is great for getting kids' creative juices flowing. They can use it to make string jewelry on wool, or to decorate a picture frame or pencil cup, for example. To dye the pasta, put a handful of pasta in a sealable plastic bag. Add several drops of food coloring. Next squirt in a few drops of rubbing alcohol and seal the bag. Shake it up so the food coloring dyes the pasta. Spread the pasta out on foil and allow it to dry.

GREASE CAKE PANS • If you're never quite sure how to handle shortening and butter when greasing a cake pan or cookie sheet, here's a tip. Place a sandwich bag over your hand, scoop up a small amount of shortening or butter from the tub and start greasing. You can leave the sandwich bag in the tub of shortening for the next time you need it.

USE AS KIDS' GLOVES • There's nothing more welcome than helping hands in the kitchen. But when they're little hands that tend to get dirty and leave prints all over the place, then something must be done. Before they start 'helping' you make those chocolate-chip cookies, place small sandwich bags over their hands. These instant gloves are disposable for easy clean-up.

MAKE A FUNNEL • That handiest of kitchen tools, the funnel, can be replicated easily with a small sandwich bag. Fill the bag with the contents you need funneled. Snip off the end and transfer the contents into the needed container. Then just toss the bag when the funneling is done.

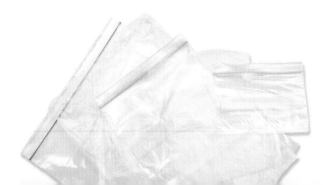

REEZER BAGS
sandwich and freezer bags

sandwich and freezer bags

for storing things

PROTECT YOUR FRAGILE BREAKABLES • If you've got a precious family heirloom—a small statue, a vase, or a trinket—that needs some extra padding during storage, here's what to do. Gently place it in a resealable bag, close the bag most of the way, blow it up with air, then finish sealing it. The air forms a protective cushion around the memento.

SAVE YOUR SWEATERS • When you're about to put away a pile of winter sweaters for the season, don't just throw them in a box without protection. Place each sweater in a large sealable plastic bag and seal. They'll be clean and moth-free when the colder weather rolls around again. Save the bags for next spring when the sweaters need to be stored again.

CREATE A SACHET

If your drawers are starting to smell musty, a sealable bag can be your dresser's best friend. Fill the bag with potpourri–dried flower petals, along with a few crushed fragrant leaves and a couple of drops of aromatic oil. Punch a collection of small holes in the bag, then place it in the drawer. Your drawers will soon smell fresh again.

ADD CEDAR TO YOUR WARDROBE • Cedar closets smell great and, more importantly, they repel moths. If you aren't lucky enough to have a cedar closet, you can easily create the next best thing. Fill a sealable bag with cedar chips—the kind you buy from a pet store to put in guinea pig cages. Zip it closed, then punch several small holes in it. Hang the bag in your closet (a pants hanger is handy for this) and let the cedar smell do its work.

MAKE A PENCIL BAG • Do the kids have trouble keeping track of their school pencils, pens, and rulers? Puncture three holes along the bottom edge of a resealable freezer bag so it will fit in a three-ring binder. Now the young scholars can zip their supplies in and out of the bag.

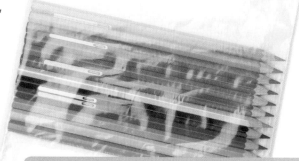

more SANDWICH AND FREEZER BAGS over →

sandwich and freezer bags
sandwich and freezer bags
SANDWICH AN

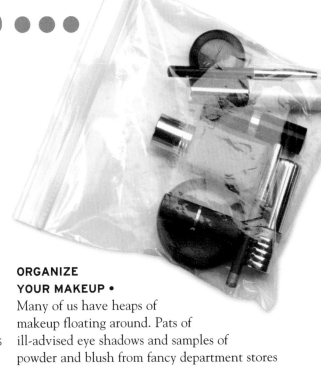

in the bath

DE-CLUTTER THE BATHROOM • Here's a quick cleanup solution. Friends are coming over and the bathroom is strewn with loofahs, razors, shaving cream, and more. Quickly gather up all the supplies in one clear sealable plastic bag. That way, you will know where the shaving supplies are, but you won't have to deal with them at the same time you're cooking dinner.

MAKE A BATH PILLOW • Ready for a nice hot bath? Want to luxuriate in the warm water with bubbles and champagne? Well, here's the perfect, and cheap, thing to make your bath experience complete. Blow up a gallon size (4 L) sealable plastic bag and you'll have a comfortable pillow for your soak.

CLEAN DENTURES • To avoid having your dentures on display in a cup by your bedside, toss them, along with their cleaner, in a resealable plastic bag in the bathroom. They'll be perfectly clean and ready to go in the morning.

ORGANIZE YOUR MAKEUP • Many of us have heaps of makeup floating around. Pats of ill-advised eye shadows and samples of powder and blush from fancy department stores fill our makeup cases. Stash everyday favorites in a resealable plastic bag so you don't have to hunt for them every morning. Clean out what you'll never use and store the rest for a special occasion.

out and about

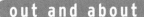

STASH DIRTY CLOTHES • Chocolate ice cream is dripping down your child's white Sunday-best shirt. If you can keep the stain from drying, it will be a lot easier to get out. Change their shirt and spray the stained shirt with stain remover if you have a small bottle handy or just soak it in water if you don't. Then seal the shirt in a ziplock bag and it will be ready for the wash when you get home.

HOLD SPARE CLOTHES • Toilet training a child? Need to be ready for meal mishaps? Put a change of clothes for your son or daughter in a resealable plastic bag and keep it in the trunk of your car. You won't have to think twice the next time there's an 'accident' and your bag will be lighter.

CARRY DETERGENT FOR WASHING • If you're planning a beach vacation and think you'll be doing a few loads of laundry while you're away, premeasure some detergent in a bag that you can pour out when the time comes. Beats lugging a big box of laundry detergent to the shore.

CARRY A WET WASHCLOTH FOR COOLING OFF • Going for a long trip on a hot and sticky day? Use a sealable bag to take along a wet washcloth that has been soaked in water and lemon juice. Carry one for each person so that everyone can get a refreshing wipe. This is a good trick for fast on-the-road, face-and-hand cleanups anytime.

CREATE A BEACH HAND CLEANER • You're sitting on the beach and it's time for lunch, but before you reach into the cooler, you'll want to get the grit off your hands. Baby powder in a resealable plastic bag is key. Place your hands in the bag, remove them and rub them together. The sand will wipe away.

APPLY INSECT REPELLENT TO YOUR FACE

It's tricky applying insect repellent to your face without squirting yourself in the eyes or getting it on your hands. Instead, throw some cotton balls into a plastic bag, squirt in the repellent, seal, and shake. Now use the cotton balls to apply the insect repellent.

CURE CAR SICKNESS • The last thing anyone wants in their car is a child vomiting. You can make a child feel better and head off the mess and stench by placing a few cotton balls in a resealable plastic bag with 2 drops of lavender oil added. If motion sickness strikes, the child can open the bag and take a few whiffs of the oil to help ease the car sickness.

KEEP YOUR VALUABLES DRY AND AFLOAT • Whoops! You tipped the canoe and got dunked. No biggie, until that sinking feeling hits—your car keys and mobile phone are at the bottom of the lake. Avoid this disaster by putting your valuables in a resealable plastic bag. Blow air into it before you seal the bag so it will float. A resealable bag can also keep valuables dry at a water park or at the beach, too.

Kids' Stuff

This is a fantastic activity if you're outdoors. Pour a small box of instant pudding mix into a resealable plastic bag and add the amount of milk recommended on the side of the box. Seal it up then reseal that bag in another sealable bag. Now you're ready to play football. Toss the bag of pudding around with your friends until it mixes and the pudding forms. Open the first bag and remove the second bag. Pour into flat-bottomed ice-cream cones and enjoy your treat.

USE AS A PORTABLE WATER DISH • When your furry best friend happily hikes alongside you during a trek in the great outdoors, don't forget that he needs water to stay hydrated, just as you do. So take a large resealable plastic bag full of water with you and hold it open for him to drink from along the way.

S 279

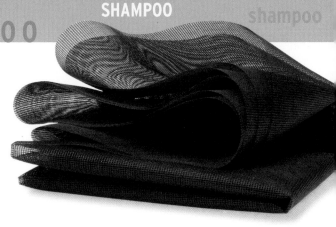

SCREENING

GET RID OF PAINT LUMPS • You want to do a touch-up paint job, but your used can of paint has some lumps in it. Instead of going through the bother of straining the paint into another container, try this. Cut a circle of screening sized to fit inside the can (use the lid as a guide for cutting). Place the screen circle on top of the paint and push it gently down to the bottom with your stirring stick. The lumps will now be trapped at the bottom of the can. Stir the paint and get to work.

PROTECT NEWLY PLANTED SEEDS • Who knows what is walking around your garden at night, so protect newly planted seeds by covering them with a sheet of screening material. It also might deter the neighborhood felines from using your nice, fluffy soil as a litter box. When the seedlings emerge, you can bend the screening to make cages.

STORE PIERCED EARRINGS • Keep your stud and hook earrings organized and ready at a glance with a spare piece of screening. Cut a square of screen with metal shears or utility scissors and cover the edges of the square with duct or cloth tape. Then push the earrings through the holes in the screen. If you like, you can hang the screen square on the wall by attaching string or floral wire to the top corners.

SHAMPOO

REVITALIZE LEATHER SHOES AND PURSES • You don't need expensive mink oil to bring life back to your leather shoes and purses. A bit of good old shampoo and a clean rag will do the job. Rub shampoo into worn areas in circles to clean and bring back the color of your accessories. It will protect your shoes from salt stains as well.

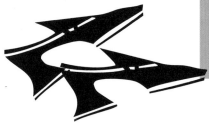

DID YOU KNOW?

One of the longest-running advertising campaigns in history, "the Breck Girl," was the brainchild of Edward Breck, a member of the family that started Breck Shampoo Co. The ads, featuring wholesome, beautiful girls with gorgeous hair, began in 1936, during the Great Depression, although they didn't go national until 1947, and then went international soon after that. Only two artists were used during the 40-year campaign. The best known was Ralph William Williams, who took over the job in 1957. Among the models for Williams's Breck girls were Cybill Shepherd, Kim Basinger, and Brooke Shields, who were all unknowns at the time. The campaign ceased soon after Williams's death in 1976.

LUBRICATE A ZIPPER • If your zipper gets stuck, don't yank on it until it breaks. Put a drop of shampoo on a cotton swab and dab it on the zipper. The shampoo will help the zipper to slide free, and any residue will come out in the wash.

RESIZE A SHRUNKEN SWEATER • If you've shrunk your favorite sweater, don't panic, you can often bring it back to full size again with baby shampoo and warm water. Fill a basin with warm water, squirt in some baby shampoo and swish once with your hand. Lay the sweater on top of the water and let it sink on its own and soak for 15 minutes. Gently take your sweater out without wringing it and put it in a container, then fill the sink again with clean water. Lay the sweater on top and let it sink again to rinse. Take the sweater out, place it on a towel and roll the towel to take out most of the moisture. Lay the sweater on a dry towel on a flat surface and gently start to reshape it. Come back to the sweater while it's drying to reshape a little more each time. Your patience will be rewarded!

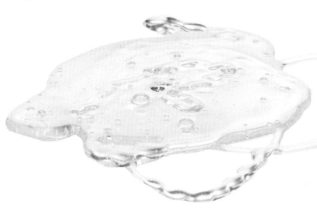

WASH HOUSEPLANT LEAVES

Houseplants get dusty, too, but unlike furniture they need to breathe. Make a soapy solution with a few drops of shampoo in a pot of water, dunk in a cloth and wring it out, then wipe those dusty leaves clean without harming them.

DID YOU KNOW?

In the early 1900s, Canadian Martha Matilda Harper invented the reclining chair used when shampooing hair at beauty salons—unfortunately, she never patented it. But Harper was still a success. She emigrated from Canada to the United States as a young girl, bringing her own recipe for a hair "tonic" (shampoo). Eventually she went from making her tonic in a shed to opening her own shop, where she offered the Harper Method. She enticed wealthy women to leave their homes for a health-conscious salon experience where they would be shampooed and pampered by professionals. She was her own best advertisement, with hair that reached down past her feet.

CLEAN YOUR CAR • The grease-cutting power of shampoo works on the family grease monkey's baby as well. Use about ¼ cup (50 ml) shampoo to a bucket of water and sponge up the car as usual. Use a dab of shampoo directly on a rag or sponge for hard-to-remove tar spots on the car's paint finish.

LUBRICATE STUBBORN NUTS AND BOLTS • Got a nut and bolt that won't come apart? If your spot lubricant isn't handy or you've run out, try a drop of shampoo instead. Let it seep into the threads and the bolt will be much more cooperative.

REMOVE STICKY GUNK FROM PET FUR • Did Rex or Fluffy step on tar or roll in what you hope is gum? Rub a tiny amount of shampoo on the spot, then gently draw out the sticky stuff towards the end of the fur. Rinse with a wet cloth.

more SHAMPOO over →

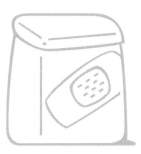

REMOVE BANDAGES PAINLESSLY

Now you don't have to say 'Ready?' when removing a bandage. Rub just a drop of shampoo on and around the bandage and let it seep through the air holes. It will come off with no mess and definitely no fuss.

REVITALIZE YOUR FEET • Give your feet a cheap and effective pick-me-up while you sleep. Rub a bit of shampoo all over your feet and put on a light pair of cotton socks. When you wake up, your feet will feel smooth and silky.

REMOVE YOUR EYE MAKEUP • You can't beat no-tears baby shampoo for a cheap eye makeup remover. Put a drop on a damp cotton pad to gently remove the makeup and rinse clear. No frills, no tears!

**GIVE YOURSELF
A BUBBLE BATH**
Shampoo makes a nice and sudsy bubble bath. And it's especially relaxing if you love the scent of your favorite shampoo. The bathtub will rinse cleaner, too.

USE IT INSTEAD OF SHAVING CREAM • If you're on the road and discover you forgot to bring your shaving cream, don't use soap. With its softening agents, shampoo is a much better alternative.

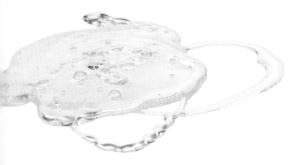

CLEAN GRIMY HANDS • In place of soap, some straight shampoo works wonders for cleaning stubborn or sticky grime from your hands. It even works well to remove water-based paint from skin.

REMOVE HAIR SPRAY FROM WALLS • If you've been using hair spray to kill flies, or you've just noticed hair spray buildup on your bathroom walls, reach for the shampoo. Put some on a wet sponge to clean, then wipe off suds with a clean, wet sponge. Shampoo is tailor-made to handle hair product buildup, wherever it occurs.

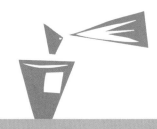

DID YOU KNOW?

Johnson & Johnson introduced the world's first shampoo made specifically for infants in 1955–containing its now-famous No More Tears formula. The company has promoted its baby shampoo to be "as gentle to the eyes as pure water." But, in fact, like most baby shampoos, Johnson's contains many of the same ingredients found in adult formulations, including citric acid, PEG-80 sorbitan laurate, and sodium trideceth sulphate. The lack of baby tears has less to do with the shampoo's purity than it does with maintaining a relatively neutral pH.

CLEAN THE TUB AND FAUCETS • Need to do a quick tub cleanup before guests arrive? Grab the handiest item—your shampoo! It does a great job on soap scum because it rinses clean. You can use it to buff a shine on your chrome faucets as well.

WASH YOUR DELICATES • Shampoo makes a great cleanser for delicate fabric items that need washing. It suds up well with just a drop, and you get two cleaning products for the price of one.

SHAVING CREAM

CLEAN YOUR HANDS • The next time your hands get dirty on a camping trip, save that hard-lugged water for cooking and drinking. Squirt a little shaving cream into your hands and rub as you would liquid soap. Then wipe your hands off with a towel.

PREVENT BATHROOM MIRROR FOG-UP • Before you shower, wipe some shaving cream on your bathroom mirror. It will stop it from fogging up so you won't waste time waiting for the mirror to clear to start shaving, or have to shave while peering through the streaks created by your towel.

REMOVE STAINS FROM CARPETING • If juice gets spilled on your carpet, put some shaving cream on the spot. Blot the stain, pat it with a wet sponge, squirt some shaving cream on it, and wipe clean with a damp sponge. Use the same technique on your clothes for small stains; shaving cream can remove that spot of breakfast you discovered you're wearing during your once-over in the bathroom.

SILENCE A SQUEAKY DOOR HINGE • A squeaky door hinge can be incredibly annoying. With its ability to seep into nooks and crannies, a little shaving cream on the hinge will cure the problem.

CLEAN BRUSHES AND COMBS • Skin oils can build up on your combs and brushes faster than you realize. And if you're tucking them into your purse or pocket, they're accumulating dust and dirt as well. Give them a fresh start in a shampoo bath. First, comb any loose hair out of the brush, then rub a little shampoo around the bristles or along the teeth of the comb. Put a small squirt of shampoo in a tall glass of water, let the comb and brush sit for a few minutes, swish, and rinse thoroughly.

DID YOU KNOW?

From the late 1920s through to the early 1960s, one of the best things about a long, tedious car ride were the signs every hundred yards or so advertising Burma-Shave, a brushless shaving cream. Here are a few of the more memorable ones:

Shaving Brushes ...
You'll Soon See 'Em ...
On The Shelf ...
In Some Museum ...
Burma-Shave.

Are Your Whiskers ...
When You Wake ...
Tougher Than ...
A Two-Bit Steak? ...
Try ... Burma-Shave.

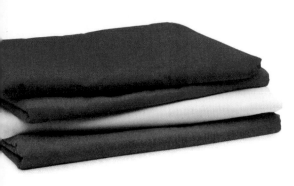

SHEETS

MAKE A BEANBAG BULL'S-EYE • On those rainy days when kids' sports games are cancelled, here's one way to ease their disappointment and let them give their pitching arms a workout. Draw a large bull's-eye on a sheet, tape the sheet to a wall, and let the kids pitch beanbags at it.

USE AS A TABLECLOTH • When it's your turn to host the whole clan for Christmas, and you don't have enough tablecloths, use a patterned sheet. They make attractive festive table coverings.

REPEL DEER FROM THE GARDEN • Circle the garden with a cord about 3 feet (1 m) above the ground, then tie strips of white sheet to it every 2 feet (60 cm); a tail-height flash of white is a danger sign to a deer.

SCOOP UP ALL THOSE AUTUMN LEAVES • Don't strain your back by lifting piles of leaves into a wheelbarrow. Just rake them onto a sheet laid on the ground. Then gather the four corners and drag the leaves to the compost heap.

WRAP UP THE OLD CHRISTMAS TREE • After removing Christmas decorations, wrap an old sheet around the tree so that you can carry or pull it out of the house without leaving a trail of pine needles.

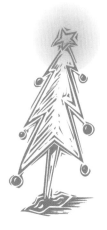

SHOE BOXES

MAKE A GIFT RIBBON DISPENSER • You will thank yourself each time you look for ribbon to wrap a present, if you use a shoe box to make this handy ribbon dispenser. Take a used broom handle or piece of a bamboo garden stake—anything you can use as a small dowel—and cut it a little longer than the length of the shoe box. Cut two holes for the dowel, one in each short end of the box, at a height where a spool of ribbon slipped on the dowel would spin freely. Slip your ribbon spools on the dowel as you poke it from one end of the shoe box through to the other. Once the dowel is in place, you can tape it at either short end to keep it from slipping out. You could also cut holes along one long side of the shoe box for each spool of ribbon, and pull a little bit of each ribbon through the hole.

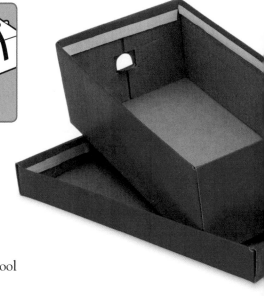

USE FOR PLAY BRICKS

Kids can get creative by using a collection of shoe boxes as building bricks. Tape the lids on for them. You can even let the little ones color the 'bricks' with poster paint.

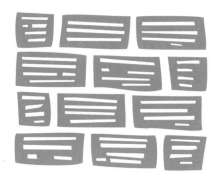

USE AS A WHELPING BOX • If there are puppies or kittens on the way at your house, reduce the risk of the mother rolling onto a newborn and smothering it by placing one or several puppies or kittens in a towel-lined shoe box while the others are being born.

GET YOUR STUFF ORGANIZED • There are lots of ways shoe boxes can help you get organized besides collecting old photos and receipts. Label the boxes and use them to store keepsakes, cancelled checks, bills to be paid, and other items you want to keep track of. For a neater appearance, cover the boxes with colored contact or any other decorative self-adhesive paper.

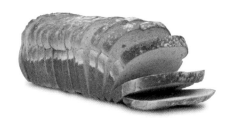

PACK YUMMY GIFTS • Shoe boxes are the perfect size for packaging loaves of homemade bread, cookies, or chocolates as special gifts for friends.

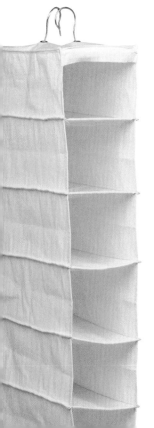

SHOE ORGANIZERS

ORGANIZE YOUR UTILITY CUPBOARD •
A hanging shoe bag is a great organizer in the utility cupboard. Use its pockets to store sponges, scrubbing brushes, and other cleaning utensils—even some bottles of cleaning products. It's also good for separating your clean, lemon-oil and lint-free rags so you'll always have the right one for the job.

ORGANIZE YOUR OFFICE AREA •
Free up some valuable drawer space in your office with an over-the-door shoe organizer. Its pockets can store lots of supplies that you need to keep handy, like scissors, staples, and markers. You can use the pockets to organize bills and other "to do" items as well.

more SHOE ORGANIZERS over →

ORGANIZE CAR-TRIP TOYS AND GAMES • Cut a shoe organizer to fit the back of your car seat and let your children make their own choices for back-seat entertainment.

LET KIDS SORT THEIR TOYS • A shoe organizer hung over the bedroom door is a great way to help your kids arrange their small toys. Whether your child likes dolls, dinosaurs, or different-colored blocks, a shoe organizer puts the toys on display so kids can sort them as they wish.

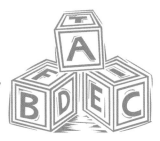

STORE BATHROOM ITEMS • A shoe organizer can keep lots of everyday bathroom items handy and neat. Brushes, shampoo, hand towels, hair spray— almost everything can be stored at your fingertips instead of cluttering the shower or vanity.

ARRANGE BEDROOM ITEMS • Instead of lifting a hanger when you need to get a belt, or rummaging for a scarf, sort your clothing accessories in a shoe organizer. The pockets can be used in the bedroom for keeping socks, gloves, and much more than shoes handy.

SHORTENING

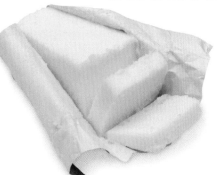

CLEAN INK STAINS • Next time a leaky pen leaves your hands full of ink, reach for some shortening. To remove ink stains from your hands and also from vinyl surfaces, rub on a dollop of shortening and wipe the stains away with a rag or paper towel.

REMOVE STICKY ADHESIVES • Don't wear down your fingernails trying to scratch off resistant sticky labels and price tags. Instead use shortening to remove them (and their dried glue and gum residue) from glass, metals, and most plastics. Simply coat the area with shortening, wait 10 minutes and scrub clean with a gentle scrub-sponge.

POLISH GALOSHES • To make dirty rubber boots shine like new again, rub on some shortening and wipe with a clean rag or cloth.

Using shortening

TIP

✳ *To take advantage of shortening for all sorts of jobs, you need to know how to store and handle it to avoid unexpected complications.*

● Keep shortening away from sunlight to prevent it from turning rancid.

● Never leave shortening unattended while frying.

● The most efficient temperature for frying with shortening is 325°F–350°F (165°C–180°C). Do not overheat shortening or it will burn. If shortening starts to smoke, turn off the heat, and let it cool.

● If shortening catches fire, cover the pan with its lid, turn off the heat, and let it cool.

● Never put water on burning or hot shortening, as it may splatter and burn you.

SOOTHE DIAPER RASH • Rub solid vegetable shortening on diaper rash for fast relief. It will soothe and moisturize sensitive skin.

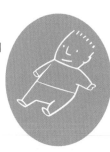

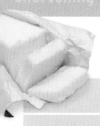

SKIN BEAUTY

REMOVE MAKEUP • Run out of your regular makeup remover? Don't fret. Just use a dab of shortening instead. Your face won't know the difference.

MOISTURIZE DRY SKIN • Why pay for fancy creams and lotions to moisturize your skin when ordinary solid vegetable shortening can do the trick at a fraction of the cost? Some hospitals even use shortening to keep skin soft and moist, and you can, too. Next time your hands are feeling dry and scaly, just rub in a bit of shortening. It's natural and fragrance-free.

REMOVE TAR FROM FABRIC • Tar stains on clothing are tough to remove, but you can make the job easier with a little help from some shortening. Scrap off as much of the tar as you can, then put a small glob of shortening over the remaining spot. Wait about 3 hours and launder as usual.

KEEP SNOW FROM STICKING TO A SHOVEL • In cold-climate areas, before you dig out the car or clear the driveway after a snowstorm, coat the blade of your shovel with shortening or liquid vegetable oil. It will not only keep snow from sticking but also make shoveling less tiring and more efficient.

REPEL SQUIRRELS • Keep annoying squirrels from getting at a bird feeder by greasing the pole with a liberal amount of shortening and the rodents won't be able to get a claw hold to climb up.

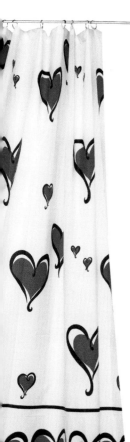

SHOWER CURTAINS

LINE CUPBOARD SHELVES • Don't discard your old vinyl shower curtains or tablecloths. Turn them into easy-to-clean shelf liners instead. Simply cut to shelf size and set in place, using some rubber cement to hold them if you prefer. When it's time for cleaning, just wipe with a damp sponge.

MAKE A PROTECTIVE APRON

For those extra messy jobs around the house, wear a homemade apron made from an old shower curtain. Make a cobbler's style apron, with a bib as well as a skirt. Use pinking shears to cut the vinyl to size, poke two holes at the top of the bib for cords or ribbons to tie around your neck and make two more holes in the sides for tying it around your waist.

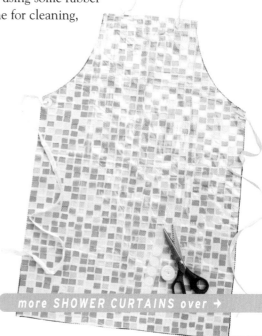

more SHOWER CURTAINS over →

S 287

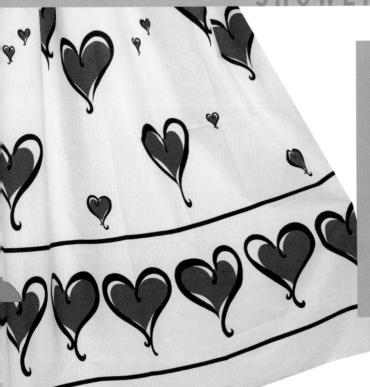

MAKE A PAINTING DROP CLOTH • Save an old shower curtain liner and use it as a drop cloth the next time you paint a room. The material is heavier and more durable than that used in commercially sold plastic drop cloths, and it's not absorbent like old bedsheets.

PROTECT THE FLOOR UNDER A HIGH CHAIR • Even the best behaved and cutest babies leave a mess on the floor when they eat. Protect your floor or carpet and make the cleanup a breeze. Cut a 36-to 48-inch (about 1-meter) square from an old shower curtain and place it under the baby's high chair. Use the leftover scraps to make bibs, too

BLOCK WEEDS IN MULCHED BEDS • Those old shower curtains will also come in handy next time you do any landscaping with gravel or bark chips. Just place the shower curtain under the mulching material and it will prevent annoying weeds from poking through the soil.

COVER PICNIC TABLES AND BENCHES • Don't let a yucky table   or sticky bench spoil your next picnic. Use an old shower curtain as a makeshift tablecloth (or as a tablecloth liner). Bring an extra shower curtain and fold it over a sticky or dirty picnic bench before you sit down to eat.

PROTECT THE TABLE WHEN CUTTING FABRIC

Next time you're cutting a pattern on your dining room table, put a shower curtain or plastic tablecloth under it before you cut. Scissors will glide easily across the surface and you'll protect the tabletop from an accidental nick or scrape.

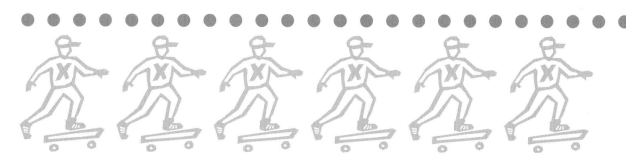

SKATEBOARDS

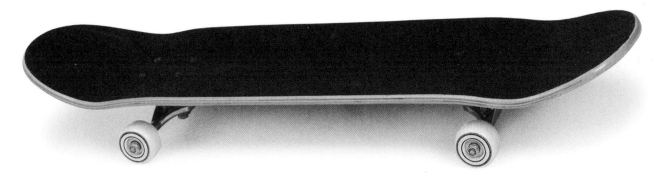

USE AS A PAINTER'S SCOOTER • Crawling along the floor to paint a baseboard can get tiring very quickly. Borrow your kid's skateboard and save your knees. Sit cross-legged on the skateboard and roll along with your paintbrush and can.

USE AS A LAUNDRY CART • If your home has a laundry chute, keep a basket on top of a skateboard directly below the chute. When you're ready to do the laundry, simply roll the load over to the washing machine.

MAKE A SHELF

Is your kid an avid skateboarder?
When he or she is ready for a new skateboard, turn the old one into a shelf for his or her room. Support it on a couple of metal shelf brackets. You can remove the wheels or leave them on.

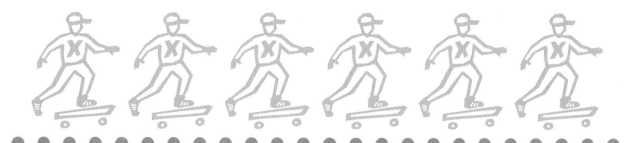

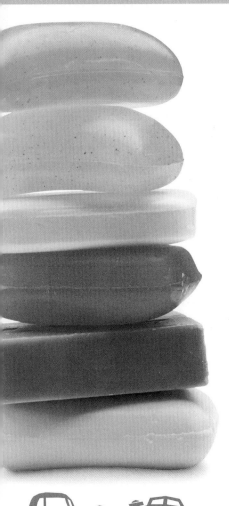

SOAP

LOOSEN STUCK ZIPPERS • If a zipper gets stuck, rub it loose with a bar of soap along the zipper's teeth. The lubrication will get it moving.

UNSTICK FURNITURE DRAWERS • If your chest of drawers or dresser drawers are sticking, rub the bottom of the drawer and the supports they rest on with a bar of soap to make them glide again.

LUBRICATE SCREWS AND SAW BLADES • A little lubrication with soap makes metal move through wood much more easily. Twist a screw into a bar of soap before driving it and rub some on your handsaw blade.

REMOVE A BROKEN LIGHTBULB • If a bulb breaks while still screwed in, don't chance nicks and cuts by trying to remove it. First, turn off the power, then insert the corner of a large, dry bar of soap into the socket. Give it a few turns and the base of the bulb will unscrew.

SAY FAREWELL TO FLEAS • Fed up with those annoying fleas? Put a few drops of dishwashing liquid and some water on a plate and place the plate on the floor next to a lamp. Fleas love light, so they will jump on the plate and drown in the liquid.

 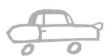

DEODORIZE YOUR CAR • Want your car to smell nice, but tired of those tree-shaped pine deodorizers? Place a little piece of your favorite-smelling soap in a mesh bag and hang it from your rearview mirror.

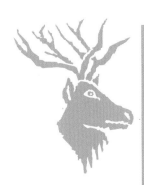

DID YOU KNOW?

Contrary to popular belief, hanging a perfumed bar of soap won't necessarily keep deer off your property. How long or how well soap works depends on a number of factors, including the type of plant you are protecting and the location of the soap. However, studies have shown that soap, especially tallow-based soap, will sometimes stop deer from making lunch out of your shrubbery. Keep in mind that local garden centers can also advise you about commercial spray repellents.

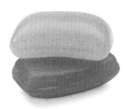

MARK A HEM • Forget store-bought marking chalk. A thin sliver of soap, like the ones left when a bar is just about finished, works just as well when you are marking a hem, and the markings wash right out.

MAKE A PIN HOLDER • Here's an easy-to-make alternative to a pincushion. Wrap a bar of soap in fabric and tie the fabric in place with a ribbon, then stick in your pins. As a bonus, the soap lubricates the pins, making them easier to insert.

PREVENT CAST-IRON MARKS • Nip cookout cleanup blues in the bud by rubbing the bottom of your cast-iron cookware with a bar of soap before cooking with it over a sooty open flame. You'll be amazed—no black cooking marks afterwards.

KEEP STORED CLOTHES FRESH • Pack a bar of your favorite scented soap when you store clothes or luggage. It will keep your clothes smelling fresh till next season and prevent musty odors in luggage.

Homemade soap

TIP

Making soap from scratch is easy to do, and it makes a special handcrafted gift for friends.

You need a solid bar of glycerine (from a drugstore); soap molds (from a craft store); a clean, dry can; a double boiler; food coloring; and essential oil. Place the glycerine in the can and put the can in a double boiler, which has water in the top as well as the bottom, and heat until the glycerine melts. For color, mix in food coloring. Spray a mold with nonstick cooking spray and fill it halfway up with melted glycerine. Add a few drops of essential oil and fill the rest with glycerine. Allow it to harden and you'll have soap.

SAVE THOSE SOAP SLIVERS • When your soap slivers get too tiny to handle, don't throw them away. Just make a small slit in a sponge and put the slivers inside. The soap will last for several more washings. Or make a washer that's easy for little hands to hold by putting the soap slivers in a sock, and let the kids get themselves clean.

SOCKS

PROTECT STORED BREAKABLES • Want to protect Grandma's precious vase or your bobble head collection? Wrap them up! Slip the item into a sock to help protect it from breaking or chipping.

COVER KIDS' SHOES WHEN PACKING • When kids insist on bringing along their favorite old sneakers on vacation, cover each one with an adult-sized sock before throwing them in the luggage, to protect the rest of the clothing from dirt and smells.

POLISH YOUR CAR

A large, old, soft sock makes a perfect hand mitt for buffing the wax on your car.

KEEP HANDS CLEAN CHANGING A TIRE • If you ever get a flat tire on your way to a fancy party or job interview, you'll thank yourself for having the foresight to throw a pair of socks in the trunk. Slip the socks on your hands while handling the tire, and they'll be clean when you arrive.

more SOCKS over →

S 291

PROTECT FLOOR SURFACES • The next time you need to move a heavy table or couch across a smooth floor, put socks over the legs and just slide the piece.

STORE YOUR WORK GOGGLES

Work goggles won't fit into glasses cases, so just slip them into a sock to protect them from getting scratched. You can even nail or screw the sock to the wall or bench so you will always know where the goggles are.

MAKE A WASH BAG FOR LINGERIE • Protect your precious delicates in the washing machine. First, slip them into a sock and tie the ends.

USE AS CLEANING MITTS • Save those old or solo socks to use as cleaning mitts. Slip them on and they'll be great for cleaning corners and crevices.

CLEAN SHUTTER AND BLIND SLATS • Don't waste money on those expensive gadgets and gizmos for cleaning venetian blind slats. Just slip a sock over your hand and gently rub the dust off. Use some dusting spray on the sock, if you like.

CLEAN ROUGH PLASTER WALLS • Use nylon or Ban-Lon socks, instead of a sponge or cloth, to clean rough plaster walls. No small pieces of material will be left behind as they'll stick to the sock fabric.

WASH SMALL STUFFED ANIMALS • Does your child's favorite stuffed fuzzy need a bath? Slip small stuffed animals into a sock and tie the end to prevent buttons, eyes, and other decorative items from coming loose.

PROTECT A WALL FROM LADDER MARKS • To prevent marks on the wall when you're leaning your ladder on it, slip socks over the ladder top ends. For obvious safety reasons, however, make sure someone is holding the ladder.

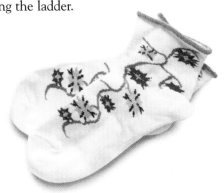

SODA POP

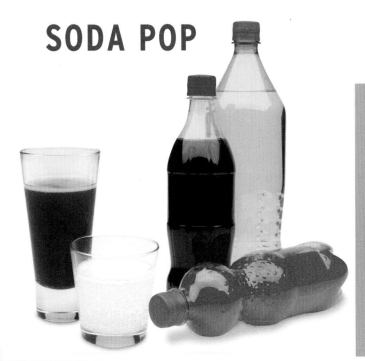

CLEAN CAR BATTERY TERMINALS • It seems hard to believe, but it's true, the acidic properties of soda pop will help to eliminate corrosion from your car battery. Nearly all carbonated soft drinks contain carbonic acid, which helps to remove stains and dissolve rust deposits. Pour some over the battery terminals and let it sit, then remove the sticky residue with a wet sponge.

LOOSEN RUSTED-ON NUTS AND BOLTS • Stop struggling with rusted-on nuts and bolts. Soda pop can help to loosen any rusted-on nuts and bolts. Soak a rag in the soda pop and wrap it around the bolt for several minutes.

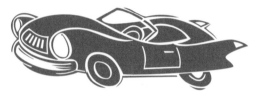

REMOVE RUST SPOTS FROM CHROME • Do you have one of those older cars with real chrome on the outside? If the chrome is developing small rust spots, you can remove them by rubbing the area with a crumpled piece of aluminium foil dipped in cola. It really works!

MAKE CUT FLOWERS LAST LONGER • Don't throw away those last drops of soda pop. Pour about ¼ cup (50 ml) into the water in a vase full of cut flowers. The sugar in the soda pop will make the blossoms last longer. But if you have a clear vase and want the water to remain clear, use a clear soda pop, such as Sprite or 7-Up.

CLEAN YOUR TOILET • Eliminate dirt and odor with a simple can of soda. Pour it into the toilet, let sit for an hour, scrub, and flush.

KEEP DRAINS FROM CLOGGING • Slow drain and no drain cleaner in the house? Pour a 32-ounce (2-L) bottle of cola down the drain to remove the clog.

MAKE A ROAST HAM MOIST • If you want to make your roast ham juicier, just add a can of cola to your traditional ham recipe. Pour it over the ham and follow regular baking instructions.

GET GUM OUT OF HAIR

It's inevitable–kids get chewing gum in their hair. Put the gummy hair section in a bowl with some cola. Let soak for a few minutes, then rinse.

CLEAN YOUR COINS • Who wants dirty money? If coin collecting is your hobby, use cola to clean your stash. Place the coins in a small dish and soak in cola for a shimmering shine. Of course, you shouldn't do this with rare and valuable coins.

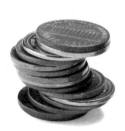
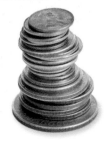

REMOVE OIL STAINS FROM CONCRETE • Gather up a small bag of clay-based cat litter, a few cans of cola, a stiff bristle broom, bucket, laundry detergent, bleach, eye protection, and rubber gloves. Cover the stain with a thin layer of cat litter and brush it in. Sweep up the litter and pour cola over the area. Work the cola in with a bristle broom and leave it for about 20 minutes. Mix ¼ cup (50 ml) laundry detergent with ¼ cup (50 ml) bleach in a gallon (4 L) of warm water and use it to mop up the mess.

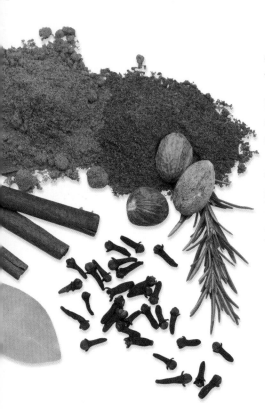

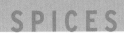

SPICES

MAKE A HAIR TONIC • You can spice up your hair care regimen with a homemade tonic that will enhance your natural color and impart shine. For dark hair, use 1 tablespoon (15 ml) crumbled sage or 1 sprig of chopped, fresh rosemary or a mixture of 1 teaspoon (5 ml) allspice, 1 teaspoon (5 ml) ground cinnamon, and ½ teaspoon (2 ml) ground cloves. For blonde hair, use 1 tablespoon (15 ml) chamomile. Pour 1 cup (250 ml) boiling water over the herb or spice mix, steep 30 minutes, strain through a coffee filter. Cool. Pour repeatedly over your hair (and into a large bowl) as a final rinse after shampooing.

TREAT MINOR CUTS • If you nick your finger while chopping vegetables for dinner, you may not even need to leave the kitchen for first aid. Alum, the old-fashioned pickling salt at the back of your spice cupboard, is an astringent. In a pinch, sprinkle some on a minor cut to staunch the flow of blood.

KEEP YOUR THERMOS FRESH • When you open a thermos bottle you haven't used for six months and the inside smells musty, give it a wash and keep it from happening the next time by placing a whole clove inside the thermos flask before capping it for storage. A teaspoon of salt works well, too. Make sure you empty and rinse the thermos before using it.

KEEP FEET SMELLING SWEET • If you have only been using sage to stuff turkeys, then you've been missing out. Sage is great for preventing food odor because it kills the odor-causing bacteria that grow on your feet in the warm, moist environment inside your shoes. Just crumble a leaf or two into you shoes before you put them on. At the end of the day, just shake the remains into the garbage.

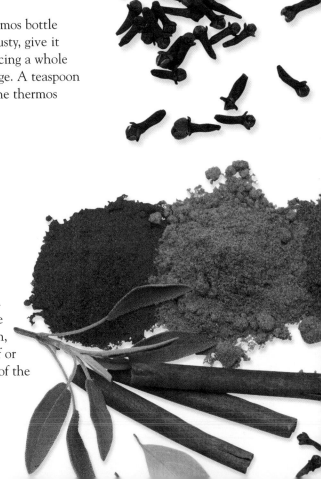

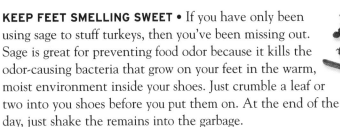

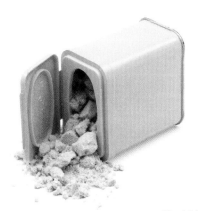

DEODORIZE BOTTLES FOR REUSE • You'd like to reuse those wonderful wide-mouthed pickle jars, but simply washing them with soap and water doesn't get rid of the pickle smell. What to do? Add 1 teaspoon (5 ml) dry mustard to a quart (1 L) of water, fill the jar, and let it soak overnight. It'll smell fresh by morning. This solution also banishes the odor of tomatoes, garlic, and other foods with strong scents.

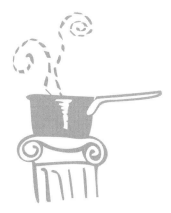

SCENT YOUR HOME

What could be more welcoming than the smell of something good cooking? Instead of using commercial air fresheners, simply toss a handful of whole cloves or a cinnamon stick in a pot of water and keep it simmering on the stove for half an hour. Or, place a teaspoon or two of the ground spices on a cookie sheet and place it in a 200°F (100°C) oven with the door ajar for 30 minutes. Either way, your house will naturally smell spicy good.

Toothache and oil of cloves

TIP

* *If you have a toothache, make an appointment to see your dentist as soon as possible. Don't wait!*

Meanwhile, oil of cloves may provide temporary relief. Place a drop directly into the aching tooth or apply it with a cotton swab. But don't put it directly on the gums. An active ingredient in the spice oil, eugenol, is a natural pain reliever.

KEEP WOOLENS WHOLE • Woolen clothing can last a lifetime if you keep the moths away. If you don't have a cedar-lined chest or closet, preserve your woolen clothing using clove sachets. Purchase some small drawstring muslin or organza bags at a craft or health food store, and fill each one with a handful of whole cloves. To prevent any transfer of oils or color to clothes and to contain any spills, put the sachet in a small plastic bag, but don't seal it. Attach it to a hanger in your wardrobe or tuck one in among your folded sweaters.

KEEP ANTS AT BAY • Flour, sugar, and paprika can all fall prey to ants. Keep these cooking essentials safe by slipping a bay leaf inside your storage containers. If you're concerned about the flour or sugar picking up a bay leaf flavor, tape the leaf to the inside of the canister lid. This trick works inside cupboards, too, where sachets of sage, bay, cinnamon sticks, or whole cloves will smell pleasant while also discouraging ants.

STAMP OUT SILVERFISH • These pests frequent places with lots of moisture, such as kitchens, bathrooms, and laundries. Hang an aromatic sachet containing apple-pie spices (cinnamon, nutmeg, allspice), sage, or bay leaves on a hook in your bathroom vanity and behind the washing machine, or keep a few in decorative baskets along baseboards.

more SPICES over →

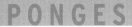

CONTROL INSECTS IN THE GARDEN • You don't have to use harsh pesticides to control a small insect infestation outdoors. If ants are swarming on your garden path, add 1 tablespoon (15 ml) ground black pepper (or another strong-smelling ground spice, such as ground cloves or dry mustard) to 1 cup (250 g) sifted white flour and sprinkle the mixture on and around the pests. They'll vanish within the hour. Sweep the dry mix into the garden instead of trying to hose it off; water will just make it gooey.

DETER PLANT-EATING ANIMALS • Everyone knows that hot peppers make your mouth burn. So if rodents are attacking your ornamental plants, the solution may be to make them too 'hot' for the pests. In fact, hot peppers are the basis for many commercial rodent repellents. Chop up the hottest pepper you can find (habañero is best) and combine it with 1 tablespoon (15 ml) ground cayenne pepper and 2 quarts (2 L) water. Boil the mix for 15 to 20 minutes, then let it cool. Strain it through cheesecloth, add 1 tablespoon (15 ml) dishwashing liquid and pour it into a spray bottle. Spray plants liberally every five days or so. The spray works best for rabbits, chipmunks, and woodchucks, but may also deter deer, especially if used in combination with commercial products.

DID YOU KNOW?

What's the difference between a spice and an herb? The basic guideline is this: If it's made from a plant's leaf, it's an herb; if it's made from the bark, fruit, seed, stem, or root, it's a spice. Parsley, basil, and coriander are typical herbs because we eat the leaves. Rosemary, often referred to as an herb, is actually a spice because it has a woody stem. Spices such as pepper and cinnamon come from the fruit and bark of trees. So what do we call salt, perhaps the most essential food enhancer but not a plant product at all? "Seasoning" is the word that describes anything used to flavor foods, regardless of its origin.

SHIELD YOUR VEGETABLE GARDEN • For centuries, gardeners have used companion planting to repel insect pests. Aromatic plants such as basil, tansy, marigolds, and sage are all said to repel pests, so try planting some near your vegetables. Mint, thyme, dill, and sage are favored near cabbage-family plants (cabbage, broccoli, cauliflower, and brussels sprouts) for their supposed ability to fend off cabbage moths. And a bonus: You can eat the savory herbs!

SPONGES

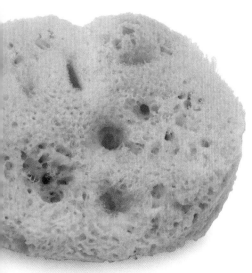

MAKE FLOWERPOTS HOLD WATER LONGER • If your potted house plants dry out too quickly after watering, when you repot them, try this simple trick for keeping the soil moist longer. Tuck a damp sponge in the bottom of the pot before filling it with soil. It'll act as a water reservoir. And it will also help prevent a gusher if you accidentally overwater.

AN 'UNWELCOME' MAT FOR THE GARDEN • Anyone who's ever cleaned a floor with ammonia knows that the smell of this strong, everyday household cleaner is overpowering. Throw browsing animals 'off the scent' of ripening vegetables in your garden by soaking old sponges in your floor-cleaning solution and distributing them wherever you expect the next garden raid.

Kids' Stuff

Making seeds grow seems magical to young children. For an easy and renewable play garden with a minimum of mess, all you need is an old soap dish, a sponge, and seeds of a plant such as lobelia, millet, flax or mustard–even birdseed will do. Cut the sponge to fit the dish, add water until it's moist but not sopping, and sprinkle the seed liberally over the top. Prop an inverted glass bowl over it until seeds begin to grow. A bright, sunny wndow spot and daily watering will keep it going for weeks.

KEEP YOUR VEGIES FRESH • Moisture that collects at the bottom of your refrigerator crisper hastens the demise of healthy vegetables. Extend their life by lining the crisper with dry sponges. When you notice that they're wet, wring them out and let them dry before putting them back in the fridge. Every now and then, between uses, let them soak in some warm water with a splash of bleach to discourage the growth of mold.

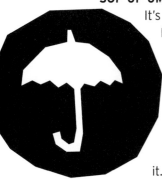

SOP UP UMBRELLA OVERRUN • It's raining and the family has been tramping in and out with umbrellas all day. Your umbrella stand has only a shallow receptacle to catch drips. Suddenly there's a waterfall coming out of it. Protect your flooring from umbrella-stand overflow with a strategically placed sponge in its base. If you forget to squirt it out, it'll dry on its own as soon as the weather clears.

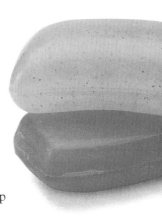

STRETCH THE LIFE OF SOAP • A shower is so refreshing in the morning—until you reach for the soap and are treated to the slimy sensation of a bar that's been left to marinate in its own suds. You'll enjoy bathing more and your soap will last longer if you park a sponge on the soap dish. It'll absorb moisture so soap can dry out.

PROTECT YOUR FRAGILE ITEMS

If you're shipping or storing small, fragile valuables that won't be harmed by a little contact with water, sponges are a clever way to cushion them. Dampen a sponge, wrap it around the delicate item and use a rubber band to secure it. As it dries, the sponge will conform to the contours of your crystal ashtray or porcelain figurine. To unpack it, just dip the item in water again. You'll even get your sponge back!

LIFT LINT FROM FABRIC • To quickly remove lint and pet fur from clothes and upholstery, give the fabric a quick wipe with a dampened and wrung-out sponge. Just run your fingers over the sponge and the unwanted fuzz will come off in a ball for easy disposal.

SPRAY BOTTLES

MIST HOUSE PLANTS • Keep your house plants healthy and happy by using an empty trigger-type spray bottle as a plant mister. Clean the bottle by filling it with equal parts water and vinegar—don't use liquid soap, as you may not be able to get it all out—let the solution sit for an hour and rinse it out thoroughly with cold water. Repeat if necessary. Then fill the bottle with lukewarm water and use it to give your plants a frequent, soothing, misty shower.

HELP WITH THE LAUNDRY • An empty spray bottle can always be put to good use around your laundry. Use clean, recycled bottles to spray water on your clothes as you're ironing. Or fill a spray bottle with stain-remover solution so that you can apply it to your garments without having to blot up drips.

KEEP CAR WINDOWS CLEAN • Be sure to include a recycled spray bottle filled with glass cleaner in the trunk of your car as part of your roadside emergency kit. Use it to clean off your car's headlights, mirrors, and, of course, windows whenever needed. In cold areas during winter months, mix in ½ teaspoon (2 ml) antifreeze and you can spray it on your windshield or mirrors to melt the ice.

SPRAY AWAY GARDEN PESTS • Keep a few recycled spray bottles on hand to use around the garden. Here are two immediate uses:

■ Fill one with undiluted white vinegar to get rid of the weeds and grass poking out of the cracks in your concrete, as well as ants and other insects—but be careful not to spray it on your plants; the high level of acidity could kill them.

■ For an effective homemade insecticide recipe that works on most soft-bodied pests, but won't harm your plants, mix several cloves of crushed garlic, ¼ cup (50 ml) canola oil, 3 tablespoons (15 ml) hot pepper sauce, and ½ teaspoon (5 ml) mild liquid soap in a gallon (4 L) of water. Pour some into your spray bottle, and shake well before using.

COOL OFF IN SUMMER • Whether you're jogging around the park, taking a breather between volleyball matches or just sitting out in the sun, a recycled spray bottle filled with water can make a great summer companion. Use it to cool off during and after your workouts, or while baking on the beach (or sitting in beach traffic).

SQUIRT BOTTLES

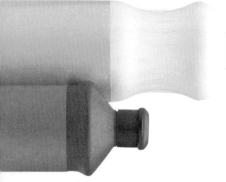

STOP COOKING OIL DRIPS • Tired of cleaning up oil spills around your kitchen? Fill a cleaned, recycled squirt bottle with olive oil or another favorite cooking oil. It's a lot easier to handle than a jar or bottle and you can pour precisely the right amount of oil over your salads or into your frying pan without having to worry about drips or spills.

SUBSTITUTE FOR A BASTER • If you can't find your kitchen baster, or one that's in working condition, a cleaned squirt bottle makes a great substitute. Simply squirt out some air first and use it to suck up the fat from your roasts and soups. You can even use it to distribute marinades and drippings over meat.

PUT THE SQUEEZE ON CONDIMENTS • Recycled squirt bottles are great for storing condiments and other foodstuffs that are typically sold in jars—such as mayonnaise, salad dressing, jams, or honey. In addition to having fewer sticky or messy jars in your refrigerator, you'll also be lightening the load in your dishwasher by eliminating the need for knives or spoons. Make sure you give the bottles a thorough cleaning before using.

CLEAN OUT CREVICES

A clean, empty squirt bottle may be just the cleaning tool you need to get the dust out of the corners of your picture frames and other tight spaces. Use it to give a good blast of air to blow out dirt you can't otherwise reach.

LET THE CHILDREN PLAY • Fill up a few clean squirt bottles with water and give them to your kids to squirt each other in the backyard on those hot summer days. It will keep them cool while they burn off some energy.

STEEL WOOL

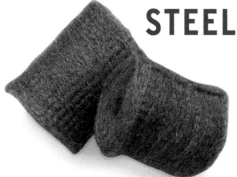

TURN NASTY SNEAKERS NICE • If your sneakers are looking so bad that the only thing you'd do in them is, well, sneak around, some steel wool may keep them out of the garbage bin. Moisten a steel wool soap pad and gently scrub away at stains and stuck-on goo. Wipe them clean with a damp sponge or put them in the washing machine and you may be able to enjoy many more months of wear.

REMOVE CRAYON MARKS FROM WALLPAPER • If a small child just created a work of crayon art on paper, and the 'paper' is your wallpaper, use a bit of steel wool soap pad to just skim the surface, making strokes in one direction instead of scrubbing in a circle. Your wall will be clean again in no time.

GET RID OF HEEL MARKS • Those black marks that rubber soles leave behind just don't come off with a mop, no matter how hard you try. To rid a vinyl floor of unsightly smudges, gently rub the surface with a moistened steel wool soap pad. When the heel mark is gone, wipe the floor clean with a damp sponge.

No steel wool on stainless steel

✳ *An oft-repeated piece of advice is to clean stainless steel items with a steel wool soap pad.*

Yet stainless steel manufacturers caution against using any abrasive on stainless steel. Steel wool may make stainless steel look better, but it scratches the surface and ultimately hastens rusting. The safest way to care for stainless steel is to wash with a sponge and mild soap and water.

TIP

more STEEL WOOL over →

SHARPEN SCISSORS

Sometimes you just want a small piece of a steel wool soap pad for a minor job. Cutting it in half with a pair or scissors will help keep the scissors sharp while giving you the pint-size pad you need for your cleaning project.

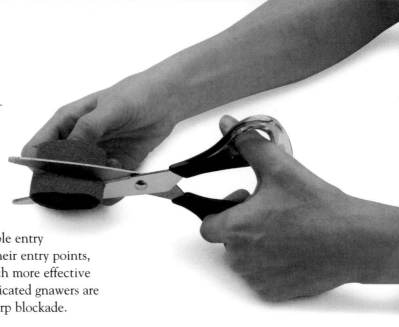

REBUFF RODENTS • Mice, squirrels, and bats are experts at finding every conceivable entry into a house. When you discover one of their entry points, stuff it full of steel wool. Steel wool is much more effective than foam or newspaper because even dedicated gnawers are unlikely to try to chew through such a sharp blockade.

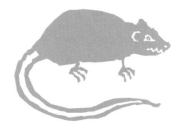

KEEP GARDEN TOOLS IN GOOD SHAPE • Nothing will extend the life of your gardening tools like a good cleaning at the end of each growing season. Grab a wad of fine steel wool from your hardware store (000, or "three-aught," would be a good choice), saturate it with the same ordinary household oil you use on squeaky door hinges, and rub rust off your shears, clippers, shovels, and anything else with metal parts. Wipe them clean with a dry rag, sharpen any blades, and reapply a bit of oil before storing them for the winter.

STRAWS

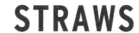

KEEP JEWELRY CHAINS UNKNOTTED • Fine gold chains always end up in a knotted, kinked mess when they're stored in open-style jewelry boxes. Before storing a chain, run it through the inside of a straw, cut to the proper length, and close the chain clasp before putting it away. It'll always be ready to wear.

GIVE FLOWERS NEEDED HEIGHT • Your flower arrangement would be just perfect, except a few of the flowers aren't tall enough. You can improve on nature by sticking each of the too-short stems into plastic straws, trimming the straw to get the desired height, and inserting them into the vase.

GET SLOW KETCHUP FLOWING • Anticipation is great, but ketchup that comes out of the bottle while your sausage and onions are still hot is even better. If your ketchup is recalcitrant, insert a straw all the way into the bottle and stir it around a little to get the flow started.

IMPROVISE WITH SOME FOAMY FUN

To make enough cheap and easy toys for even a large group of children, cut the ends of some plastic straws at a sharp angle and set out a shallow pan of dishwashing liquid diluted with a little bit of water. Dip a straw in the soap and blow through the other end. Little kids love the piles of bubbles that result.

DID YOU KNOW?

The quest for a perfectly cold mint julep led to the invention of the drinking straw. Mint juleps are served chilled, and their flavor diminishes as they warm up. Holding a glass heats the contents, so the custom was to drink mint juleps through natural straws made from a section of hollow plant stem, usually rye grass. But the rye imparted an undesirable 'grassy' flavor. In 1888, Marvin Stone, a Washington, D.C. manufacturer of paper cigarette holders, fashioned a paper tube through which to sip his favorite drink– a mint julep. When other mint julep aficionados began clamoring for paper straws, he realized he had a hot new product on his hands.

MAKE A PULL-TOY PROTECTOR • Pull toys are perennial favorites with young children, but you can spend all day untying the knots that a toddler will inevitably put in the pull string. By running the string through a plastic straw (or a series of them), you can keep it untangled.

MAKE EASY-TO-CARRY SEASONING HOLDERS • If you're on a low-sodium diet and need potassium salt, which most restaurants don't keep on the table, or perhaps you want salt and pepper to season your packed lunch just before you eat it, straws provide an easy way to take along small amounts of dry seasonings. Fold one end over and tape it shut, fill it and fold and tape the other end. If moisture is a concern, use a plastic straw.

FIX LOOSE VENEER • The veneer from a favorite piece of furniture has lost its grip near the edge of the piece. A bit of yellow carpenter's glue is the obvious solution for re-adhering the veneer, but how do you get the glue under there? Veneer can be very brittle, and you don't want to break off a piece by lifting it up. The solution is to cut a length of plastic drinking straw and press it to flatten it somewhat. Fold it in half and fill one half with glue, slowly dripping the glue in from the top. Slip the filled half under the veneer and gently blow in the glue. Wipe off any excess, cover the area with wax paper and a wood block, and clamp it overnight.

STRING

POLISH SILVERWARE MORE EASILY • The rich shine of polished silverware is part of what makes it look so beautiful in formal dinner settings. To get your silverware looking that good, run a length of string through some silver polish, and then use the string to get at those hard-to-reach spots between fork tines.

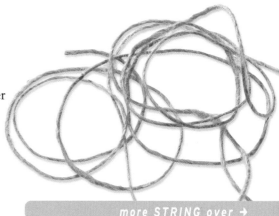

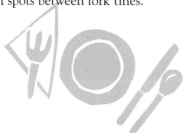

more STRING over →

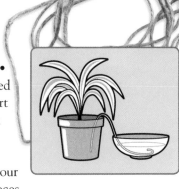

FOR GREEN THUMBS...

OUTLINE GARDEN FEATURES • When you're making a new garden, lay common bright, white string on the ground to outline paths and beds. From an upstairs window or other high vantage point, you'll be able to tell at a glance if borders are straight and whether the layout is pleasing.

USE AS A STRAIGHT-LINE GUIDE • Trimming a long hedge straight is a near-impossible feat unless you use a visual guide. Drive two stakes into the ground, one at each end of the hedge. Measure the height you want for the trimmed hedge, then run the string between the two stakes, tying it to each one at that exact height. As you clip away, cut down to the string line but no further. The top of your hedge will be straight as an arrow.

PLANT PERFECTLY STRAIGHT ROWS • It's harder than it looks to make straight garden rows. Use string two ways to keep plants in line:

☐ For planting heavy seeds such as beans, put sticks in the ground at each end of a planting row and run a piece of string between the sticks to guide you as you plant.

☐ To plant dozens of lightweight seeds in a jiffy, cut string to the length of a row, wet it thoroughly, then sprinkle the seed directly on it. The moisture will make seeds stick long enough to lay the string in a prepared furrow. Just cover the string with soil and you're done!

MAKE WICKS FOR WATERING PLANTS • Keeping plants watered while you're on a short trip is easier than you think. Fill a large container with water and place it next to your potted plants. Cut pieces of string so they're long enough to hang down to the bottom of the container at one end and be buried a few inches deep in the soil of the pots at the other. Soak the strings until they're thoroughly wet and put them in position. As the soil begins to dry, capillary action will draw water from the reservoir to the pots through the strings.

STOP THE SOUND OF A DRIPPING FAUCET • If a leaky faucet is keeping you awake at night, there's a way to silence it until the plumber arrives. Tie a piece of string to the fixture with one end right where the water is coming out and the other end hanging down to the bottom of the sink basin. Water droplets will travel down the string silently instead of driving you to distraction while you're trying to go to sleep.

MAKE A QUICK PACKAGE OPENER • Next time you're preparing a box for mailing, take a second to make it easier for the recipient to open. Place a piece of string along the center and side seams before you tape, allowing a tiny bit to hang free at one end. That way, the recipient just needs to pull the strings to sever the tape without resorting to sharp blades that might damage delicate contents. Do the same for packing boxes when you move.

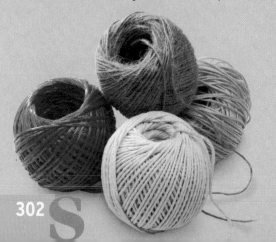

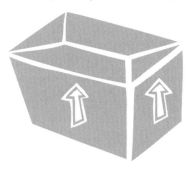

STOP SLAMMING DOORS • Is a slamming door getting on your nerves? Here are two ideas for using string to control the way a door closes:

■ A piece of light string tied to both sides of a knob and running around the door edge provides just enough friction to slow it down and prevent a loud slam when it shuts.

■ Use thicker rope the same way to temporarily prop open a door that automatically locks when it closes or to make sure pets don't get trapped in one room of the house when the door slams shut.

MEASURE IRREGULAR OBJECTS • A cloth tape measure is the ideal tool for measuring unusual-shaped objects, but you may not have one if you don't sew. Wrap a plain piece of string around the item instead, then hold it up to a ruler to get the measurement you need.

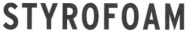

STYROFOAM

MAKE YOUR OWN SHIPPING PELLETS • You'd like to use foam to ship some fragile things, but all you've got is sheets or blocks of foam, not pellets. No problem. Just break up what you have into pieces small enough to fit in a blender and pulse it on and off to shred the foam into perfect packing material.

HOLD TREATS FOR FUTURE EATING • To prepare a quantity of snow cones or ice-cream cones in advance, cut a foam block to size so it will fit flat in your freezer. Cut holes just large enough and close enough to hold cones so they won't touch, fall over, or poke through the bottom. Fill the cones and slip them into the waiting holes. Then pop the whole thing into the freezer, ready for serving at a moment's notice.

KEEP NAIL POLISH LOOKING GOOD • When applying nail polish, a foam pellet or a small chunk cut from a block of foam packaging placed between each finger or toe will help spread them apart and keep the polish unblemished until it can dry.

MAKE A KICKBOARD

A sharp kitchen knife is all you need to cut a scrap of Styrofoam insulation into an instant kickboard for your swimming pool.

more STYROFOAM over →

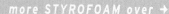

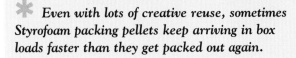

MAKE A BUOYANT TRAY FOR THE POOL •
Styrofoam is nearly unsinkable. You can use the scraps from a construction project to make a drink holder or a tray that will float in your pool (but remember only use plastic cups, never glass):

■ To make a soda can holder, cut two pieces to the size you want the finished holder to be, then cut holes the same size as a soda can in one piece. Glue the piece with holes on top of the other piece, using a hot-glue gun.

■ To make a tray with a rim, just glue small strips of foam that are at least 1-inch (2.5-cm) high around the edge of a larger, tray-sized section of the material.

Recycling foam pellets

TIP

* *Even with lots of creative reuse, sometimes Styrofoam packing pellets keep arriving in box loads faster than they get packed out again.*

If you've got more than you can handle, remember that packing and shipping businesses often accept clean pellets for reuse. Just call first, to confirm with them before you start delivering.

HELP SHRUBS WITHSTAND WINTER • Sometimes shrubs need a little help to survive winter's ravages. Leftover sheets of extruded tongue-and-groove Styrofoam insulation are perfect for the job. They're rigid, waterproof, and block wind. Here are two ways to use the material:

■ To give moderate protection, cut two Styrofoam sheets and lash them together to form a pup tent over the plant. To hold the pieces in place, drive bamboo garden stakes through the bottom of each piece into the ground.

■ For something more substantial, fit pieces together to box in your less hardy garden plants on four sides. Put a stake inside each corner and join the pieces with duct or packing tape.

■ Plants in containers that overwinter outdoors are more likely to survive with Styrofoam protection, too.

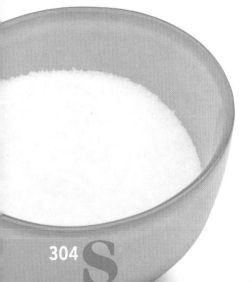

SUGAR

KEEP CUT FLOWERS FRESH • Make your own preservative to keep cut flowers fresh longer. Dissolve 3 tablespoons (45 ml) sugar and 2 tablespoons (30 ml) white vinegar per quart (1 L) warm water. When you fill the vase, make sure the cut stems are covered by 3 to 4 inches (7–10 cm) of the water mixture. The sugar nourishes the plants, while the vinegar inhibits bacterial growth. You'll be surprised how long the arrangement stays fresh!

RID THE GARDEN OF NEMATODES • If your outdoor plants look unhealthy, with ugly knots at the roots, chances are they've been victims of an attack of the nematodes! The nematode worm, nemesis of many an otherwise healthy garden, is a microscopic parasite that pierces the roots of plants and causes knots. You can prevent nematode attacks by using sugar to create an inhospitable environment for the tiny worms. Apply 5 pounds (2 kg) sugar for every 250 square feet (25 m²) of garden. Microorganisms feeding on the sugar will increase the organic matter in the soil, eliminating those nasty nematodes.

CLEAN GREASY, GRIMY HANDS • To clean filthy hands of grease, grime, or paint easily and thoroughly, pour equal amounts of olive oil and sugar into the cupped palm of one hand, and gently rub your hands together for several minutes. Rinse thoroughly and dry. The grit of the sugar acts as an abrasive to help the oil remove grease, paint, and grime. Your hands will look and feel clean, soft, and moisturized.

MAKE A NONTOXIC FLY TRAP • Keep your kitchen free of flies with a homemade fly trap that uses no toxic chemicals. In a small saucepan, simmer 2 cups (500 ml) milk, ¼ pound (115 g) raw sugar and ¼ cup (50 g) ground pepper for about 10 minutes, stirring occasionally. Pour into shallow dishes or bowls and set them around the kitchen, patio or anywhere the flies are a problem. The insects will flock to the bowls and drown!

EXTERMINATE ROACHES • If you hate noxious pesticides as much as you loathe cockroaches, don't call an exterminator. Instead, when you have a roach infestation, scatter a mixture of equal parts sugar and borax powder over the infested area. The sugar will attract the roaches and the borax will kill them. Replace it frequently with a fresh mixture to prevent future infestations.
WARNING: Keep this mixture away from pets and small children, as it is poisonous if ingested.

Kids' Stuff

Here's an easy way to make old-fashioned rock candy with the kids, with no strings, paperclips, sticks, or thermometers needed. Make the syrup by stirring 2½ cups (625 g) sugar into 1 cup (500 ml) hot water. Pour the syrup into several open dishes and set aside. Add a grain of sugar to act as a seed crystal in each container. Within days or weeks you should be able to collect glittering crystals of rock. Use a spoon to scoop it out. Rinse and dry the rock before you eat it.

SOOTHE A BURNED TONGUE

That slice of piping-hot pizza looked great, but ouch! You burned your tongue when you bit into it. To relieve a tongue burned by hot pizza, coffee, tea, or soup, reach for the sugar bowl and sprinkle a pinch or two of sugar over the affected area. The pain will begin to subside immediately.

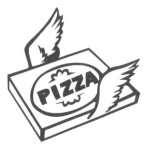

KEEP DESSERTS FRESH • You used sugar to make the cake batter; now use it to keep the finished cake fresh and moist. Store the cake in an airtight container with a couple of sugar cubes and it will stay fresh for days longer. You can store a few lumps of sugar in with your cheeses the same way to prevent the cheese from getting moldy.

TALCUM POWDER

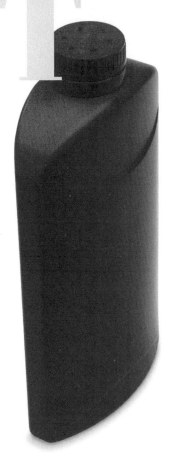

KEEP ANTS AWAY • For an effective ant repellent, scatter talcum powder liberally around house foundations and known points of entry, such as doors and windows. Other effective organic repellents include cream of tartar, borax, powdered sulphur, and oil of cloves. You can also try planting mint around the house foundations.

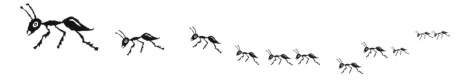

FIX A SQUEAKY FLOOR • Don't let squeaky floorboards drive you crazy. For a quick fix, sprinkle talcum powder or powdered graphite between the boards that squeak. If that doesn't do the trick, squirt in some liquid wax.

REMOVE BLOODSTAINS FROM FABRIC • To remove fresh bloodstains from fabric, make a paste of water and talcum powder and apply it to the spot. When it dries, brush away the stain. Use cornstarch or polenta instead if you're out of talcum powder.

CAUTION: Health care experts warn that scented talcum powder may cause skin allergies and worsen body odors. They recommend only unscented powder, used on dry skin. Women are advised not to use talcum powder in the vaginal or anal areas, where excessive powdering has been linked to an increased risk of ovarian cancer.

GET RID OF GREASY CARPET STAINS • A greasy stain can spoil the look of the most luxurious carpeting. You can remove greasy stains from a carpet with a combination of talcum powder and patience. Just cover the affected area with talcum powder, wait at least 6 hours for the talcum powder to absorb the grease, and vacuum the stain away. Baking soda, polenta, or cornstarch may be substituted for the talcum powder.

DEGREASE POLYESTER STAINS • Your favorite polyester shirt or blouse may come back into style someday, but you'll have to get rid of that ugly grease stain before you wear it. To get rid of grease stains on polyester, sprinkle some talcum powder directly on the spot and rub it in with your fingers. Wait 24 hours, then gently brush. Repeat as necessary until the stain is completely gone.

LOOSEN TANGLES AND KNOTS • Don't break a fingernail trying to untie that knot in your shoelace. Sprinkle talcum powder on shoelaces (or any knotted cords) and the knots will pull apart more easily. Use talcum powder to help untangle chain necklaces, too.

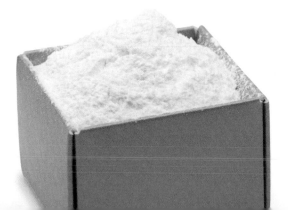

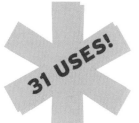

TAPE

in the kitchen and dining room

PICK UP GLASS SHARDS SAFELY • Why risk cutting yourself picking up bits of broken glass from the kitchen floor? Just hold a long piece of transparent tape tightly at each end and use it to blot up all the shards.

CREATE A NO-FLY ZONE • Make your own fly and pest strips that are free of polluting toxic chemicals and poisons. Cover empty paper towel or toilet paper rolls with transparent tape, sticky side out, and hang them in the kitchen or wherever else you need them.

MARK THE START OF A PLASTIC-WRAP ROLL • If you've ever had trouble finding the beginning of a roll of plastic food wrap, you'll appreciate this time-saving trick. Put a piece of transparent tape on your finger, sticky side out, and dab your finger on the roll until you find the edge. Use a short piece of tape to lift the edge and pull gently.

PREVENT SALT AND PEPPER SPILLS • Many salt and pepper shakers, especially ceramic ones, have to be filled through a hole in the bottom. Before you refill one of these shakers, tape over the holes on top. That way you won't have any wasteful spills when you turn the shaker upside down to fill it. Also, remember to tape the tops when moving to a new home, or even when you're just transporting the shakers to and from a picnic.

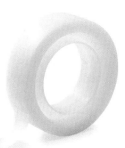

KEEP HANDS FREE WHEN SHOPPING

Next time you go food shopping, bring some tape with you and use it to attach your shopping list to the handle of your shopping cart. This will free both your hands and you won't keep misplacing or dropping your list.

MAKE CANDLES FIT SNUGLY • Don't let loose candles spoil the romantic mood or cause a fire at your next candlelight dinner. If the candles don't fit snugly into the holder, wrap layers of tape around their bottom edges until they fit snugly.

around the house

• • •

CODE YOUR KEYS • Are you always groping around to find the right key when you get home in the dark? Just wrap some tape around the top of your house key, and you'll be able to feel for the right key when it is too dark to see. Or if you have several similar-looking keys that you can't tell apart, color-code them with different-colored tapes.

KEEP SPARE BATTERIES HANDY • You won't be behind the times for long if you remember to tape extra batteries to the back of your wall clock. When the clock stops and it's time to replace the batteries, they'll be readily at hand.

more TAPE over →

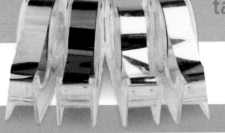

DID YOU KNOW?

Scotch tape got its name from an insult hurled at Richard Drew, the 3M company engineer who invented it. In 1925, five years before he invented the world's first and best-known transparent cellophane tape, Drew invented masking tape. He was field-testing his first masking-tape samples to find the right amount of adhesive when a frustrated body-shop painter exclaimed, "Take this tape back to those Scotch bosses of yours and tell them to put more adhesive on it!"

PREVENT JEWELRY TANGLES • To keep fine chains from tangling when you travel, cover both sides of each chain with transparent tape. You can also use tape to keep a pair of earrings from separating.

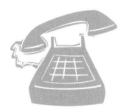

MARK A PHONE NUMBER FOR QUICK REFERENCE

Use transparent tape to highlight numbers in the phone book that you often look up. The tape will make the page easier to find and you will also be able to find the number easily without having to search the whole page.

CONTAIN GREASE STAINS ON PAPER • You may never be able to get rid of grease spots on books or important papers, but you can keep them from spreading with a little help from some transparent tape. Fix tape over both sides of the spot to keep the grease from seeping through to other pages or papers.

KEEP PAPERS FROM BLOWING IN THE WIND • If you have to make a speech or accept an award at an outdoor event, bring a roll of transparent tape with you. When it's your turn to talk, place some tape on the lectern, sticky side out, to prevent your papers from blowing away.

FIND YOUR FAVORITE PHOTO NEGATIVE • Before framing a favorite photograph, tape the negative to the back of the picture. If you ever want to make copies of the photo, you won't have to go searching through piles of old negatives to find the right one.

DETER CATS FROM SCRATCHING • Stop naughty cats and kittens from scratching your fine furniture! Sprinkle ground red pepper or hot paprika on a strip of tape and attach it to the areas you don't want them to scratch. They hate the smell and they'll quickly get the message.

SEW WHAT!

MAKE SEWING EASIER • Let transparent tape simplify your sewing. Use it to hold a zipper in place when you're making a garment. (You can sew through the tape and remove it when you're done.) Keep badges, patches, or name tags in place when sewing them onto shirts, uniforms, or caps. Tape hooks, eyes, and snaps to garments when sewing so they won't slip. Just pull the tape off when you're done. Tape a pattern to the material; when you cut the pattern, you'll have a reinforced edge.

END LOOSE ENDS ON THREAD SPOOLS • Put an end to time-wasting, frustrating searches for loose ends of thread. Just tape the ends to the top or bottom of the spool when you're done sewing and they'll be at your fingertips and ready to use next time you sew.

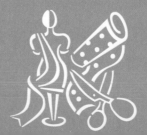

KEEP FLOWERS UPRIGHT IN A VASE • To keep cut flowers from sagging in their vase, crisscross several pieces of transparent tape across the mouth of the vase, leaving spaces where you can insert the flowers. The flowers will look perky and fresh for a few extra days.

REMOVE LIPSTICK FROM SILK • Why pay an expensive dry cleaning bill to remove a lipstick spot from a silk scarf or dress when you can do it yourself for free? Just place a piece of transparent tape (or masking tape) over the spot and yank it off. If you can still see some of the lipstick color, sprinkle on some talcum powder or chalk and dab until the powder and the remaining lipstick disappear.

CLEAN YOUR NAIL FILE • Clean a nail file easily and effectively. Simply place a piece of transparent tape over it, press, and pull off. The tape will pick up all the dirt embedded in the surface of the file.

DID YOU KNOW?

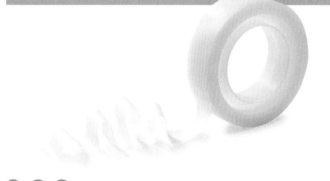

Transparent tape is made from an acetate film derived from wood pulp or cotton fibers. It is formed into paper-thin sheets and wound onto giant rolls before being coated with adhesive. Twenty-nine raw materials go into the adhesive used in transparent tape. Even after the film and adhesive have been produced, 10 separate steps remain to be done before a roll of tape is manufactured.

for the do-it-yourselfer

STOP PICTURE NAILS FROM DAMAGING A WALL • Before driving a nail into a wall, put a piece of tape on the wall at the site. This will prevent the paint from peeling off if you have to remove the nail and it will stop the wall from cracking, too.

KEEP SCREWS HANDY • When doing household repairs, place loose screws, nuts, and bolts directly on a piece of transparent tape so they won't roll around and get lost. Stick some double-sided tape on your workbench and use it to hold screws and other bits in place while you're working on a project.

MEND A BROKEN PLANT STEM • Use transparent tape to add support to a broken plant stem. Just wrap the stem in tape at the damaged area and leave the tape on until it mends. The taped plant will keep growing as long as moisture can travel up the stem.

MAKE A SEED STRIP • Make your own seed strip to create perfectly straight rows in your garden with almost no effort. Sprinkle some seeds on a piece of wax or parchment paper and use your fingers to arrange and align them. After removing the excess, take a strip of transparent tape and place it over the seeds. Then just bury the tape in the garden and you will soon have perfect rows.

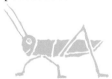

CATCH INVADING CRICKETS • If noisy crickets have invaded your cellar or garage, try trapping them with packaging tape. Take a strip of the tape and place it on the floor, sticky side up. Later, release your catch into the wild or feed them to a cricket-eating pet.

more TAPE over →

for safety's sake

SAFETY MARKERS FOR A CAR EMERGENCY • You'll be a lot safer when your car breaks down at night if you have safety markers on hand to warn oncoming drivers. You can make your own safety markers easily at home. Just put strips of brightly colored reflector tape on some old coffee cans. Keep them in the trunk of your car for use in an emergency.

MAKE PETS VISIBLE AT NIGHT • Don't let your beloved family pet get hit by a car during the night. Put reflector tape on your dog's collar so drivers will be able to see him easily in the dark.

MARK DARK STAIRWAYS • Stop stumbling on those poorly lit cellar or outdoor stairways or worrying about guests tripping and falling. Simply apply reflector tape along the edges of the steps and you and your guests will be able to see exactly where you're stepping.

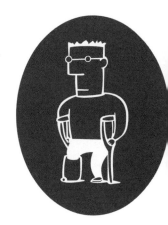

for the kids

SECURE A BABY'S BIB • Stop bits of food from getting under a baby's bib by taping the edges of the bib to the baby's clothes.

MAKESHIFT CHILDPROOFING • If you bring a baby or small child with you when visiting a home that isn't childproofed, bring a roll of transparent tape along, too. Use it to cover electrical outlets as a temporary safety measure. Although it will not give a lot of protection, it could give you the extra time you need to remove a child from a potentially hazardous situation.

MAKE MULTICOLORED DESIGNS • Tape a few different-colored markers or pencils together and give them to the kids to draw multicolored designs. Be careful not to use too many, so the children can maintain control of the drawings.

Kids' Stuff

Kids will be delighted and amazed when you do this easy party trick at a birthday gathering. Secretly place a piece of transparent tape over an area of a blown-up balloon. When you are ready, get the children's attention and hold up the balloon in one hand and a pin in the other. For added effect, tell them to cover their ears. Pierce the balloon with the pin at the taped spot and remove it. The balloon will not pop! Then pop the balloon in another area. Guaranteed to leave them laughing and scratching their heads.

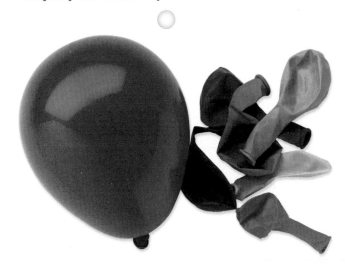

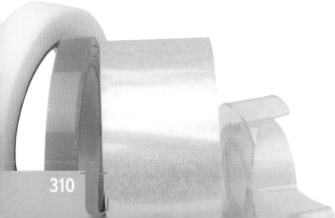

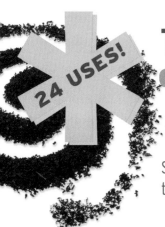

24 USES!

TEA
for health and beauty

RELIEVE TIRED EYES

Revitalize tired, achy, or puffy eyes. Soak two tea bags in warm water and place them over your closed eyes for 20 minutes. The tannins in the tea act to reduce puffiness and soothe tired eyes.

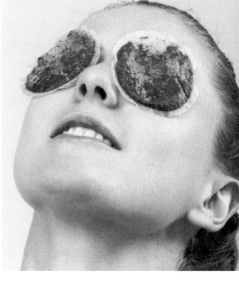

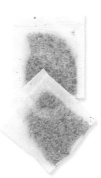

COOL SUNBURNED SKIN • What can you do when you forget to use sunscreen and have to pay the price with a painful burn? A few wet tea bags applied to the affected skin will take out the sting. This works well for other types of minor burns (e.g., from a teapot or steam iron), too. If the sunburn is too widespread to treat this way, put some tea bags in your bath water and soak your whole body in the tub.

REDUCE RAZOR BURN • If you forget to replace a razor blade before you start shaving, it'll probably hurt when the blade is dragged across your skin. To soothe razor burn and relieve painful nicks and cuts, apply a wet tea bag to the affected area. And don't forget to replace the blade before your next shave.

GET THE GRAY OUT • Turn gray hair dark again without an expensive trip to the salon or the use of chemical hair dyes. Make your own natural dye using brewed tea and herbs. Steep 3 tea bags in 1 cup (250 ml) boiling water. Add 1 tablespoon (15 ml) each rosemary and sage (fresh or dried) and let it stand overnight before straining. To use, shampoo as usual, then pour or spray the mixture on your hair, making sure to saturate it thoroughly. Take care not to stain clothes. Blot with a towel; do not rinse. You may need to do this several times to achieve your desired result.

CONDITION DRY HAIR • To give a natural shine to dry hair, use a quart (1 L) warm, unsweetened tea, freshly brewed or from a tea bag, as a final rinse after your regular shampoo.

TAN YOUR SKIN WITH TEA • Give pale skin a healthy tanned appearance without exposure to dangerous ultraviolet rays. Brew 2 cups (500 ml) strong black tea, let it cool, and pour into a plastic spray bottle. Make sure your skin is clean and dry. Spray the tea directly onto your skin and let it air-dry. Repeat as desired for a healthy-looking glowing tan. This will also work to give a man's face a more natural look after shaving off a beard.

more TEA over →

DID YOU KNOW?

Legend has it that tea originated some 5,000 years ago with the Chinese emperor Shen Nung. A wise ruler and creative scientist, the emperor insisted that all drinking water be boiled as a health precaution. One summer day, during a rest stop in a distant region, servants began to boil water for the royal entourage to drink when some dried leaves from a nearby bush fell into the pot. As the water boiled, it turned brown. The emperor's scientific curiosity was aroused, and he insisted on tasting the liquid. It was just his cup of tea.

DRAIN A BOIL • Drain a boil with a boiled tea bag! Cover a boil with a wet tea bag overnight and the boil should drain without pain by the time you wake up the next morning.

SOOTHE SORE NIPPLES FROM BREASTFEEDING • If feeding your baby leaves your nipples sore, treat them to an ice-cold bag of tea. Just brew a cup of tea, remove the bag, and place it in a cup of ice for about a minute. Then place the wet tea bag on the sore nipple and cover it with a nursing pad under your bra for several minutes while you enjoy a cup of tea. The tannic acid in the wet tea leaves will soothe and help heal the nipple skin.

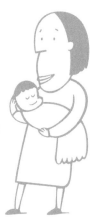

SOOTHE BLEEDING GUMS • A child may be all smiles later when the tooth fairy arrives, but bleeding gums are no fun whatsoever. To stop the bleeding and soothe the pain from a lost or recently pulled tooth, wet a tea bag with cool water and press it directly on the empty tooth site.

RELIEVE BABY'S PAIN FROM INJECTION • If your baby is still crying from a recent immunization injection, try wetting a tea bag and placing it over the site of the injection. Hold it gently in place until the crying stops. The tannic acid in the tea will soothe the soreness. It's worth trying it on yourself the next time an injection leaves your arm sore.

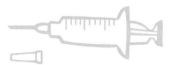

DRY POISON IVY RASH • Dry a weepy poison ivy rash with strongly brewed tea. Simply dip a cotton ball into the tea, dab it on the affected area and let it air-dry. Repeat as needed.

STOP FOOT ODOR

Put an end to smelly feet by giving them a daily tea bath. Just soak your tootsies in strongly brewed tea for 20 minutes a day and say goodbye to offensive odors.

MAKE A SOOTHING MOUTHWASH • To ease mouth or toothache pain, rinse with a cup of hot peppermint tea mixed with a pinch or two of salt. Peppermint is an antiseptic and contains menthol, which alleviates pain on contact with skin surfaces. To make peppermint tea, boil 1 tablespoon (15 ml) fresh peppermint leaves in 1 cup (250 ml) water. Steep for several minutes.

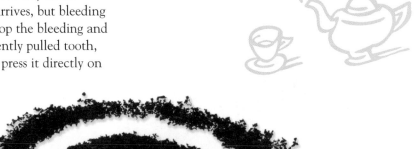

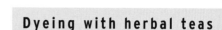

around the house

TENDERIZE TOUGH MEAT • Even the toughest cuts of meat will melt in your mouth after you marinate them in plain old black tea. Place 4 tablespoons (60 ml) black tea leaves in a pot of warm (not boiling) water and steep for 5 minutes. Strain to remove the leaves and stir in ½ cup (125 g) brown sugar until it dissolves, then set aside. Season up to 3 pounds (1.5 kg) of meat with salt, pepper, onion, and garlic powder, and place it in a casserole dish with a lid. Pour the liquid over the seasoned meat and cook it in a preheated 325°F (165°C) oven until the meat is fork tender—about 90 minutes.

CLEAN WOODEN FURNITURE AND FLOORS • Freshly brewed tea is great for cleaning wooden furniture and floors. Just boil a couple of tea-bags in a quart (1 L) of water and let it cool. Dip a soft cloth in the tea, wring out the excess, and use it to wipe away dirt and grime. Buff dry with a clean, soft cloth.

CREATE AN 'ANTIQUE' LOOK • Soak white lace or garments in a tea bath to create an antique beige, ecru, or ivory look. Use 3 tea bags for every 2 cups (500 ml) boiling water and steep for about 20 minutes. Let it cool for a few minutes before soaking the material for 10 minutes or so. The longer you let it soak, the darker the shade you will get.

SHINE YOUR MIRRORS • To make mirrors shine, brew a pot of strong tea, let it cool, then use it to clean the mirrors. Dampen a soft cloth in the tea and wipe it all over the surface of the mirrors. Buff with a soft, dry cloth for a sparkly, streak-free shine.

in the garden

GIVE ROSES A BOOST • Sprinkle new or used tea leaves (loose or in tea bags) around your rosebushes and cover them with mulch to give them a midsummer boost. When you water the plants, the nutrients from the tea will be released into the soil, spurring growth. Roses love the tannic acid that occurs naturally in tea.

TIP

Dyeing with herbal teas

Using plain old tea leaves to dye fabrics is a technique that has been around for a long time, and was first used to hide stains on linens.

But you can also use herbal teas to dye fabric different colors and to create subtle hues. Try using hibiscus leaves to achieve red tones and darker herbal teas like licorice for soft brown tints. You should always experiment using fabric scraps until you obtain the desired results.

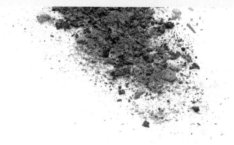

CONTROL DUST FROM FIREPLACE ASH • To keep dust from rising from the ash when you clean out your fireplace, sprinkle wet tea leaves over the area before you begin cleaning. The tea will keep the ash from spreading all over as you lift it out.

PERFUME A SACHET • Next time you make a sachet, try perfuming it with the fragrant aroma of your favorite herbal tea. Just open a few used herbal tea bags and spread the wet tea on some old newspapers to dry. Then use the dry tea as stuffing for the sachet.

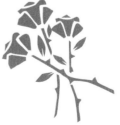

more TEA over →

FEED YOUR FERNS • Schedule an occasional tea time for your ferns and other acid-loving houseplants. Substitute brewed tea when watering the plants. Work wet tea leaves into the soil around houseplants to give them a lush, luxuriant look.

PREPARE PLANTER FOR POTTING • For healthier potted plants, place a few used tea bags on top of the drainage layer at the bottom of the planter before potting. The tea bags will retain water and leach nutrients into the soil.

TENNIS BALLS

FLUFF DOWN-FILLED CLOTHES AND COMFORTERS

Down-filled items like jackets, vests, quilts, and pillows get flat and soggy when you wash them. You can fluff them up again by tossing a couple of tennis balls with them in the dryer.

SAND CURVES IN FURNITURE • Wrap a tennis ball in sandpaper and use it to sand curves when you're refinishing furniture. The tennis ball is just the right size and shape to fit comfortably in your hand.

COVER YOUR TRAILER HITCH • To protect a chrome trailer hitch from scratches and rust, cut a tennis ball and slip it over the hitching ball. The tennis ball will keep moisture and rust away.

MASSAGE YOUR BACK • Give yourself a relaxing and therapeutic back massage. Simply fill a long tube sock with a few tennis balls, tie the end, and stretch your homemade massager around your back just as you would a towel after a shower or bath.

ENHANCE YOUR COMPOST PILE • To speed up the decomposition process and enrich your compost, pour in a few cups of strongly brewed tea. The liquid tea will hasten decomposition and draw acid-producing bacteria, creating desirable, acid-rich compost.

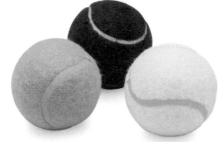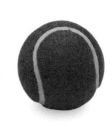

KEEP A SWIMMING POOL OIL-FREE • Float a couple of tennis balls in your swimming pool to absorb body oils from swimmers. Replace the balls every couple of weeks during periods of high use.

MAKE A BIKE KICKSTAND FOR SOFT SOIL • To prevent a bicycle kickstand from sinking into soft grass, sand, or mud, cut a slit in a tennis ball and put it on the end of the kickstand.

STORE YOUR VALUABLES AT THE GYM • Here's a great way to hide and store your valuables when you are working out at the gym. Make a 2-inch (5-cm) slit along one seam of a tennis ball and insert the valuables inside. Keep the ball in your gym bag among other sporting gear. Just remember not to use your doctored ball next time you're playing tennis!

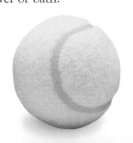

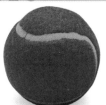

SCIENCE **WORKS!**

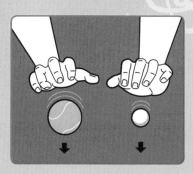

Teach kids about gravity.

Stand on a chair holding two tennis balls, one in each hand, and extend your arms so they're at the same distance from the floor. Ask the kids to observe as you release both balls at once. Did they hit the floor at the same time? Now repeat using a tennis ball and a much lighter ping-pong ball. Again ask which will land first. Most will guess the heavier tennis ball, but they'll land at the same time because gravity exerts the same force on all objects regardless of their weight. Of course, if you try this with a ball and a feather, the kids will also learn that less dense objects fall more slowly due to air resistance.

GET PARKING RIGHT

Make parking your car in the garage easier. Hang a tennis ball on a string from the garage ceiling so it will hit the windshield at the spot where you should stop the car. You'll always know exactly where to park.

MASSAGE YOUR SORE FEET • For a simple, but amazingly enjoyable and therapeutic foot massage, take your shoes off, place a tennis ball on the floor, and roll it around under your feet.

GET A BETTER GRIP ON BOTTLE CAPS • If your hands are weakened by arthritis or other ailments, you probably have a difficult time removing twist-off bottle caps. An old tennis ball may help. Simply cut a ball in half and use one of the halves to enhance your grip.

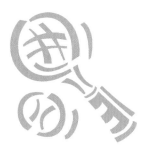

TIRES

MAKE A CLASSIC TIRE SWING • A swing made from an old tire is a timeless source of pleasure for children of all ages. To make one in your backyard, drill a few drainage holes in the bottom of the tire. Drill two holes for bolts in the top, bolt two chains to the tire, and suspend it by the chains from a healthy branch of a hardwood tree. Use ¾-inch (18-mm) playground chain. Put some wood chips or other soft material under and around the swing to cushion falls.

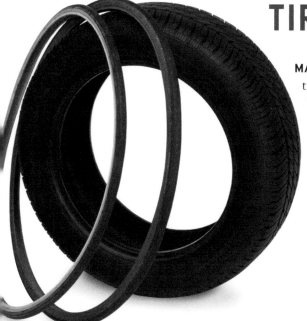

more *TIRES* over →

STORE PLUMBING SNAKES • An old bicycle tire is just the right size to store metal snakes used to clean plumbing lines or "fish wires" used to run electric cables inside walls. Lay the snake or fish wire inside the tire, where it will expand to the shape of the tire and become encased within it. Then you can hang the tire conveniently on a hook in your workshop, garage, or shed.

PROTECT YOUR VEGETABLES • Plant your peppers, tomatoes, potatoes, eggplants, or other vegetables inside tires laid on the ground. The tires will protect the plants from harsh winds and the dark rubber of the tire will absorb heat from the sun, warming the surrounding soil.

MAKE A WADING POOL FOR THE KIDS • To make an improptu wading pool for toddlers, drape a shower curtain over the center of a large truck tire and fill it with water.

Tire check-up

TIP

✳ *Spending 5 minutes a month to check your tires can protect against avoidable breakdowns and crashes, improve vehicle handling, increase gas mileage, and extend the life of your tires. Here are some basic guidelines:*

● Check the tire air pressure at least once a month and before going on a long road trip. Don't forget to check the spare while you're at it.

● Inspect for uneven wear on tire treads, cracks, foreign objects, or other signs of wear or trauma. Remove bits of glass and other objects wedged in the tread of the tire.

● Make sure your tire valves have caps.

● Do not overload your vehicle.

TOMATO JUICE

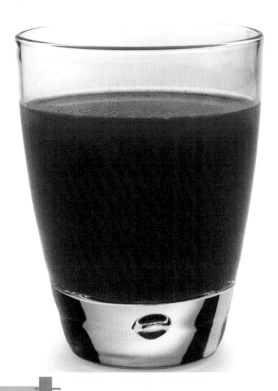

REMOVE BAD DOG SMELLS • Is there a dog alive that hasn't rolled in something foul and stinky? If your dog does this, douse the affected area thoroughly with undiluted tomato juice. Be sure to sponge some of the juice over your pet's face, too, avoiding his eyes. Wait a few minutes for the acids from the tomatoes to neutralize the smell, then give him a shampoo or scrub with soap and water. Repeat as necessary over several days until the smell is completely gone.

GET RID OF FRIDGE ODORS • If a power failure causes the food in your fridge to spoil and become malodorous, you can get rid of those smells in your refrigerator and freezer with the help of some tomato juice. Dispose of the offending food and thoroughly wipe inside the fridge and freezer with a sponge or washcloth doused in undiluted tomato juice. Rinse with warm, soapy water and wipe dry. If traces of smell remain, repeat the procedure or substitute vinegar for the tomato juice.

RESTORE BLONDE HAIR COLOR • If you're a blonde who has ever gone swimming in a chlorine-treated pool, you know it can sometimes give your hair an unappealing green tint. To restore the blonde color to your hair, saturate it with undiluted tomato juice, cover it with a shower cap, and wait 10 to 15 minutes. Shampoo, rinse thoroughly, and soon you'll be ready to have more fun.

DEODORIZE PLASTIC CONTAINERS • To remove foul odor from a plastic container, pour a little tomato juice on a sponge and wipe it around the inside of the container. Wash the container and lid in warm, soapy water, dry well, and store them separated in the freezer for a couple of days. The container will be stench-free and ready to use again.

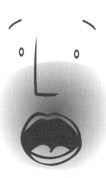

RELIEVE A SORE THROAT

For temporary relief of sore throat symptoms, gargle with a mixture of ½ cup (125 ml) tomato juice, ½ cup (125 ml) hot water, and about 10 drops Tabasco sauce.

TOOTHBRUSHES

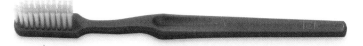

USE AS ALL-PURPOSE CLEANERS • You can use old toothbrushes to clean a host of diverse items and small or hard-to-reach areas and crevices. Use them to clean artificial flowers and plants, costume jewelry, combs, shower tracks, crevices between tiles, and around faucets. They're good for computer keyboards, can opener blades, and around stove burners. And don't forget the seams on shoes where the leather meets the sole.

BRUSH YOUR CHEESE GRATER • Give the teeth of a cheese grater a good brushing with an old toothbrush before you wash the grater or put it in the dishwasher. This will make it easier to wash and will prevent clogs in your dishwasher drain by getting rid of bits of cheese or any other food you may have grated.

REMOVE TOUGH STAINS • Removing a stain can be a pain, especially one that has soaked deep down into soft fibers. To remove those deep stains, try using a soft-bristled nylon toothbrush, dabbing it gently to work in the stain-removing agent (bleach or vinegar, for example) until the stain is gone.

CLEAN SILK FROM EARS OF CORN • Before cooking shucked corn, take an old toothbrush and gently rub down the ear to brush away the remaining clingy strands of silk. Then you won't have to brush them out from between your teeth after you eat the corn!

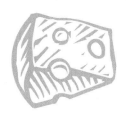

more TOOTHBRUSHES over →

CLEAN AND OIL YOUR WAFFLE IRON • A clean, soft toothbrush is just the right utensil to clean crumbs and burned batter from the nooks and crannies of a waffle iron. Use it to spread oil evenly on the waffle iron surface before the next use, too.

APPLY HAIR DYE • Dyeing your hair at home? Use an old toothbrush as an applicator. It's the perfect size.

CLEAN GUNK FROM APPLIANCES • Dip an old toothbrush in soapy water and use it to clean between appliance knobs and buttons, and raised-letter nameplates.

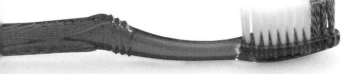

TOOTHPASTE

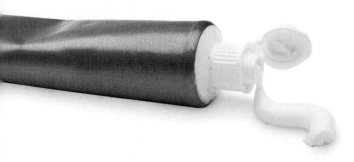

REMOVE SCUFFS FROM SHOES • A little toothpaste does an amazing job of removing scuffs from leather shoes. Just squirt a dab on the scuffed area, rub with a soft cloth, and wipe clean with a damp cloth. The leather will look like new.

CLEAN YOUR PIANO KEYS • Has tickling the ivories left them a bit dingy? Clean them with toothpaste and a toothbrush and wipe them down with a damp cloth. Makes sense, since ivory is essentially elephant teeth. However, toothpaste will work just as well on modern pianos that usually have keys covered with plastic rather than real ivory.

SPIFF UP YOUR SNEAKERS

Want to clean and whiten the rubber part of your sneakers? Get out the non-gel toothpaste and an old toothbrush. After scrubbing, clean off the toothpaste with a damp cloth.

CLEAN YOUR CLOTHES IRON • The mild abrasive in non-gel toothpaste is just the ticket for scrubbing the gunk off the sole plate of your clothes iron. Apply the toothpaste to the cool iron, scrub with a rag, and rinse clean.

POLISH A DIAMOND RING • Put a little toothpaste on an old toothbrush and use it to make your diamond ring sparkle instead of your teeth. Clean off the residue with a damp cloth.

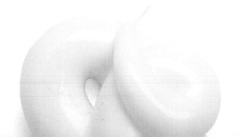

DEODORIZE BABY BOTTLES • Well-used baby bottles inevitably pick up a sour-milk smell. However, toothpaste will remove the odor in a jiffy. Just put some on your bottlebrush and scrub away. Make sure you rinse off the toothpaste thoroughly.

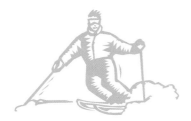

PREVENT FOGGED GOGGLES

Whether you are woodworking or going skiing or scuba diving, nothing is more frustrating (and sometimes dangerous) than fogged goggles. Prevent the problem by coating the goggles with toothpaste and wiping them off.

REMOVE CRAYON FROM WALLS • If children leave crayon marks on your walls, roll up your sleeves and grab a tube of non-gel toothpaste and a rag or, better yet, a scrubbing brush. Squirt the toothpaste on the wall and start scrubbing. The fine abrasive in toothpaste will rub away the crayon every time. Rinse the wall with water.

REMOVE INK OR LIPSTICK STAINS ON FABRIC • If a pen opens up in the pocket of your favorite shirt, don't panic. This may or may not work, depending on the fabric and the ink, but it is certainly worth a try before consigning the shirt to the scrap heap. Put non-gel toothpaste on the stain and rub the fabric vigorously together and rinse with water. Most or all of the ink should have come out. Repeat the process a few more times until you get rid of all the ink. Works for lipstick, too.

BATHROOM BLISS

NO-FOGGING BATHROOM MIRRORS • Ouch! You cut yourself shaving and it's no wonder—you can't see your face clearly in that fogged-up bathroom mirror. Next time, coat the mirror with non-gel toothpaste and wipe it off before you get in the shower. When you get out, the mirror won't be fogged.

SHINE BATHROOM AND KITCHEN CHROME • They make commercial cleaners with a very fine abrasive designed to shine up chrome, but if you don't have any handy, the fine abrasive in non-gel toothpaste works just as well. Just smear on the toothpaste and polish with a soft, dry cloth.

CLEAN THE BATHROOM SINK • Non-gel toothpaste works as well as anything else to clean the bathroom sink. The tube's sitting right there, so squirt some in, scrub with a sponge, and rinse it out. The toothpaste will also kill any odors emanating from the drain trap.

REMOVE WATERMARKS FROM FURNITURE • You leave coasters around, but some people just won't use them. To get rid of those telltale watermark rings left by sweating beverages, gently rub some non-gel toothpaste on the wood with a soft cloth. Wipe it off with a damp cloth and let it dry before applying your regular furniture polish.

CAUTION: All toothpaste, including gel, contains abrasives. The amount varies, but too much can damage your tooth enamel. People with sensitive teeth in particular should use a low-abrasive toothpaste. Ask your dentist which is the best toothpaste for you.

more TOOTHPASTE over →

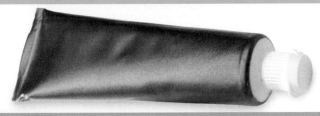

REMOVE BEACH OR ROAD TAR • Getting black beach tar or road tar on your feet can put a damper on a vacation, but it is easy enough to remove. Just rub it with some non-gel toothpaste and rinse.

CLEAR UP PIMPLES • When your teenager moans about a prominent pimple, have him or her dab a bit of non-gel, nonwhitening toothpaste on the offending spot and it should be dried up by morning. The toothpaste dehydrates the pimple and absorbs the oil. This pimple-clearing remedy works best on spots that have come to a head.
WARNING: This remedy may be irritating to sensitive skin. Try it on a small area of skin first.

CLEAN SMELLS FROM HANDS • The ingredients in toothpaste that deodorize your mouth will work on your hands as well. If you've managed to get into something stinky, wash your hands with toothpaste instead of soap and they'll smell great.

DID YOU KNOW?

Ancient Egyptians used a mixture of ox-hoof ash, burned eggshells, myrrh, pumice, and water to clean their teeth. For most of history, tooth-cleaning concoctions were used mostly by the wealthy. That began to change in 1850, when Dr. Washington Sheffield, of New London, Connecticut, developed a formula we would recognize as toothpaste. He called it Dr. Sheffield's Creme Dentifrice. It was his son, Dr. Lucius Sheffield, who observed collapsible metal tubes of paint and thought, 'Why not toothpaste?' To this day, Sheffield Laboratories, the company Dr. Washington Sheffield founded in 1850, continues to make toothpaste and put it in tubes.

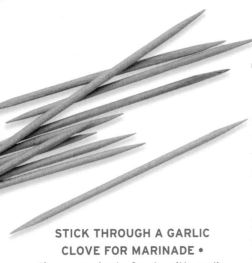

TOOTHPICKS

MARK RARE, MEDIUM, AND WELL DONE STEAKS • When guests want their steaks done differently at a barbecue, how do you keep track of who gets what? Easy. Just use different-colored toothpicks to mark them rare, medium, and well done, and get ready for the accolades.

KEEP SAUCEPANS FROM BOILING OVER • It seems as though all you have to do is turn around for a minute and the saucepan is boiling over, making a mess on the stovetop. Next time, just stick a toothpick, laid flat, between the saucepan and lid. The little space will allow enough steam to escape to prevent the saucepan from boiling over. This also works with a casserole dish that's cooking in the oven.

STICK THROUGH A GARLIC CLOVE FOR MARINADE •
If you marinate foods with garlic cloves, stick a toothpick through the clove so you can remove it easily when you are ready to serve the food.

MICROWAVE POTATOES FASTER • The next time you microwave a potato, stick four toothpick 'legs' in one side. The suspended potato will cook much faster because the microwaves will reach the bottom as well as the top and sides.

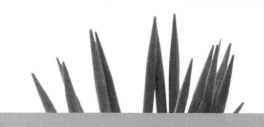

CONTROL YOUR USE OF SALAD DRESSING •
Restrict your intake of carbohydrates and calories from salad dressing by removing the foil seal when you open the bottle and punching several holes in the foil, using a toothpick. This will help prevent overuse of the dressing and make it last longer.

KEEP SAUSAGES FROM ROLLING AROUND • When cooking sausages, insert toothpicks between pairs to make turning them over easy and keep them from rolling around in the pan. They'll cook more evenly and only need to be turned over once.

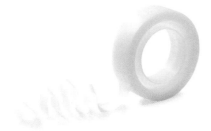

DID YOU KNOW?

■ Buddhist monks used toothpicks as far back as the 8th century, and researchers have even found toothpick grooves in the teeth of prehistoric humans.

■ Toothpicks were first used in the U.S. at the Union Oyster House, the oldest restaurant in Boston, which opened in 1826.

■ In 1872, Silas Noble and J.P. Cooley patented the first toothpick-manufacturing machine.

■ One cord of white birch wood (known as the toothpick tree) can make up to 7.5 million toothpicks.

MARK THE START OF A TAPE ROLL • Instead of wasting time trying to find the beginning of a tape roll, just wrap it around a toothpick whenever you have finished using the tape and the start of the roll will always be easy to find. No more frustration, and you can use the time you just saved to attack something else on your to-do list.

SEW EASY

APPLY GLUE TO SEQUINS • If you're working on a project that calls for gluing on sequins or buttons, squirt a little bit of glue onto a piece of paper and dip in a toothpick to apply small dabs of the glue. That way, you won't make a mess and you won't waste the glue.

MAKE SEWING EASIER • Make sewing projects easier and complete them faster, by using a round toothpick to push fabrics, lace, or gatherings under the presser foot as you sew.

CLEAN CRACKS AND CREVICES • To get rid of dirt, grime, and cobwebs in hard-to-reach cracks or crevices, dip an ordinary toothpick in some alcohol and run it through the affected area. You can also use this to clean the keys on your computer.

TOUCH UP FURNITURE CREVICES • The secret to a good touch-up paint job is to use as little paint as possible, because even if you do have the right paint, the stuff in the can may not exactly match the sun-faded or dirty paint on the furniture. The solution is to dip the end of a toothpick in the paint and use it to touch up just the crevice. Unlike a brush, the toothpick won't apply more paint than you need and you won't have a brush to clean.

REPAIR SMALL HOLES IN WOOD • Did you drive a finish nail or brad into the wrong spot in your pine project? Don't panic. Dip the tip of a toothpick into white or yellow glue. Stick the toothpick in the hole and break it off. Sand the toothpick flush to the surface and you will never notice the repair.

more TOOTHPICKS over →

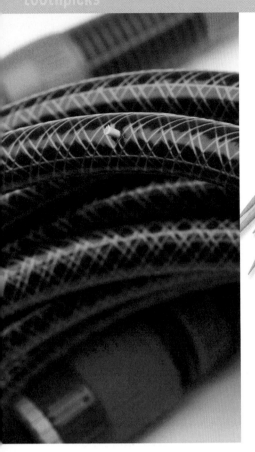

USE THEM TO LIGHT CANDLES • When a candle has burned down and the wick is hard to reach, don't burn your fingers trying to use a small match to light it. Instead, light a wooden toothpick and use it to light the burned-down wick.

GET RID OF CUTWORMS • Cutworms kill seedlings by encircling the stem and severing it. To protect your seedlings, stick a toothpick in the soil about ¼ inch (6 mm) from each stem. This prevents a cutworm from encircling it.

FIX A LOOSE HINGE SCREW • If you take a door off and remove the hinges before you paint it, you may find the screw just turns without tightening when you reattach the hinges, and that the hole is stripped. It's an easy problem to fix. Just put some glue on the end of a toothpick, stick it in the hole, and break it off. Add one or two more toothpicks with glue until the hole is tightly filled, breaking each one off. Re-drill the hole and you're ready to screw the hinge in place.

REPAIR A BENT PLANT STEM • If the stem of your favorite plant has folded over, it doesn't mean the plant is doomed. Straighten the stem and support it by placing a toothpick against the stem and wrapping the toothpick on with tape. Water the plant and keep an eye on it—depending on how fast it grows, the stem will regain its strength and you'll need to remove the splint so you don't strangle the stem.

REPAIR A LEAKY GARDEN HOSE

If your garden hose springs a leak, don't go out and buy another one. Just find the hole and insert a toothpick into it. Cut off the excess part of the toothpick. The water will make the wood swell, plugging up the leak every time.

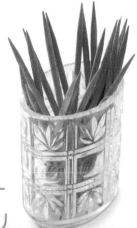

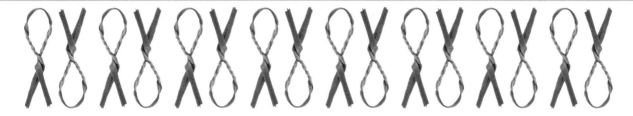

TWIST TIES

ORGANIZE ELECTRICAL CORDS • Does the top of your computer desk look like wild vines have taken over? Is there a thicket of wires behind your rapidly expanding entertainment center? Tame the jungle of electrical wires by rolling each one up neatly and securing the extra length with a twist tie.

STITCH HOLDERS FOR KNITTERS • Those little plastic store-bought stitch holders are expensive and have a habit of wandering off. You won't care if you have a supply of twist ties. To know where you left off, thread a twist tie through your stitches and twist it together. Use colored ties for diferent projects and needle sizes, and use them to hold the stitches you're not working on.

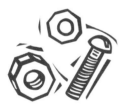

SMALL-STUFF WRANGLER • There are always stray washers, bolts, and other little do-dads that you try to keep together in the workshop. Twist ties can loop them together so you can find them when needed. Stash them in a drawer or hang them each on their own hook on the wall above your workbench.

MAKE A TRELLIS • To make a trellis for climbing annual vines such as peas or morning glories, all you need are some twist ties and some of those plastic rings from soda six-packs. Use the twist ties to join together as many of the six-pack rings as you need. Attach the trellis between two stakes, also using twist ties. You can even add sections to the trellis as the plant grows so that it looks like the plant is climbing on its own. At the end of the season, just roll the trellis up for storage and you can use it again next year.

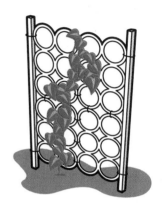

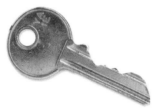

CODE YOUR KEYS

Do you have several similar-looking keys on your chain? You can quickly identify them by inserting twist ties of different colors secured through the existing holes in your keys.

more TWIST TIES over →

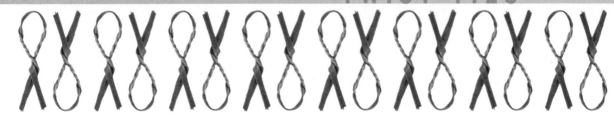

TIE UP PLANT STEMS • Twist ties are handy for securing a droopy plant stem to a stake or holding vines to a trellis. Don't twist the ties too tightly, however, because you don't want injure the stem or restrict its growth.

LIGHTWEIGHT PICTURE HANGER • A big metal picture hanger is overkill if you want to display a photo, document, or other lightweight object. Secure the ends of a twist tie together to form a loop and attach it to the back of whatever you want to hang. Now you can use a thumbtack or small nail that won't make a big hole in the wall.

TEMPORARILY REPAIR EYEGLASSES • Whoops! Your specs slip off because that tiny screw that holds the arm fell out. Secure the arm temporarily with a twist tie. Trim the edges of the tie so that you just have the center wire. After you insert and tie it off, snip the excess with scissors.

USE AS AN EMERGENCY SHOELACE • If you don't have a replacement shoelace handy, try using twist ties. Use one tie across each opposing pair of eyelets.

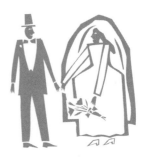

MAKE AN EMERGENCY CUFF LINK • Wardrobe malfunctions always seem to happen at the last minute. If you forget to pack your cuff links for an out-of-town wedding, it's not a disaster. Secure the cuffs with twist ties. Pull the ties through so the twist is discreetly hidden inside the cuff.

BIND LOOSE-LEAF PAPER • Sheets of loose-leaf paper can be easily held together by simply inserting twist ties through the holes.

CLEAN RAZORS AND ELECTRIC SHAVERS • Shaving is always better with a fresh razor or clean blade. If that little brush that comes with an electric razor is missing in action, a twist tie is the perfect replacement. It's just the right size for getting at all that dried shaving cream and little whiskers. You can also save on buying disposable razors by cleaning the space between the razor and the blade.

HANG CHRISTMAS TREE ORNAMENTS. • Some of those Christmas tree ornaments have been in the family for generations. As extra insurance against breakage, secure them to the tree with twist ties.

UMBRELLAS

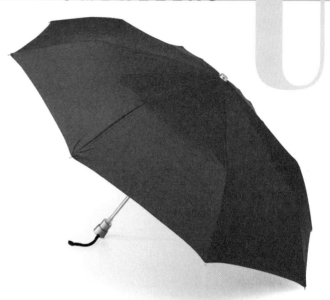

USE AS A DRYING RACK • An old umbrella makes a handy drying rack. Just strip off the fabric and hang the frame upside down from your shower-curtain bar. Attach wet clothing with clothespins. Plus, your new drying rack easily folds up for storage.

CLEAN A CHANDELIER • The next time you climb up high to clean the chandelier or ceiling fan, bring an old umbrella with you. Open the umbrella and hook its handle on the fixture so that it hangs upside down to catch any drips or dust.

COVER YOUR PICNIC FOOD • To keep flies from feasting on your picnic before you do, open an old umbrella and cut off the handle. Place the umbrella over the picnic dishes. It will shield your lunchtime treats from the sun, too.

SIGNAL IN A CROWD • The next time you and friends go to a crowded event, carry a couple of identical, brightly-colored umbrellas. If you get separated, you can hold the umbrellas over your head and open them up to find each other in a flash.

BLOCK PLANT OVERSPRAY • Houseplants love to be misted with water, but your walls don't love to get soaked with overspray. Stick an open umbrella between the plants and the wall and give your plants a no-holds-barred shower.

MAKE PLANT STAKES • If the wind caught your umbrella, turned it inside out, and ripped the fabric, don't just toss it into the trash. Remove the umbrella's ribs first, as they make excellent supports for top-heavy garden plants, such as peonies.

MAKE AN INSTANT TRELLIS • Remove the fabric from an old umbrella and insert the handle into the ground to support climbing vines, such as morning glories or sweet peas. The umbrella's shape, covered with flowers, will look terrific in the garden.

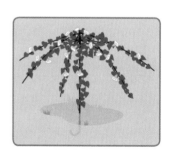

SHIELD YOUR SEEDLINGS • If you waited long enough before planting your seedlings outside but a frost is unexpectedly predicted, you can use an old umbrella to save the seedlings. Open the umbrella, and cut off the handle. Place the umbrella over the seedlings to keep the frost off them.

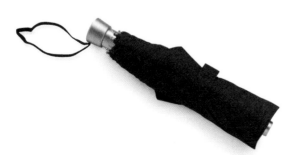

VANILLA EXTRACT

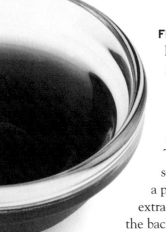

FRESHEN UP THE FRIDGE • If you're having trouble getting rid of a bad odor in your refrigerator, even after scrubbing it out, try wiping down the inside of the fridge with vanilla extract. To prolong the fresh vanilla scent, soak a cotton ball or a piece of sponge with vanilla extract and leave it on one of the back shelves.

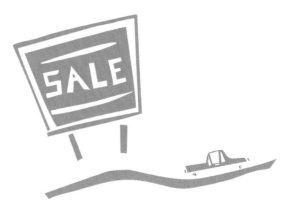

SWEETEN THE SMELL OF YOUR HOME

It's an old real estate agent's trick. Put a drop or two of vanilla extract on a light bulb, turn on the light and your house will be filled with the appealing scent of baked goods in the oven.

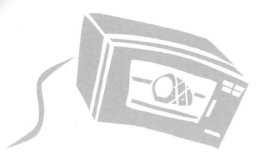

DEODORIZE YOUR MICROWAVE • Is the odor of fish, or some other strong or unpleasant smell, lingering in your microwave oven? Pour a bit of vanilla extract in a bowl and microwave it on *High* for 1 minute. That bad odor will be history.

USE IT AS PERFUME • Try it! Just put a dab of vanilla extract on each wrist. You'll smell delicious, and many people find the scent of vanilla to be very relaxing.

REPEL INSECTS • Everybody likes the smell of vanilla. Everybody but insects, that is. Dilute 1 tablespoon (15 ml) vanilla extract into 1 cup (250 ml) water and wipe the mixture on any exposed skin to discourage mosquitoes, blackflies, and ticks.

NEUTRALIZE THE SMELL OF FRESH PAINT • If you don't like the unpleasant smell of fresh paint in your house, mix 1 tablespoon (15 ml) vanilla extract in the paint can when you open it. The house will smell great and it won't affect the paint!

RELIEVE MINOR BURNS • Yee-oow! When you accidentally grab a hot saucepan or get splattered with grease in the kitchen, grab the vanilla extract for quick pain relief. The evaporation of the alcohol in the vanilla extract cools the burn.

vegetable oil
vegetable oil
vegetable oil
vegetable oil
vegetable oil
VEGETABLE OIL

VEGETABLE OIL

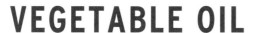

TIP

HELP REMOVE A SPLINTER

If a stubborn splinter won't come out, take a break from poking at your finger for a few minutes and soak it in vegetable oil. The oil will soften up your skin, perhaps just enough to ease that splinter out with your tweezers.

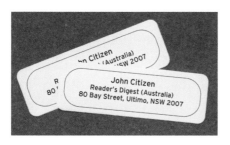

CONQUER GRASS CLIPPINGS

The next time you flip your lawn mower over to remove those stuck-on grass clippings, rub some vegetable oil under the housing and on the blade. It will take longer for those clippings to build up next time.

Oiling cutting boards

✳ *To restore and preserve dried-out wooden kitchen items such as cutting boards, salad bowls, and tongs, use medical-quality mineral oil—a food-safe oil that won't get rancid and is designed to protect wood that will come into contact with food. Don't use regular vegetable oil. Of course, it will soak into the dried-out wood and make it look much better, but it never really dries and can turn rancid once it's in the wood.*

REMOVE LABELS AND STICKERS • Used jars—both plastic and glass—are always handy to have around. But removing the old labels usually leaves a stubborn, sticky residue. Soak the label with vegetable oil and the label will slide right off. Works well for address labels and sticky price tags, too.

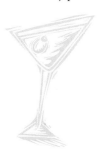

SEPARATE STUCK GLASSES • When stacked drinking glasses get stuck, it seems like nothing you can do will get them apart. But the solution is simple; just pour a little vegetable oil around the rim of the bottom glass and the glasses will pull apart with ease.

more VEGETABLE OIL over →

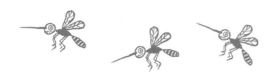

CONTROL MOSQUITOES IN THE BIRDBATH • It's so satisfying to watch birds enjoying a garden bath, but still water is a perfect breeding ground for mosquitoes. Floating a few tablespoons of vegetable oil on the surface of the water keeps mosquitoes from using the water, and it won't bother the birds. But it's still important to change the water twice a week so any larvae don't have time to hatch.

SEASON CAST-IRON COOKWARE • After washing and thoroughly drying a cast-iron frying pan or wok, use a paper towel to wipe it down with vegetable oil. Just leave a very thin layer of oil behind after wiping. It will prevent the pan from rusting and also season it for the next time you use it.

SMOOTH YOUR FEET • Rub your feet with a few drops of vegetable oil before you go to bed then put on a pair of socks. When you wake up, your feet will feel silky-smooth and soft.

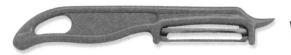

VEGETABLE PEELERS

SLICE SLIVERS OF CHEESE OR CHOCOLATE

When you need cheese slivers that are thinner than you can cut with a knife, or you want to decorate a cake with fine curlicues of chocolate, reach for the vegetable peeler.

SOFTEN HARD BUTTER QUICKLY • You're ready to add the butter to your cake mix when you discover that the only butter you have is as hard as a rock. When you need to soften cold, hard butter in a hurry, shave off what you need with a vegetable peeler. You'll have soft butter in seconds.

SHARPEN YOUR PENCILS • No pencil sharpener handy? A vegetable peeler will do a top job of bringing your pencil to a point.

RENEW SCENTED SOAPS • Ornamental scented soaps are a great addition to the guest bathroom because they make the room smell great as well as lending a decorative touch. But after a while, the surface of exposed ornamental soaps dries out, causing the scent to fade. To renew the scent, use a vegetable peeler to skim off a thin layer, revealing a new moist and fragrant surface.

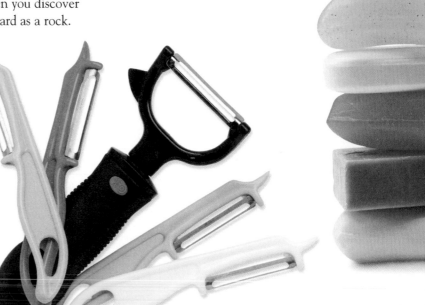

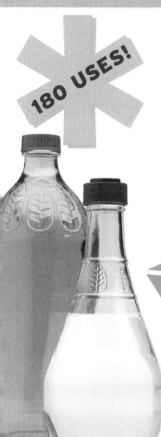

180 USES!

VINEGAR

around the house

CLEAR DIRT OFF COMPUTERS AND PERIPHERALS • Your computer, printer, and other home-office gear will work better if you keep them clean and dust-free. Before you start cleaning, make sure that all your equipment is turned off. Now mix equal parts white vinegar and water in a bucket. Dampen a clean cloth in the solution—never use a spray bottle; you don't want to get liquid on the circuits inside—then squeeze it out as hard as you can and start wiping. Keep a few cotton swabs on hand for getting to the buildups in tight spaces (like around the keys of your computer's keyboard).

CLEAN YOUR COMPUTER MOUSE • If you have a mouse with a removable tracking ball, use a 50:50 vinegar–water solution to clean it. First, remove the ball from underneath the mouse by twisting off the cover over it. Use a cloth, dampened with the solution and wrung out, to wipe the ball clean and to remove fingerprints and dirt from the mouse itself. Then use a moistened cotton swab to clean out the gunk and debris from inside the ball chamber (let it dry for a couple of hours before reinserting the ball).

CLEAN YOUR WINDOW BLINDS • You can make the job of cleaning mini-blinds or venetians much less torturous by giving them the 'white glove' treatment. Just put on a white cotton glove—the kind sold for gardening is perfect—and moisten the fingers in a solution made of equal parts white vinegar and hot tap water. Now simply slide your fingers across both sides of each slat. Use clean water to periodically wash off the glove.

GET RID OF SMOKE ODOR • If you've recently burned a steak or something else, remove the lingering smoky odor by placing a shallow bowl about three-quarters full of white or cider vinegar in the room where the scent is strongest. Use several bowls if the smell permeates your entire home. The odor should be gone in less than a day. You can also quickly dispense of the smell of fresh cigarette smoke inside a room by moistening a cloth with vinegar and waving it around a bit.

TIP

Buying vinegar

Vinegar comes in a surprising number of varieties—including herbal organic blends, Champagne, rice, and wine—not to mention bottle sizes and prices.

For household chores, however, plain distilled white vinegar is the best and least expensive choice, and you can buy it in 1 gallon (4 L) jugs to save even more money. Apple cider vinegar runs a close second in terms of practicality and is also widely used in cooking and home remedies. All other types of vinegar are strictly for ingestion and can vary wildly in price as well.

more VINEGAR over →

UNCLOG AND DEODORIZE DRAINS • The combination of vinegar and baking soda is one of the most effective mixtures for unclogging and deodorizing drains. It's also far gentler on your pipes than commercial drain cleaners.

■ To clear clogs in sink and tub drains, use a funnel to pour in ½ cup (125 g) baking soda followed by 1 cup (250 ml) vinegar. When the foaming subsides, flush with hot tap water. Wait 5 minutes and flush again with cold water. Besides clearing blockages, this technique also washes away odor-causing bacteria.

■ To speed up a slow drain, pour in ½ cup (125 g) salt followed by 2 cups (500 ml) boiling vinegar, and follow by flushing with hot and cold tap water.

WIPE AWAY MILDEW • When you want to remove mildew stains, reach for white vinegar first. It can be safely used without additional ventilation and also be applied to almost any surface—bathroom fixtures and tiles, clothing, furniture, painted surfaces, plastic curtains, and more. To eliminate heavy mildew accumulations, use it full strength. For light stains, dilute with an equal amount of water. You can also prevent mildew from forming on the bottoms of rugs and carpeting by misting the backs with full-strength white vinegar from a spray bottle.

ERASE BALLPOINT-PEN MARKS

Has a budding young artist just decorated a painted wall in your home with a ballpoint original? Don't lose your cool. Instead, dab some full-strength white vinegar on the 'masterpiece' using a cloth or a sponge. Repeat until the marks are gone. Then go out and buy your child a nice big sketch pad.

CLEAN AND POLISH

CLEAN CHROME AND STAINLESS STEEL • To clean chrome and stainless steel fixtures around your home, apply a light misting of undiluted white vinegar from a recycled spray bottle. Buff with a soft cloth to bring out the brightness.

SHINE YOUR SILVER • Make your silverware—as well as your pure silver bracelets, rings, and other jewelry—shine like new by soaking them in a mixture of 1/2 cup (125 ml) white vinegar and 2 tablespoons (30 ml) baking soda for 2 to 3 hours. Rinse them under cold water, then dry thoroughly with a soft cloth.

POLISH BRASS AND COPPER ITEMS • Put the shimmer back in your brass, bronze, and copper objects by making a paste of equal parts white vinegar and salt, or vinegar and baking soda (wait for the fizzing to stop before using). Use a clean, soft cloth or paper towel to rub the paste into the item until the tarnish is gone. Then rinse with cool water and polish with a soft towel until dry.

CAUTION: Do not apply vinegar to items of jewelry containing pearls or gemstones because it can damage their finish or, in the case of pearls, actually disintegrate them. Also, do not attempt to remove tarnish from the surface of antiques, because it could diminish their value significantly.

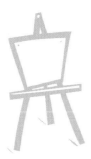

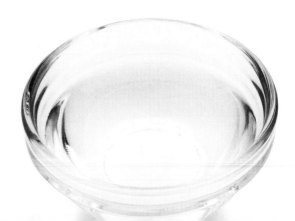

UNGLUE STICKERS, DECALS, AND PRICE TAGS • To remove a sticker or decal fixed to painted furniture or a painted wall, simply saturate the corners and sides of the sticker with full-strength white vinegar and carefully scrape it off (using an expired credit card or a plastic phone card). Remove any sticky remains by pouring on a bit more vinegar. Let it sit for a minute or two and wipe with a clean cloth. This approach is equally effective for removing price tags and other stickers from glass, plastic, and other glossy surfaces.

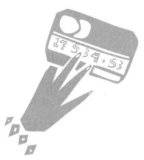

BURNISH YOUR SCISSORS • When your scissor blades get sticky or grimy, don't use water to wash them off; you're far more likely to rust the fastener that holds the blades together—or even the blades—than get them clean. Instead, wipe down the blades with a cloth dipped in full-strength white vinegar, and dry them off with a rag or dish towel.

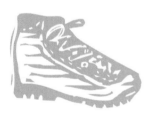

GET THE SALT OFF YOUR SHOES • Getting ice and snow on your shoes and boots is bad enough, but worse still is the rock salt that's used to melt it in some cold areas. In addition to leaving unsightly white stains, salt can actually cause footwear to crack and even disintegrate if it's left on indefinitely. To remove it and prevent long-term damage, wipe fresh stains with a cloth dipped in undiluted white vinegar.

CLEAN YOUR PIANO KEYS • Here's an easy and efficient way to get those grimy fingerprints and stains off your piano keys. Dip a soft cloth into a solution of ½ cup (125 ml) white vinegar and 2 cups (500 ml) water, squeeze it out until there are no drips, then gently wipe off each key. Use a second cloth to dry off the keys as you move along. Leave the keyboard uncovered for 24 hours.

DEODORIZE LUNCH BOXES, GYM LOCKERS, AND CAR TRUNKS • Does your old gym locker smell like, well, an old gym locker? Or perhaps your child's lunch box has taken on the bouquet of week-old tuna? What about that musty car trunk? Stop holding your breath every time you open it. Instead, soak a slice of white bread in white vinegar and leave it in the malodorous space overnight. The smell should be gone by morning.

FRESHEN A MUSTY CLOSET • Got a closet that doesn't smell as fresh as you'd like? First, remove the contents, then wash down the walls, ceiling, and floor with a cloth dampened in a solution of 1 cup (250 ml) each vinegar and ammonia and ¼ cup (50 g) baking soda in a gallon (4 L) of water. Keep the closet door open and let the interior dry before replacing your clothes and other stuff. If the smell persists, place a small tray of cat litter inside. Replenish it every few days until the odor is gone.

BRIGHTEN UP BRICKWORK • How's this for an effortless way to clean your brick floors without breaking out the polish? Just go over them with a damp mop dipped in 1 cup (250 ml) white vinegar mixed in a gallon (4 L) warm water. Your floors will look so good you'll never clean them with anything else. You can also use this same solution to brighten the bricks around your fireplace.

more VINEGAR over →

TIP

REVITALIZE WOOD PANELING • Does the wood paneling in your study look dull and dreary? Liven it up with this simple homemade remedy. Mix 2 cups (500 ml) warm water, 4 tablespoons (60 ml) white or apple cider vinegar and 2 tablespoons (30 ml) olive oil in a container, give it a couple of shakes and apply to wood with a clean cloth. Let the mixture soak in for several minutes, then polish with a dry cloth.

RESTORE WORN RUGS • If your rugs or carpets are looking worn and dingy from too much foot traffic or an excess of kids' building blocks, toy trucks and such, bring them back to life by brushing them with a clean broom dipped in a solution of 1 cup (250 ml) white vinegar in a gallon (4 L) water. Your faded threads will perk up, and you won't even need to rinse off the solution.

REMOVE CARPET STAINS • You can lift out many stains from your carpet with vinegar:

■ Rub light carpet stains with 2 tablespoons (30 ml) salt dissolved in ½ cup (125 ml) white vinegar. Let the solution dry and vacuum.

■ For larger or darker stains, add 2 tablespoons (30 ml) borax to the mixture and use it in the same way.

Vinegar and floor cleaning

❋ *Using a damp mop with a mild vinegar solution is widely recommended as a way to clean wooden and wax-free vinyl or laminate flooring.*

But, if at all possible, check with your flooring manufacturer first. Even when diluted, vinegar's acidity can ruin some floor finishes, and too much water will damage most wooden floors. If you want to try vinegar on your floors, use ½ cup (125 ml) white vinegar mixed in a gallon (4 L) warm water. Use a trial application in an inconspicuous area. Before applying the vinegar–water solution, squeeze out the mop thoroughly (or just use a spray bottle to moisten the mop head directly).

■ For tough, ground-in dirt and stains, make a paste of 1 tablespoon (15 ml) vinegar with 1 tablespoon (15 ml) cornstarch and rub into the stain using a dry cloth. Let it set for two days and vacuum.

■ To make a spray-on spot-and-stain remover, fill a spray bottle with 5 parts water and 1 part vinegar. Fill a second spray bottle with 1 part nonsudsy ammonia and 5 parts water. Saturate a stain with the vinegar solution, let it settle for a few minutes, and blot thoroughly with a clean, dry cloth. Then spray and blot using the ammonia solution. Repeat until the stain is completely gone.

in the garage ● ● ●

REMOVE BUMPER STICKERS • If those tattered old bumper stickers on your car make you feel more nauseated than nostalgic, it's time to break out the vinegar. Saturate the top and sides of the sticker with undiluted distilled vinegar and wait 10 to 15 minutes for the vinegar to soak through. Then use an expired credit card to scrape it off. Use more full-strength vinegar to get rid of any remaining gluey residue. Use the same technique to detach those cute decals your children use to decorate the back windshields.

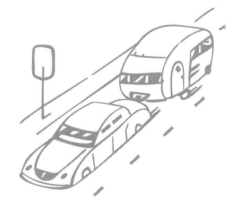

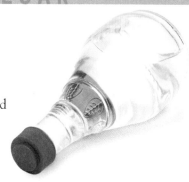

CLEAN WINDSHIELD WIPER BLADES • When your windshield actually gets blurrier after you turn on your wipers during a rainstorm, it usually means that your wiper blades are dirty. To make them as good as new, dampen a cloth or rag with some full-strength white vinegar and run it down the full length of each blade once or twice.

KEEP CAR WINDOWS FROST-FREE • If you park your car outdoors during the cold winter months, a smart and simple way to stop frost from forming on your windows is by wiping (or, better yet, spraying) the outsides of the windows with a solution of 3 parts white vinegar to 1 part water. Each coating may last up to several weeks—although, unfortunately, if you live in a cold-climate area it won't do much in the way of warding off a heavy snowfall.

CARE FOR CAR CARPET • A good vacuuming will get up the sand and other loose debris from your car's carpeting, but it won't do much for stains or ground-in dirt. For that, mix up a solution of equal parts water and white vinegar and sponge it into the carpet. Give the mixture a couple of minutes to sink in, then blot it up with a cloth or paper towel. This technique will also eliminate salt residues left on car carpets during the winter months in snow areas.

for furniture care ● ● ●

REMOVE CANDLE WAX • Candles are great for intimate dinners, but the mood can quickly sour if you wind up getting melted candle wax on your wooden furniture. To remove it, first soften the wax using a blow-dryer on its hottest setting and blot up as much as you can with paper towels. Remove what's left by rubbing with a cloth soaked in a solution made of equal parts white vinegar and water. Wipe clean with a soft, absorbent cloth.

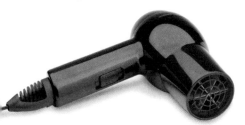

GIVE GREASE STAINS THE SLIP • Eliminate grease stains from your kitchen table or countertop by wiping them down with a cloth dampened in a solution of equal parts white vinegar and water. In addition to removing the grease, the vinegar will neutralize any odors on the surface (once its own pungent aroma has evaporated, that is).

CAUTION: Don't use vinegar—or alcohol or lemon juice—on marble tabletops, countertops, or floors. Vinegar's acidity can dull or even pit the protective coating—and possibly damage the stone itself. Also, avoid using vinegar on travertine and limestone; the acid eats through the calcium in the stonework.

CONCEAL SCRATCHES IN WOODEN FURNITURE

Got a scratch on a wooden tabletop that grabs your attention every time you look at it? To make it much less noticeable, mix some distilled or cider vinegar and iodine in a small jar and paint over the scratch with a small artist's brush. Use more iodine for darker woods; more vinegar for lighter shades.

more VINEGAR over →

GET RID OF WATER RINGS ON FURNITURE • To remove white rings left by wet glasses on wooden furniture, mix equal parts vinegar and olive oil and apply the mixture with a soft cloth while moving with the wood grain. Use another clean, soft cloth to shine it up. To get white water rings off leather furniture, dab them with a sponge soaked in full-strength white vinegar.

WIPE OFF WAX OR POLISH BUILDUP • When furniture polish or wax builds up on wood furniture or leather tabletops, get rid of it with diluted white vinegar. For wood furniture, dip a cloth in equal parts vinegar and water and squeeze it out well. Then, moving with the grain, clean away the polish. Wipe dry with a soft towel or cloth. For leather tabletops, simply wipe them down with a soft cloth dipped in ¼ cup (50 ml) vinegar and ½ cup (125 ml) water. Use a clean towel to dry off any remaining liquid.

REVITALIZE LEATHER FURNITURE • Has your leather couch or easy chair lost its luster? To restore it to its former glory, mix equal parts white vinegar and boiled linseed oil in a recycled spray bottle, shake it up well, and spray it on. Spread it evenly over your furniture using a soft cloth, give it a couple of minutes to settle in, and rub it off with a clean cloth.

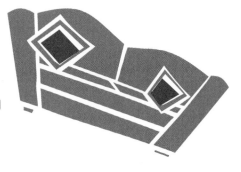

DID YOU KNOW?

Taken literally, vinegar is nothing more than wine that's gone bad. The word derives from the French *vin* (wine) and *aigre* (sour). But, in fact, anything used to make alcohol can be turned into vinegar, including apples, honey, malted barley, molasses, rice, sugarcane, even coconuts. Vinegar's acidic, solvent properties were well known even in ancient times. According to one popular legend, Cleopatra is said to have wagered she could dispose of a fortune in the course of a single meal. She won the bet by dissolving a handful of pearls in a cup of vinegar...and then consuming it.

in the kitchen

FRESHEN YOUR REFRIGERATOR • Did you know that vinegar might be an even more effective, safer cleanser for your refrigerator than baking soda? Use equal parts white vinegar and water to wash both the interior and exterior of your fridge, including the door gasket and the fronts of the fruit and vegetable crispers. To prevent mildew growth, wash the inside walls and crisper interiors with some full-strength vinegar on a cloth. Also use undiluted vinegar to wipe off accumulated dust and grime on top of your refrigerator. And don't forget to put that box of baking soda inside your fridge to keep it smelling clean when you're done.

STEAM-CLEAN YOUR MICROWAVE • To clean your microwave, place a glass bowl filled with a solution of ¼ cup (50 ml) vinegar in 1 cup (250 ml) water inside and zap the mixture for 5 minutes on *High*. Once the bowl cools, dip a clean cloth or sponge into the liquid and use it to wipe away those persistent stains and splatters on the interior walls.

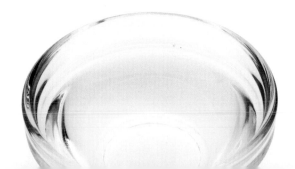

DISINFECT CUTTING BOARDS • To disinfect and clean your wooden cutting boards or a butcher block countertop, wipe them with full-strength white 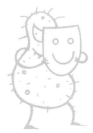 vinegar after each use. The acetic acid in the vinegar is a good disinfectant, effective against such harmful bugs as *E. coli*, salmonella and staphylococcus. Never use water and dishwashing liquid, because it can weaken surface wood fibers. When wooden cutting surfaces also need deodorizing, spread some baking soda over them and spray on undiluted white vinegar. Let it foam and bubble for 5 to 10 minutes, then rinse with a cloth dipped in clean, cold water.

DEODORIZE YOUR KITCHEN SINK

Here's an incredibly easy way to keep your sink drain sanitized and smelling clean. Mix equal parts water and vinegar in a bowl, pour the solution into an ice-cube tray and freeze it. Then simply drop a couple of 'vinegar cubes' into the sink every week or so, let them melt into the drain, and follow with a cold-water rinse.

WASH OUT YOUR DISHWASHER • To remove built-up soap film in your dishwasher, pour 1 cup (250 ml) undiluted white vinegar into the bottom of the unit—or in a bowl on the top rack. Then run the machine through a full cycle without any dishes or detergent. Do this once a month, especially if you live in a hard-water area. However, if there's no mention of vinegar in your dishwasher owner's manual, check with the manufacturer first.

CLEAN CHINA, CRYSTAL, AND GLASSWARE • Put the sparkle back in your glassware by adding vinegar to your rinse water or dishwater.

■ To keep everyday glassware gleaming, add ¼ cup (50 ml) vinegar to your dishwasher's rinse cycle.

■ To rid drinking glasses of cloudiness or spots caused by hard water, heat up a pot of equal parts white vinegar and water (use full-strength vinegar if your glasses are very cloudy), and let them soak in it for 15 to 30 minutes. Give them a good scrubbing with a bottlebrush and rinse clean.

■ Add 2 tablespoons (30 ml) vinegar to your dishwater when cleaning your good crystal glasses. Rinse them in a solution of 3 parts warm water to 1 part vinegar and allow them to air-dry. You can also wash delicate crystal and fine china by adding 1 cup (250 ml) vinegar to a basin of warm water. Gently dunk the glasses in the solution and allow to dry.

■ To get coffee stains and other discolorations off china dishes and teacups, try scrubbing them with equal parts vinegar and salt, followed by rinsing them under warm water.

CLEAN A DRIP-FILTER COFFEEMAKER • If your coffee consistently comes out weak or bitter, odds are your drip coffeemaker needs cleaning. Fill the decanter with 2 cups (500 ml) white vinegar and 1 cup (250 ml) water. Place a filter in the machine and pour the solution into the coffeemaker's water chamber. Turn on the coffeemaker and let it run through a full brew cycle. Remove the filter and replace it with a fresh one. Then run clean water through the machine for two full cycles, replacing the filter again for the second brew. If you have soft water, clean your coffeemaker after 80 brew cycles. If you have hard water, clean it after 40 brew cycles.

more VINEGAR over →

CLEAN A KETTLE • To eliminate lime and tough mineral deposits in your kettle, bring 3 cups (750 ml) full-strength white vinegar to a full boil for 5 minutes and leave the vinegar in the kettle overnight. Rinse out with cold water the next day.

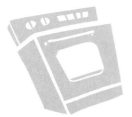

USE AS A GREASE CUTTER • Every professional cook knows that distilled vinegar is one of the best grease cutters around. It even works on seriously greasy surfaces such as the fry vats used in many food outlets. But you don't need to have a deep fryer to find plenty of ways to put vinegar to good use:

■ When you've finished frying, clean up grease splatters from your stovetop, walls, range hood, and surrounding countertop by washing them with a sponge dipped in undiluted white vinegar. Use another sponge soaked in cold tap water to rinse, and wipe dry with a soft cloth.

■ Pour 3–4 tablespoons (45–60 ml) white vinegar into your favorite brand (especially bargain brands) of dishwashing liquid and give it a few shakes. The added vinegar will increase detergent's grease-fighting capabilities and provide you with more dishwashing liquid for your money, because you'll need less of it to clean your dishes.

■ Boiling 2 cups (500 ml) vinegar in a frying pan for 10 minutes will help keep food from sticking to it for several months at a time.

■ Remove burned-on grease and food stains from stainless steel cookware by mixing 1 cup (250 ml) distilled vinegar in enough water to cover the stains (if they're near the top of a large pot, you may need to increase the vinegar). Let it boil for 5 minutes. The stains should come off with some mild scrubbing.

■ Get that blackened, cooked-on grease off your broiler pan by softening it up with a solution of 1 cup (250 ml) apple cider vinegar and 2 tablespoons (30 ml) sugar. Apply the mixture while the tray is still hot, and let it sit for an hour or so. Give it a light scrubbing and watch the grime slide off easily.

■ Got a hot plate that looks more like a grease pan? Whip it back into shape by washing it with a sponge dipped in full-strength white vinegar.

■ Fight grease build up in your oven by wiping down the inside with a rag or sponge soaked in full-strength white vinegar once a week. The same treatment gets grease off the grates in gas stoves.

Homemade wine vinegar

✳ *Contrary to popular belief, old wine rarely turns into vinegar; usually a half-empty bottle of wine just spoils due to oxidation.*

To create vinegar, you need the presence of *Acetobacter*, a specific type of bacteria. You can make your own wine vinegar, though, by mixing 1 part leftover red, white, or rosé wine with 2 parts cider vinegar. Pour the mixture into a clean, recycled wine bottle and store it in a dark cupboard. It just might taste as good, if not better, on your salads than some of those expensive wine vinegars that are sold at upscale food stores.

BRUSH-CLEAN CAN OPENER BLADES • Does that dirty wheel blade of your electric can opener look like it's seen at least one can too many? To clean and sanitize it, dip an old toothbrush in white vinegar, and position the bristles of the brush around the side and edge of the wheel. Turn on the appliance and let the blade scrub itself clean.

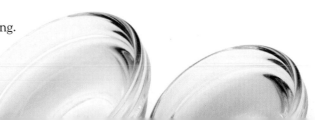

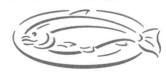

REMOVE STAINS FROM POTS, PANS, AND OVENWARE • Nothing will do a better job than vinegar when it comes to removing stubborn stains on your cookware. Here's how to put the power of vinegar to use:

■ Give the dark stains on your aluminium cookware (caused by cooking acidic foods) the heave-ho by mixing in 1 teaspoon (5 ml) white vinegar for every 1 cup (250 ml) water needed to cover stains. Let boil for a couple of minutes and rinse with cold water.

■ To remove stains from your stainless steel pots and pans, soak them in 2 cups (500 ml) white vinegar for 30 minutes and rinse them with hot, soapy water, followed by a cold-water rinse.

■ To clean cooked-on food stains on glass ovenware, fill them with 1 part vinegar and 4 parts water, heat the mixture to a slow boil and let it boil at a low level for 5 minutes. The stains should come off with some mild scrubbing once the mixture cools.

■ No cookware is completely stainproof. For mineral stains on your nonstick cookware, rub the utensil with a cloth dipped in undiluted distilled vinegar. To loosen up stubborn stains, mix 2 tablespoons (30 ml) baking soda, ½ cup (125 ml) vinegar, and 1 cup (250 ml) water and let it boil for 10 minutes.

REFRESH YOUR ICE CUBE TRAYS • If your plastic ice cube trays are covered with hard water stains—or if it's been a while since you've cleaned them—a few cups of white vinegar can help you, in either case. To remove the spots or disinfect your trays, let them soak in undiluted vinegar for 4 to 5 hours, then rinse well under cold water and allow to dry.

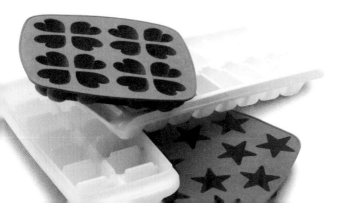

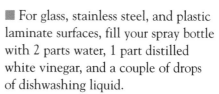

CLEAR THE AIR IN YOUR KITCHEN • If the smell of yesterday's cooked cabbage or fish stew is hanging around your kitchen longer than you'd like, mix ½ cup (125 ml) white vinegar with 1 cup (250 ml) water in a saucepan. Let it boil until the liquid is almost gone. You'll be breathing easier in no time.

MAKE ALL-PURPOSE CLEANERS • For fast cleanups around the kitchen, keep two recycled spray bottles filled with these vinegar-based solutions:

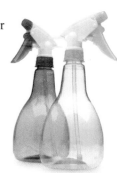

■ For glass, stainless steel, and plastic laminate surfaces, fill your spray bottle with 2 parts water, 1 part distilled white vinegar, and a couple of drops of dishwashing liquid.

■ For cleaning walls and other painted surfaces, mix ½ cup (125 ml) white vinegar, 1 cup (250 ml) ammonia, and ¼ cup (50 g) baking soda in a gallon (4 L) of water and pour into a spray bottle. Spray it on spots and stains. Wipe off with a clean dishtowel.

MAKE AN ALL-PURPOSE SCRUB FOR POTS AND PANS

How would you like an effective scouring mix that costs a few pennies, and can be safely used on all of your metal cookware–including expensive copper pots and pans? Want even better news? You probably already have this 'miracle mix' in your kitchen. Simply combine equal parts salt and flour and add just enough vinegar to make a paste. Work the paste around the cooking surface and the outside of the utensil, and rinse off with warm water. Dry thoroughly with a soft dish towel.

more VINEGAR over →

SANITIZE JARS, CONTAINERS, AND VASES •
Do you cringe at the thought of cleaning out a mayonnaise, peanut butter, or mustard jar to reuse it? Or worse, getting the residue out of a slimy vase, decanter, or container? There is an easy way to handle these jobs. Fill the item with equal parts vinegar and warm, soapy water and let it stand for 10 to 15 minutes. If you're cleaning a bottle or jar, close it and give it a few good shakes or use a bottle brush to scrape off the remains before thoroughly rinsing.

CLEAN A DIRTY THERMOS •
To get a thermos flask clean, fill it with warm water and ¼ cup (50 ml) white vinegar. If you see any residue, add some uncooked rice, which will act as an abrasive to scrape it off. Close, shake well, rinse, and let air-dry.

PURGE BUGS FROM YOUR PANTRY •
Do you have moths or other insects in your cupboard or pantry? Fill a small bowl with 1½ cups (375 ml) apple cider vinegar and add a couple of drops of dishwashing liquid. Leave it in there for a week; it will attract the bugs, which will fall into the bowl and drown. Then empty the shelves and give the interior a thorough washing with dishwashing liquid or 2 cups (500 g) baking soda in a quart (1 L) of water. Discard all wheat products (breads, pasta, flour, etc.), and clean canned goods before putting them back.

TRAP FRUIT FLIES •
Fruit flies often make the trip home with you from the supermarket. Make a trap for them wherever they appear by filling an old jar about halfway with apple cider. Punch a few holes in the lid, screw it back on, and they'll dive right in.

for the cook

TENDERIZE AND PURIFY MEATS AND SEAFOOD •
Soaking a lean or inexpensive cut of red meat in a couple of cups of vinegar breaks down tough fibers to make it more tender—and in addition, kills off any potentially harmful bacteria. You can also use vinegar to tenderize seafood steaks. Let the meat or fish soak in full-strength vinegar overnight. Experiment with different vinegar varieties for added flavor, or simply use apple cider or distilled vinegar if you intend to rinse it off before cooking.

KEEP CORNED BEEF FROM SHRINKING •
Ever notice how the corned beef that comes out of the pot is always smaller than the one that went in? Stop your meat from shrinking by adding a couple tablespoons of apple cider vinegar to the water next time you boil beef.

MAKE BETTER BOILED OR POACHED EGGS •
Vinegar does fantastic things for eggs. Here are the two most useful 'egg-samples':

■ When you are making hard-boiled eggs, adding 2 tablespoons (30 ml) distilled vinegar for every quart (liter) of water will keep the eggs from cracking and make them easier to shell.

■ When you are poaching eggs, adding a couple of tablespoons of vinegar to the water will keep your eggs in tight shape by preventing the egg whites from spreading.

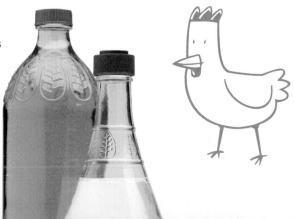

WASH STORE-BOUGHT PRODUCE

You can't be too careful these days when it comes to handling the foods you eat. Before serving your fruits and vegetables, a great way to eliminate the hidden dirt, pesticides, even insects, is to rinse them in 4 tablespoons (60 ml) apple cider vinegar dissolved in a gallon (4 L) cold water.

REMOVE ODORS FROM YOUR HANDS • It's often difficult to get strong onion, garlic, or fish odors off your hands after preparing a meal. But you'll find these scents are a lot easier to wash off if you rub some distilled vinegar on your hands before and after you slice vegetables or clean fish.

GET RID OF BERRY STAINS • You can use undiluted white vinegar on your hands to remove stains from berries and other fruits.

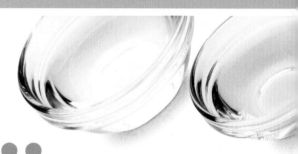

DID YOU KNOW?

Authentic balsamic vinegar comes solely from Modena in Italy, and is made from Trebbiano grapes, a particularly sweet white variety grown in the surrounding hills. Italian law mandates that the vinegar be aged in wooden barrels made of chestnut, juniper, mulberry, or oak. There are only two grades of true balsamic vinegar—which typically sells for $100-200 for about 3.5-ounces (100 ml): tradizionale vecchio, vinegar that is at least 12 years old and tradizionale extra vecchio, vinegar that's aged for at least 25 years (some balsamic vinegars are known to have been aged for more than 100 years).

in the medicine cabinet

CONTROL DANDRUFF • To get rid of dandruff, follow each shampoo with a rinse of 2 cups (500 ml) apple cider vinegar mixed with 2 cups (500 ml) cold water. You can also fight dandruff by applying 3 tablespoons (45 ml) vinegar on your hair and massaging into your scalp before shampooing. Wait a few minutes, rinse it out, and wash as usual.

CONDITION YOUR HAIR • Want to put the life back into limp or damaged hair? You can whip up a terrific hair conditioner by combining 1 teaspoon (5 ml) apple cider vinegar with 2 tablespoons (30 ml) olive oil, and 3 egg whites. Rub the mixture into your hair, and keep it covered for 30 minutes using plastic wrap or a shower cap. Shampoo and rinse as usual.

PROTECT BLONDE HAIR FROM CHLORINE • Keep your golden locks from turning green in a chlorinated pool by rubbing ¼ cup (50 ml) cider vinegar into your hair. Let it set for 15 minutes before diving in.

APPLY AS AN ANTIPERSPIRANT • Why not put the deodorizing power of vinegar to use where it matters most? That's right, you don't need a roll-on or spray to keep your underarms smelling fresh. Instead, splash a little white vinegar under each arm in the morning and let it dry. In addition to combating perspiration odor, this method also does away with those deodorant stains on your garments.

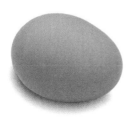

more VINEGAR over →

SOAK AWAY ACHING MUSCLES •
Got a sore back, a strained tendon in your shoulder or calf, or maybe you're just feeling a bit rundown? Adding 2 cups (500 ml) apple cider vinegar to your bathwater is a great way to soothe away aches and pains, or simply to take the edge off a stressful day. Adding a few drops of peppermint oil to your bath can also help to give you a lift.

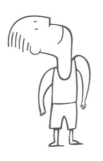

FRESHEN YOUR BREATH • After eating garlic or onions, a quick and easy way to sweeten your breath is to rinse your mouth with a solution made by dissolving 2 tablespoons (30 ml) apple cider vinegar and 1 teaspoon (5 ml) salt in a glass of warm water.

EASE SUNBURN AND ITCHING • You can cool a bad sunburn by gently dabbing the area with a cotton ball or soft cloth saturated with white or cider vinegar. (This treatment is especially effective if it's applied before the burn starts to sting.) The same technique works to instantly stop the itch of mosquito and other insect bites, as well as the rashes caused by exposure to poison ivy and poison oak.

BANISH BRUISES

If you or someone you care about has a nasty fall, you can speed healing and prevent black-and-blue marks by soaking a piece of cotton gauze in white or apple cider vinegar and leaving it on the injured area for 1 hour.

SOOTHE A SORE THROAT • Here are three easy ways to make a sore throat feel better:

1 • If your throat is left raw by a bad cough, or even a speaking or singing engagement, you'll find fast relief by gargling with 1 tablespoon (15 ml) apple cider vinegar and 1 teaspoon (5 ml) salt dissolved in a glass of warm water. Use the gargle several times a day if needed.

2 • For sore throats from a cold or the flu, combine ¼ cup (50 ml) cider vinegar and ¼ cup (50 ml) honey. Take 1 tablespoon (15 ml) every 4 hours.

3 • To soothe both a cough and a sore throat, mix ½ cup (125 ml) vinegar, ½ cup (125 ml) water, 4 teaspoons (20 ml) honey, and 1 teaspoon (5 ml) Tabasco sauce. Swallow 1 tablespoon (15 ml) four to five times a day, including one dose before bedtime. **WARNING: Children under the age of one year should never be given honey.**

FEET FIRST

MAKE A POULTICE FOR CORNS AND CALLUSES • Here's an old-fashioned, time-proven method to treat corns and calluses. Saturate a piece of white or stale bread with 1/4 cup (50 ml) white vinegar. Let the bread soak in the vinegar for 30 minutes, then break off a piece big enough to completely cover the corn. Keep the poultice in place with gauze or adhesive tape and leave it on overnight. The next morning, hard, calloused skin will be dissolved and the corn should be easy to remove. Older, thicker calluses may require several treatments.

GET THE JUMP ON ATHLETE'S FOOT • A bad case of athlete's foot can drive you hopping mad. But you can often quell the infection, and quickly ease the itching, by rinsing your feet three or four times a day for a few days with undiluted apple cider vinegar. As an added precaution, soak your socks or stockings in a mixture of 1 part vinegar and 4 parts water for 30 minutes before laundering them.

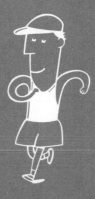

V

BREATHE EASIER • Adding ¼ cup (50 ml) white vinegar to the water in a hot-steam vaporizer can help ease congestion caused by a chest cold or sinus infection. It can also be good for your vaporizer, as the vinegar will clear away any mineral deposits in the water tubes resulting from the use of hard water. Note: Check with the manufacturer before adding vinegar to a cool-mist vaporizer.

TREAT AN ACTIVE COLD SORE • The only thing worse than a bad cold is a bad cold sore. Fortunately, you can usually dry up a cold sore in short order by dabbing it with a cotton ball saturated in white vinegar three times a day. The vinegar will quickly soothe the pain and swelling.

PAMPER YOUR SKIN • Using vinegar as a skin toner dates back to the time of Helen of Troy. And it's just as effective today. After washing your face, mix 1 tablespoon (15 ml) apple cider vinegar with 2 cups (500 ml) water as a finishing rinse to cleanse and tighten your skin. You can also make your own facial treatment by mixing ¼ cup (50 ml) cider vinegar with ¼ cup (50 ml) water. Gently apply the solution to your face and let it dry.

SAY GOODBYE TO AGE OR SUN SPOTS • Before you take any drastic measures to remove or cover up those brown spots on your skin caused by exposure to the sun or hormonal changes, give vinegar a try. Simply pour some full-strength apple cider vinegar onto a cotton ball and apply it to the spots for 10 minutes at least twice a day. The spots should fade or disappear within a few weeks.

SOFTEN YOUR CUTICLES • You can soften the cuticles on your fingers and toes before manicuring them by soaking your digits in a bowl of undiluted white vinegar for 5 minutes.

MAKE NAIL POLISH LAST LONGER • Your nail polish will have a longer life expectancy if you first dampen your nails with vinegar on a cotton ball and let it dry before applying your nail polish.

DID YOU KNOW?

The world's only museum dedicated to vinegar, the International Vinegar Museum (www.internationalvinegarmusem.com), is located in Roslyn, South Dakota. Housed in a building that was the former town hall, the museum is operated by Dr. Lawrence J. Diggs, an international vinegar consultant also known as the Vinegar Man. The museum showcases hundreds of vinegars from around the world, has displays on the various methods used to make vinegar, and lets visitors sample different types of vinegars. Visitors can even see paper and ceramic made from vinegar!

CLEAN YOUR GLASSES • When it's more difficult to see with your glasses on than it is with them off, it's a clear indication that they're in need of a good cleaning. Applying a few drops of white vinegar to the lenses and wiping them with a soft cloth will easily remove dirt, sweat, and fingerprints, and leave them spotless. Don't use vinegar on modern plastic lenses, though.

TREAT A JELLYFISH OR BEE STING • A jellyfish can pack a nasty sting. If you have an encounter with one, pouring some undiluted vinegar on the sting will take away the pain in no time and let you scrape out the stinger with a plastic credit card. The same treatment can also be used to treat bee stings. Using vinegar on stings inflicted by the jellyfish's cousin—the Portuguese man-of-war—is now discouraged because vinegar may actually increase the amount of toxin released under the skin. **WARNING: If you have difficulty breathing or the sting area becomes inflamed and swollen, seek medical attention immediately; you could be having an allergic reaction.**

more VINEGAR over →

341

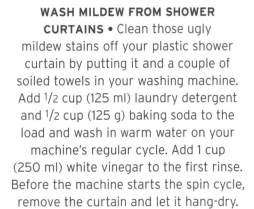

in the bathroom ● ● ●

WASH MILDEW FROM SHOWER CURTAINS • Clean those ugly mildew stains off your plastic shower curtain by putting it and a couple of soiled towels in your washing machine. Add 1/2 cup (125 ml) laundry detergent and 1/2 cup (125 g) baking soda to the load and wash in warm water on your machine's regular cycle. Add 1 cup (250 ml) white vinegar to the first rinse. Before the machine starts the spin cycle, remove the curtain and let it hang-dry.

CLEAN SINKS AND BATHTUBS • Put the shine back in your porcelain sinks and bathtub by scrubbing them with full-strength white vinegar, followed by a rinse of clean, cold water. To remove hard water stains from your tub, pour in 3 cups (750 ml) white vinegar under running hot tap water. Let the tub fill to cover the stains and allow it to soak for 4 hours. When the water drains out, you should be able to easily scrub off the stains.

SHINE UP YOUR SHOWER DOORS • To leave your glass shower doors sparkling clean—and to remove all of those annoying water spots—wipe them down with a cloth dipped in a solution of 1/2 cup (125 ml) white vinegar, 1 cup (250 ml) ammonia and 1/4 cup (50 g) baking soda in a gallon (4 L) of warm water.

DISINFECT SHOWER DOOR TRACKS • Use vinegar to remove accumulated dirt and grime from the tracks of your shower doors. Fill the tracks with about 2 cups (500 ml) full-strength white vinegar and let it sit for 3 to 5 hours. (If the tracks are really dirty, heat the vinegar in a glass container for 30 seconds in your microwave first.) Then pour some hot water over the track to flush away the gunk. You may need to use a small scrubbing brush, or even a recycled toothbrush, to get up tough stains.

SHINE CERAMIC TILES • If soap scum or water spots have dulled the ceramic tiles in your bathroom, bring back the brightness by scrubbing them with 1/2 cup (125 ml) white vinegar, 1/2 cup (125 ml) ammonia and 1/4 cup (50 g) borax mixed in a gallon (4 L) warm water. Rinse well with cool water and air-dry.

WHITEN YOUR GROUT • Has the grout between the tiles of your shower or bathtub enclosure become stained or discolored? Restore it to its original shade of white by using a toothbrush dipped in undiluted white vinegar to scrub away the dinginess.

REMOVE MINERAL DEPOSITS ON SHOWERHEADS • Wash away blockages and mineral deposits from removable showerheads by placing them in a quart (1 L) boiling water with 1/2 cup (125 ml) distilled vinegar for 10 minutes (use hot, not boiling, liquid for plastic showerheads). When you remove it from the solution, obstructions should be gone. If you have a non-removable showerhead, fill a small plastic bag half full with vinegar and tape it over the fixture. Let it sit for about 1 hour, then remove the bag and wipe off any remaining vinegar from the showerhead.

WIPE DOWN BATHROOM FIXTURES • Don't stop at the shower when you're cleaning with vinegar! Pour a bit of undiluted white vinegar onto a soft cloth and use it to wipe your chrome faucets, towel bars, bathroom mirrors, and doorknobs–anything that might need a cleaning. It'll leave them gleaming.

> **CAUTION:** Combining vinegar with bleach—or any other product containing chlorine, such as chlorinated lime (sold as bleaching powder)—may produce chlorine gas. In low concentrations, this toxic, acrid-smelling gas can cause damage to your eyes, skin, or respiratory system. High concentrations of the gas are often fatal.

Some researchers believe vinegar will ultimately be adopted as a simple and inexpensive way to diagnose cervical cancer in women—especially those living in impoverished nations. In tests conducted over a two-year period, midwives in Zimbabwe used a vinegar solution to detect more than 75 percent of potential cancers in 10,000 women (the solution turns tissue containing pre-cancerous cells white). Although the test is not as accurate as a Pap smear, doctors believe it will soon be an important screening tool in developing countries, where only 5 percent of women are currently tested for this often fatal disease.

FIGHT MOLD AND MILDEW • To remove and retard bathroom mold and mildew, pour a solution of 3 tablespoons (45 ml) white vinegar, 1 teaspoon (5 ml) borax, and 2 cups (500 ml) hot water into a clean, recycled spray bottle and shake well. Spray the mixture on painted surfaces, tiles, windows, wherever you see mold or mildew spots. Use a soft scrub brush on the stains or just let it soak in.

in the laundry ● ● ●

SOFTEN FABRICS, KILL BACTERIA, ELIMINATE STATIC, AND MORE • There are so many benefits to be reaped by adding 1 cup (250 ml) white vinegar to your washing machine's rinse cycle that it's surprising you don't find it prominently mentioned inside the owner's manual of every washing machine sold. Here are the main ones:

■ A single cup of vinegar will kill off any bacteria that may be present in your wash load, especially if it includes cloth diapers and other items that are in contact with germs, such as dishtowels.

DISINFECT TOILET BOWLS • An easy way to keep your toilet looking and smelling clean is to pour 2 cups (500 ml) white vinegar into the bowl and let the solution soak overnight before flushing. Including this vinegar soak in your weekly cleaning regimen will also help keep away those ugly water rings that typically appear just above water level.

CLEAN YOUR TOOTHBRUSH HOLDER • Get the grime, bacteria, and caked-on toothpaste drippings out of the grooves of your bathroom toothbrush holder by cleaning the openings with cotton swabs moistened with white vinegar.

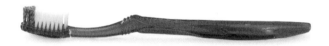

WASH OUT YOUR RINSE CUP • If several people in your home use the same rinse cup after brushing their teeth, give it a weekly cleaning by filling it with equal parts water and white vinegar, or just full-strength vinegar, and let it sit overnight. Rinse thoroughly with cold water before using again.

■ A cup of vinegar will keep your clothes coming out of the wash soft and smelling fresh—so you can kiss your liquid fabric softeners and sheets goodbye.

■ A cup of vinegar will brighten small loads of white clothes, sheets, and towels.

■ Added to the last rinse, a cup of vinegar will keep your clothes lint- and static-free.

■ Adding a cupful of vinegar to the last rinse will set the color of your newly dyed fabrics.

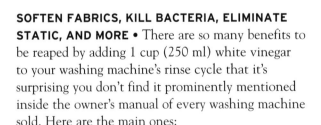

more VINEGAR over →

CLEAN YOUR WASHING MACHINE • An easy way to periodically clean out soap scum and disinfect your washing machine is to add 2 cups (500 ml) white vinegar, and run the machine through a full cycle without any clothes or detergent. If your machine is particularly dirty, fill it with very hot water, add 2 gallons (7.5 L) vinegar and let the agitator run for 8 to 10 minutes. Turn off the machine and let stand overnight. Next day, drain, then run the machine through a complete cycle.

STOP REDS FROM RUNNING

Unless you have a fondness for pink-tinted clothing, take one simple precaution to prevent red–or other brightly dyed–washable clothes from ruining your wash loads. Soak your new garments in a few cups of undiluted white vinegar for 10 to 15 minutes before their first washing. You'll never have to worry about running colors again!

BRIGHTEN WASHING LOADS • Why waste money on that costly all-color bleach when you can get the same results using vinegar? Just add ½ cup (125 ml) white vinegar to your machine's wash cycle to brighten up the colors in each load.

MAKE NEW CLOTHES READY TO WEAR • Get the chemicals, dust, odor, and whatever else out of your brand-new or secondhand clothes by pouring 1 cup (250 ml) white vinegar into the wash cycle the first time you launder them.

WHITEN DINGY SOCKS • If it's getting harder to identify the white socks in your sock drawer, here's a simple way to make them so bright you can't miss them. Start by adding 1 cup (250 ml) vinegar to 2 quarts (2 L) tap water in a large pot. Bring the solution to a boil, pour into a bucket, and drop in the dingy socks. Let them soak overnight. The next day, wash them as you normally would.

IRONING BORED?

FLUSH YOUR IRON'S INTERIOR • To eliminate mineral deposits and prevent corrosion on your steam iron, give it an occasional cleaning by filling the reservoir with undiluted white vinegar. Place the iron in an upright position, switch on the steam setting and let the vinegar steam through it for 5 to 10 minutes. Refill the chamber with clean water and repeat. Finally, give the water chamber a good rinsing with cold, clean water.

CLEAN YOUR IRON'S SOLE PLATE • To remove scorch marks from the sole plate of your iron, scrub it with a paste made by heating equal parts vinegar and salt in a small saucepan. Use a rag dipped in clean water to wipe away the remaining residue.

SHARPEN YOUR CREASES • You'll find the creases in freshly ironed clothes will come out a lot neater if you lightly spray them with equal parts water and vinegar before ironing them. For truly sharp creases in slacks and dress shirts, first dampen the garment using a cloth moistened in a solution of 1 part white vinegar and 2 parts water. Then place a brown paper bag over the crease and start ironing.

ERASE SCORCH MARKS • If your iron gets too hot while pressing a collar, or perhaps a sleeve or pant leg, you can often eliminate slight scorch marks by rubbing the spot with a cloth dampened with white vinegar, and blotting it with a clean towel. Repeat if necessary.

MAKE OLD HEMLINES DISAPPEAR • When you want to make unsightly needle marks from an old hemline disappear for good, simply moisten the area with a cloth dipped in equal parts vinegar and water, and place it under the garment before you start ironing.

SPRAY AWAY WRINKLES • In a perfect world, laundry would emerge from the dryer freshly pressed. Until that day, you can often get the wrinkles out of clothes after drying by misting them with a solution of 1 part vinegar to 3 parts water. Once you're sure you didn't miss a spot, hang it up, and let it air-dry. You may find this approach works better for some clothes than ironing and it's certainly a lot gentler on the garment fabric.

GET THE YELLOW OUT OF CLOTHING • To restore yellowed clothing, let the garments soak overnight in a solution of 12 parts warm water to 1 part vinegar, then wash them the following morning.

SOFTEN YOUR BLANKETS • Add 2 cups (500 ml) white vinegar to your machine's rinse water (or a laundry tub filled with water) to remove soap residue from cotton and wool blankets before drying. This will also leave them feeling fresh and soft as new.

DULL THE SHINE IN YOUR PANTS' SEAT • Want to get rid of that shiny seat on your dark pants or skirt? Just brush the area lightly with a soft recycled toothbrush dipped in equal parts white vinegar and water, and pat dry with a soft towel.

> **CAUTION:** Keep apple cider vinegar out of the laundry. Using it to pretreat clothes or adding it to wash or rinse water may actually create stains rather than remove them. Use only distilled white vinegar for laundering.

REMOVE CIGARETTE SMELL FROM SUITS • If you find yourself heading home with the lingering smell of cigarette smoke on your good suit or dress, you can remove the odor without having to take your clothes to the dry cleaner. Just add 1 cup (250 ml) vinegar to a bathtub filled with the hottest tap water your can get. Close the door and hang your garments above the steam. The smell should be gone after several hours.

RESHAPE YOUR WOOLENS • Shrunken woolen sweaters and other items can sometimes be stretched back to their former size or shape after boiling them in a solution of 1 part vinegar to 2 parts water for around 25 minutes. Allow the garment to air-dry after you've finished stretching it.

for removing stains

BRUSH OFF SUEDE STAINS • To eliminate a fresh grease spot on a suede jacket or skirt, gently brush it with a soft toothbrush dipped in white vinegar. Let the spot air-dry, then brush with a suede brush. Repeat if necessary. You can also generally tone up suede items by lightly wiping them with a sponge dipped in vinegar.

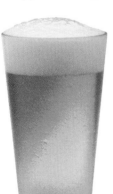

PAT AWAY WATER-SOLUBLE STAINS • You can lift out many water-soluble stains—including beer, orange, and other fruit juices, black coffee or tea, and vomit—from your cotton-blend clothing by patting the spot with a cloth or towel moistened with undiluted white vinegar just before placing it in the wash. For large stains, you may want to soak the garment overnight in a solution of 3 parts vinegar to 1 part cold water before washing.

UNSET OLD STAINS • Older, set-in stains will often come out in the wash after being pre-treated with a solution of 3 tablespoons (45 ml) white vinegar and 2 tablespoons (30 ml) dishwashing liquid in a quart (1 L) of warm water. Rub the solution into the stain and blot it dry before washing.

more VINEGAR over →

SPONGE OUT PERSISTENT STAINS • Cola, hair dye, tomato sauce, and wine stains on washable cotton blends should be treated as soon as possible (that is, within 24 hours). Sponge the area with undiluted vinegar first, then launder immediately afterwards. For severe stains, add 1 to 2 cups (250–500 ml) vinegar to the wash cycle as well.

GET RUST STAINS OUT OF COTTON CLOTHING • To remove a rust stain from your cotton workclothes (or any cotton item with rust stains), first moisten the rust spot with some full-strength vinegar and rub in a bit of salt. If it's warm outdoors, let it dry in the sunlight (otherwise a sunny window will do), then toss it into the wash.

CLEAR AWAY CRAYON STAINS • Somehow or other, kids often manage to get crayon marks on their clothing. You can easily get these stains off by rubbing them with a recycled toothbrush soaked in undiluted vinegar before washing them.

REMOVE RINGS FROM COLLARS AND CUFFS • If you're tired of seeing those sweat rings around your shirt collars and annoying discoloration along the edges of your cuffs, just give them the boot by scrubbing the stained fabric with a paste made from 2 parts white vinegar to 3 parts baking soda. Let the paste set for half an hour before washing. This approach also works to remove light mildew stains from clothing.

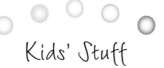

Kids' Stuff

Tie-dying T-shirts, socks, and anything else you can think of, is tons of fun for kids of all ages. Start with a few plain white T-shirts, then use as many colors as allowed by your supermarket's selection of Kool-Aid drink mixes.

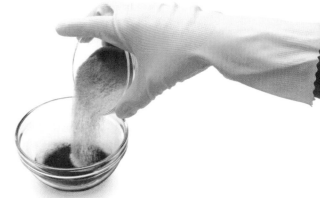

1 Dissolve each package of drink mix into 2 tablespoons (30 ml) vinegar in its own bowl.

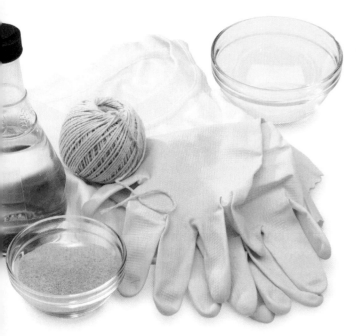

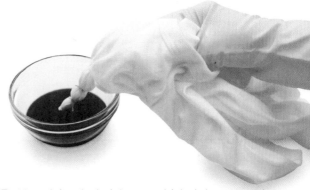

2 Use string to twist your shirts into unusual shapes, then dip them into the bowls (first, put on a pair of rubber gloves).

PRETREAT PERSPIRATION STAINS • To get rid of sweat marks from shirts and other sweat-stained garments, just pour a bit of vinegar directly on the stain and rub it into the fabric before placing the item in the wash. You can also remove deodorant stains from your washable shirts and blouses by gently rubbing the spot with undiluted vinegar before laundering.

MAKE PEN INK DISAPPEAR • If you discover a pen-ink stain in a shirt pocket, treat the stain by first wetting it with some white vinegar, then rub in a paste of 2 parts vinegar to 3 parts cornstarch. Let the paste thoroughly dry before washing the shirt.

3 After drying, set your colors by placing a pillowcase or thin dishtowel over each shirt and ironing it with a medium-hot iron. Wait at least 24 hours, then wash each T-shirt separately. For a greater array of colors, of course, use real fabric dyes or strong vegetable dyes.

SOAK OUT BLOODSTAINS • Whether you nick yourselfshaving or receive an unexpected scratch, it's important to treat bloodstains on your clothing as soon as possible. Bloodstains are relatively easy to remove before they set but can be nearly impossible to wash out after 24 hours. If you can get to the stain before it sets, treat it by pouring full-strength white vinegar on the spot. Let it soak in for 5 to 10 minutes and blot well with a cloth or towel. Repeat if necessary, then wash immediately.

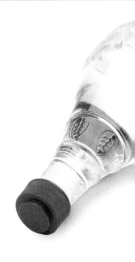

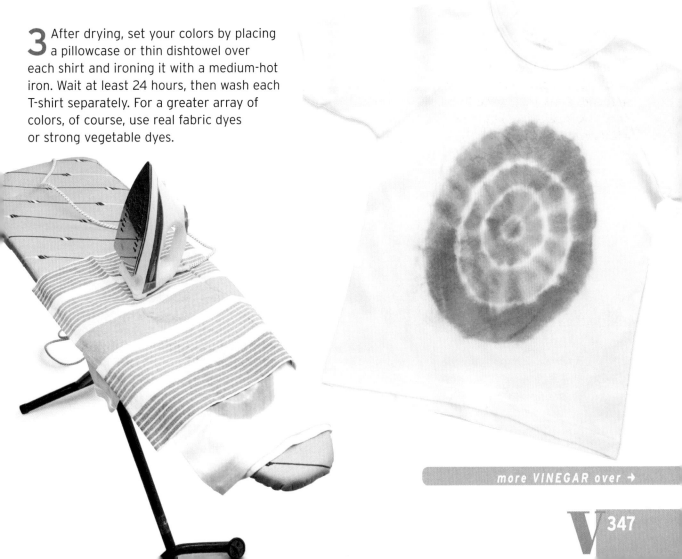

more VINEGAR over →

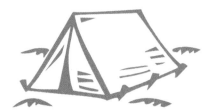

USE AS INSECT REPELLENT • Next time you're planning a camping trip, remember this old trick to keep away the ticks and mosquitoes. Approximately three days before you leave, start taking 1 tablespoon (15 ml) apple cider vinegar three times a day. Continue using the vinegar throughout your trek, and you just might return home without a bite. Another approach is to moisten a cloth or cotton ball with white vinegar and rub it over your exposed skin.

MAINTAIN FRESH WATER WHEN HIKING • Keep your water supply fresh and clean tasting when hiking or camping by adding a few drops of apple cider vinegar to your canteen or water bottle. It's also a good idea to use a half-vinegar, half-water rinse to clean out your water container at the end of each trip to kill bacteria and remove residue.

CLEAN OUTDOOR FURNITURE AND DECKS • If you live in a hot, humid climate, you're probably no stranger to seeing mildew on your wooden decks and patio furniture. But before you reach for the bleach, try these milder vinegar-based solutions:

■ Keep some full-strength white vinegar in a recycled spray bottle and use it wherever you see any mildew growth. The stain will wipe right off most surfaces and the vinegar will keep it from coming back for a while.

■ Remove mildew from wooden decks and wooden patio furniture by sponging them off with a solution of 1 cup (250 ml) ammonia, ½ cup (125 ml) white vinegar, and ¼ cup (50 g) baking soda mixed in a gallon (4 L) water. Use an old toothbrush to work the solution into corners and other tight spaces.

■ To deodorize and inhibit mildew growth on outdoor plastic-mesh furniture and patio umbrellas, mix 2 cups (500 ml) white vinegar and 2 tablespoons (30 ml) dishwashing liquid in a bucket of hot water. Use a soft brush for scrubbing seat pads and umbrella fabric. Rinse with cold water and dry in the sun.

MAKE A TRAP FOR FLYING INSECTS
Who wants to play host to a bunch of gnats, flies, mosquitoes, or other six-legged pests when you're trying to have a barbecue in your backyard? Keep the flying gate-crashers at bay by giving them their own VIP section. Place a bowl filled with apple cider vinegar near some food, but away from you and your guests. By the evening's end, most of your uninvited guests will be floating inside the bowl.

GIVE ANTS THE BOOT • Get rid of household ants once and for all by pouring equal parts water and white vinegar into a spray bottle, and spraying it on anthills and around areas where you see the insects. Ants hate the smell of vinegar, so it won't take long for them to move on to better-smelling quarters. Also keep the spray bottle handy for outdoor trips or to keep ants away from picnic or children's play areas. If you have lots of anthills around your property, try pouring full-strength vinegar over them to hasten the insects' departure.

CLEAN BIRD DROPPINGS • Have birds been using your patio or driveway for target practice again? Make those messy droppings disappear by spraying them with full-strength apple cider vinegar. Or pour the vinegar on a rag and wipe the droppings off.

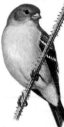

in the garden ● ● ●

TEST SOIL ACIDITY OR ALKALINITY • To do a quick test for excess alkalinity in the soil in your garden, place a handful of soil in a container and pour in ½ cup (125 ml) white vinegar. If the soil fizzes or bubbles, it's definitely alkaline. Similarly, to see if your soil has a high acidity, mix soil with ½ cup (125 ml) water and 1½ cups (375 g) baking soda. This time, fizzing would indicate acid in the soil. To find the exact pH level of your soil, have it tested or pick up a simple, do-it-yourself kit from a garden center.

CLEAN A HUMMINGBIRD FEEDER

Humingbirds are innately discriminating creatures, so don't expect to see them flocking around a dirty, sticky or crusted-over sugar-water feeder. Regularly clean your feeders by thoroughly washing them in equal parts apple cider vinegar and hot water. Rinse well with cold water after washing and air-dry them outdoors in full sunlight before refilling them with food (but never with honey, as it can spread disease).

SPEED GERMINATION OF FLOWER SEEDS • You can get woody seeds, such as passionfruit, morning glory, pumpkin, and gourds, off to a healthier start by scarifying them—lightly rubbing them between a couple of sheets of fine sandpaper—and soaking them overnight in ½ cup (125 ml) apple cider vinegar and 1 cup (500 ml) warm water. Next day, remove the seeds, rinse them off, and plant them. You can use this solution (minus the sandpaper treatment) to start many herb and vegetable seeds.

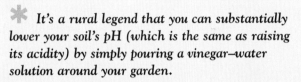

A myth about vinegar

It's a rural legend that you can substantially lower your soil's pH (which is the same as raising its acidity) by simply pouring a vinegar–water solution around your garden.

In fact, it takes a lot of hard work to lower the pH of high-alkaline soil. You can, however, use vinegar around the garden to help existing plants (*see the tips below and on page 350 for treating plant diseases and encouraging blooms on azaleas and gardenias*). But even that takes diligence—and repeated applications. Also, vinegar loses most of its potency after a rainfall. So you'll need to reapply any treatments after those surprise downpours.

KEEP CUT FLOWERS FRESH • Everyone likes to keep cut flowers around as long as possible and there are several good methods to achieve this. One way is to mix 2 tablespoons (30 ml) apple cider vinegar and 2 tablespoons (30 ml) sugar with the vase water before adding the flowers. Make sure you change the water (with more vinegar and sugar, of course) every few days to enhance your flowers' longevity.

WIPE AWAY MEALYBUGS • They're among the most insidious and common pests on both houseplants and in the garden. But you can nip a mealybug invasion in the bud by dabbing the insects with a cotton swab dipped in full-strength white vinegar. You may need to use a handful of swabs, but the vinegar will kill the fluffy monsters and any eggs left behind. Be vigilant for missed targets and break out more vinegar-soaked swabs if you spot more pests.

more VINEGAR over ➜

ELIMINATE INSECTS AROUND THE GARDEN • If insects are feasting on the fruits and vegetables in your garden, give them the boot with this simple, nonpoisonous trap. Fill a 2-quart (2-L) soda bottle with 1 cup (250 ml) apple cider vinegar and 1 cup (250 g) sugar. Slice up a banana peel into small pieces, put them in the bottle, add 1 cup (250 ml) cold water, and shake it up. Tie a piece of string around the neck of the bottle and hang it from a low tree branch, or place it on the ground, to trap the freeloaders. Replace used traps with new ones as needed.

ENCOURAGE BLOOMS ON AZALEAS AND GARDENIAS • A little bit of acid goes a long way towards bringing out the blooms on your azalea and gardenia bushes—especially if you have hard water. Both bushes do best in acidic soils (with pH levels between 4 and 5.5). To keep them healthy and to produce more flowers, water them every week or so with 3 tablespoons (45 ml) white vinegar mixed in a gallon (4 L) water. Don't apply the solution while the bush is in bloom, though; it may shorten the life of the flowers or harm the plant.

STOP YELLOW LEAVES ON PLANTS • The appearance of yellow leaves on plants accustomed to acidic soils—such as azaleas, hydrangeas, and gardenias—could signal a drop in the plant's iron intake or a shift in the ground's pH above a comfortable 5.0 level. Either problem can be resolved by watering the soil around the afflicted plants once a week for three weeks with 1 cup (250 ml) of a solution made with 2 tablespoons (30 ml) apple cider vinegar in a quart (1 L) water.

TREAT RUST AND OTHER PLANT DISEASES • You can use vinegar to treat a host of plant diseases, including rust, black spot, and powdery mildew. Mix 2 tablespoons (30 ml) apple cider vinegar in 2 quarts (2 L) of water and pour some into a spray bottle. Spray the solution on your affected plants in the morning or early evening (when temperatures are relatively cool and there's no direct light on the plant) until the condition is cured.

CLEAN YOUR LAWN MOWER BLADES • Grass, especially when it's damp, has a tendency to accumulate on your lawn mower blades after you cut the lawn—sometimes with grubs hiding inside. Wipe down the blades with a cloth dampened with undiluted white vinegar. It will clean off leftover grass on the blades, as well as any pests that are stuck to the blades.

SCIENCE **WORKS!**

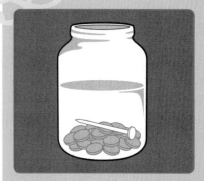

Mix together 1/2 cup (125 ml) white vinegar and 1/4 teaspoon (1 ml) salt in a glass jar.

Add 25 old copper coins to the solution, and let them sit for 5 minutes. While you're waiting, take a large iron nail and clean it off with some baking soda sprinkled on a damp sponge. Rinse off the nail and place it into the solution. After 15 minutes, the nail will be coated with copper, while the coins will shine like new. This is a result of the acetic acid in the vinegar combining with the copper on the coins to form copper acetate, which then accumulates on the iron nail.

KEEP OUT FOUR-LEGGED PESTS • Some animals—including cats, deer, dogs, rabbits, and racoons—can't stand the scent of vinegar even after it has dried. You can keep these unauthorized visitors out of your garden by soaking several recycled rags in white vinegar and placing them on stakes around your veggies. Resoak the rags every 7 to 10 days.

EXTERMINATE DANDELIONS AND UNWANTED GRASS • Are dandelions sprouting up in the cracks of your driveway or along the fringes of your patio? Make them disappear for good by spraying them with full-strength white or apple cider vinegar. Early in the season, give each plant a single spray of vinegar in its midsection, or in the middle of the flower before the plants go to seed. Aim another shot near the stem at ground level so the vinegar can soak down to the roots. Keep an eye on the weather, though; if it rains the next day, you'll need to give the weeds another spraying.

DID YOU KNOW?

Looking for a nontoxic alternative to commercial weed killers? Vinegar is the way to go. In studies at the Agricultural Research Service in Beltsville, Maryland, researchers proved vinegar effective at killing five common weeds within their first two weeks above ground. The vinegar was sprayed by hand in concentrations between 5 and 10 percent. But that's old news to seasoned gardeners who've been using full-strength apple cider vinegar for ages to kill everything from poison ivy to crabgrass (and, the occasional ornamental plant that grew too close to the target).

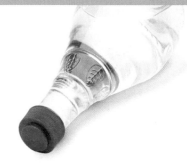

for pet care

KEEP CATS AWAY • If you want to keep cats out of the kids' playroom, or discourage them from using your favorite easy chair as a scratching post, sprinkle some full-strength distilled white vinegar around the area or on the object itself. Cats don't like the smell of vinegar and will avoid it.

UNMARK YOUR PET'S SPOTS • When house-training a puppy or kitten, it'll often wet previously soiled spots. After cleaning up the mess, it's essential to remove the scent from your floor, carpeting, or couch. And nothing does that better than vinegar:

■ On a floor, blot up as much of the stain as possible, then mop with equal parts white vinegar and warm water. (On a wood or vinyl floor, test a few drops of vinegar in an inconspicuous area first, to make sure that it won't harm the floor's finish.) Dry with a cloth or paper towel.

■ For urine stains on carpets, rugs, and upholstery, thoroughly blot the area with a towel or some rags, then pour a bit of undiluted vinegar over the spot. Blot it up with a towel, reapply the vinegar, and let it air-dry. Once the vinegar dries, the spot should be completely deodorized.

ADD TO PET'S DRINKING WATER • Adding a teaspoon of apple cider vinegar to your dog or cat's drinking water provides needed nutrients to its diet, gives it a shinier, healthier-looking coat, and also acts as a natural deterrent to fleas and ticks.

more VINEGAR over →

PROTECT AGAINST FLEAS AND TICKS • To give your dog effective flea and tick protection, fill a spray bottle with equal parts water and vinegar and apply it directly to the dog's coat and rub it in well. You may have more trouble doing this with cats, because they really hate the smell of the stuff.

CLEAN YOUR PET'S EARS • If you've noticed that Rover has been scratching around his ears a lot more than usual lately, a bit of vinegar could bring some relief. Swabbing your pet's ears with a cotton ball or soft cloth dabbed in a solution of 2 parts vinegar and 1 part water will keep them clean and help deter ear mites and bacteria. It also soothes minor itches from mosquito bites. **WARNING: Do not apply undiluted vinegar to open lacerations. If you see a cut in your pet's ears, seek veterinary treatment.**

REMOVE STINKY ODORS • If your dog has rolled in something unpleasant, here are some ways to help him get rid of the smell:

■ Bathe your pet in a mixture of ½ cup (125 ml) white vinegar, ¼ cup (50 g) baking soda, and 1 teaspoon (5 ml) liquid soap in 1 quart (1 L) of 3 percent hydrogen peroxide. Work the solution deep into his coat, give it a few minutes to soak in, then rinse the mixture out thoroughly with clean water.

■ Bathe your pet in equal parts water and vinegar (preferably outdoors), then repeat using 1 part vinegar to 2 parts water, followed by a good rinsing.

■ If cleaning the dog means you also get the rotten smell of whatever he's rolled in on you, use undiluted vinegar to get the smell out of your own clothes. Let the affected clothing soak in the vinegar overnight.

for the do-it-yourselfer

WASH CONCRETE OFF YOUR SKIN • Even though you wear rubber gloves when working with concrete, some of the stuff inevitably splashes on your skin. Prolonged contact with wet concrete can cause your skin to crack, and may even lead to eczema. Use undiluted white vinegar to wash dried concrete or mortar off your skin, then wash with warm, soapy water.

DEGREASE GRATES, FANS, AND AIR-CONDITIONER GRILLES • Even in the cleanest of homes, air-conditioner grilles, heating grates, and fan blades eventually develop a layer of dust and grease and grime. To clean them, wipe them over with full-strength white vinegar. Use an old toothbrush to work the vinegar into the tight spaces on air-conditioner grilles and exhaust fans.

REMOVE PAINT FUMES • Place a couple of shallow dishes filled with undiluted white vinegar around a freshly painted room to get rid of the strong smell.

DID YOU KNOW?

You just came across an old, unopened bottle of vinegar and you wonder if it's still any good. The answer is an unqualified yes. In fact, vinegar has a practically limitless shelf life. Its acid content makes it self-preserving and even negates the need for refrigeration (although many people mistakenly believe in refrigerating their open bottles). You won't see any changes in white vinegar over time, but some other types may change slightly in color or develop a hazy appearance or a bit of sediment. However, these are strictly cosmetic changes; the vinegar itself will remain virtually unchanged.

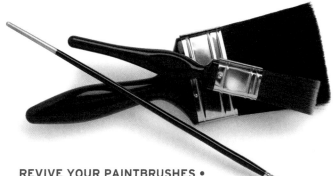

DISINFECT AIR-CONDITIONER AND HUMIDIFIER FILTERS • An air-conditioner or humidifier filter can quickly become inundated with dust, soot, pet hair, and even potentially harmful bacteria. Every 10 days or so, clean your filter in equal parts white vinegar and warm water. Let the filter soak in the solution for an hour and simply squeeze it dry before using. If your filters are particularly dirty, let them soak overnight to dislodge stubborn grime.

KEEP THE PAINT ON YOUR CEMENT FLOORS • Painted cement floors have a tendency to peel after a while. But you can keep the paint stuck to the cement longer by giving the floor an initial coat of white vinegar before you paint it. Wait until the vinegar has dried, then begin painting. This same technique will also help keep paint fixed to galvanized metal.

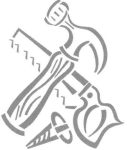

GET RID OF RUST

If you want to clean up those rusted old tools you recently unearthed under your house or picked up at a garage sale, soak them in full-strength white vinegar for several days. The same treatment is equally effective at removing the rust from corroded nuts and bolts. And you can pour vinegar on rusted hinges and screws to loosen them up for removal.

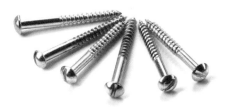

REVIVE YOUR PAINTBRUSHES • To remove dried-on paint from a synthetic-bristle paintbrush, soak it in full-strength white vinegar until the paint dissolves and the bristles are soft and pliable, and wash in hot, soapy water. Does a paintbrush seem beyond hope? Before tossing it, try boiling in 1 to 2 cups (250-500 ml) vinegar for 10 minutes, followed by a thorough washing in soapy water.

PEEL OFF WALLPAPER • Removing old wallpaper can be messy, but you can make it peel off easily by soaking it with a vinegar solution. Spray equal parts white vinegar and water on the wallpaper until it is saturated and wait a few minutes. Then zip the stuff off the wall with a wallpaper scraper. If it is stubborn, try carefully scoring the wallpaper with the scraper before you spray on the vinegar solution.

SLOW HARDENING OF PLASTER • Want to keep your plaster pliable a bit longer to get it all smoothed out? Just add a couple tablespoons of white vinegar to your plaster mix. It will slow down the hardening process to give you the extra time you need.

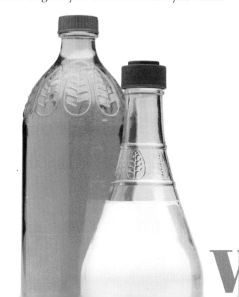

VODKA

MAKE YOUR OWN VANILLA EXTRACT • Here's an unusual homemade treat you can use to spice up a gift basket, and it takes only minutes to make. Get one real dried vanilla bean (available from specialty food stores) and slice it open from top to bottom. Place in a glass jar and cover with ¾ cup (175 ml) vodka. Seal the jar and let it rest in a cupboard for 4–6 months and shake occasionally. Filter your homemade vanilla extract through an unbleached coffee filter or cheesecloth into a decorative bottle and watch the face of your favorite cook light up with pleasure!

CLEAN GLASS AND JEWELRY • In a pinch, a few drops of vodka will clean any glass or jewelry with crystalline gemstones. So although people might look at you askance, you could dip a napkin into your vodka on the rocks to wipe away the grime on your glasses or dunk your diamond ring for a few minutes to get it sparkling again. But don't try this with contact lenses! And avoid getting alcohol on any gemstone that's not a crystal. Only diamonds, emeralds, and the like will benefit from a vodka bath.

USE AS A HYGIENIC SOAK • Vodka is an alcohol, and like any alcohol, it kills germs. If you don't have ordinary rubbing alcohol on hand, use vodka instead. You can use it to soak razor blades you plan to reuse, as well as to clean hairbrushes, toothbrushes, and pet brushes, or on anything else that might spread germs from person to person or animal to animal.

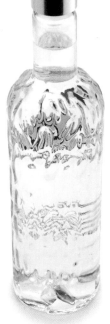

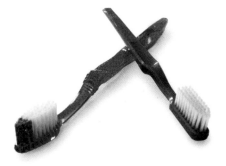

KILL WEEDS IN THE GARDEN • For a quick and easy weed killer, mix 2 tablespoons (30 ml) vodka, a few drops of dishwashing liquid, and 2 cups (500 ml) water in a spray bottle. Spray it on the weed leaves until the mixture runs off. Apply it at midday on a sunny day to weeds growing in direct sunlight, because the alcohol breaks down the waxy cuticle covering on leaves, leaving them susceptible to dehydration in sunlight. It won't work in shade.

KEEP CUT FLOWERS FRESH • The secret to keep cut flowers looking good as long as possible is to minimize the growth of bacteria in the water and to provide nourishment to replace what the flower would have had if it had not been cut. Add a few drops of vodka (or any clear spirit) to the vase water for antibacterial action along with 1 teaspoon (5 ml) sugar. Change the water every other day, refreshing the vodka and sugar each time.

DID YOU KNOW?

Essential to James Bond's martini—and so intrinsic to Russian culture that its name derives from the Russian word for water (voda)—vodka was first made in the 1400s as an antiseptic and painkiller before it was drunk as a beverage. But what exactly is it? Classically, vodka starts as a soupy mixture of ground wheat or rye that's fermented (sugars in the grain are converted into alcohol by yeast), then distilled (heated until the alcohol evaporates and then condenses). Flavorings such as citrus were originally added to mask the taste of impurities, but are used today for enhancement and brand identification.

WALLPAPER

LINE DRAWERS • Wallpaper remnants can be a great substitute for shelf liner paper when used to line chests of drawers or wardrobe shelves—especially designs with raised patterns or fabrics, which may add a bit of friction to prevent things from moving around. Cut the wallpaper into appropriate-sized strips to accommodate the space you're lining.

RESTORE A FOLDING SCREEN • If you have an old folding screen that's become torn or stained over the years, give it a new, younger look by covering it with leftover wallpaper. Use masking tape to hold the strips at top and bottom if you don't want to glue it on top of the original material.

PROTECT SCHOOLBOOKS • If your child goes through book covers on textbooks on a regular basis, get your hands on some old rolls of wallpaper. Book covers made of wallpaper are typically more rugged than even the traditional brown paper bag sleeves. They can hold their own against pens and pencils, and are much better at handling the elements, especially rain and dust.

MAKE A JIGSAW PUZZLE • What to do with your leftover wallpaper? Why not use a piece to make a jigsaw puzzle? Simply cut off a medium-sized rectangular piece and glue it onto a piece of thin cardboard. Once it's dried, cut it up into a bunch of curvy and angular shapes. It'll give you, or the kids, something to do on a rainy day.

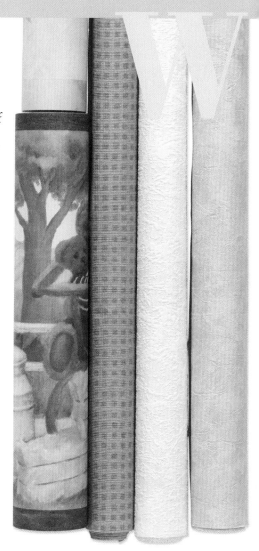

WAX PAPER

FAIL-SAFE CAKE DECORATING • Can you pipe out 'Happy Birthday' in icing on the first try? Not many of us can, so try this trick to make it easier. Cut a piece of waxed paper or parchment paper the same size as your cake, using the cake pan as a guide. Then pipe the name and the message on the paper and freeze it. After just half an hour it should be easy to handle. Loosen the icing and slide it off onto the cake using a spatula. It's so easy and it really works. Everyone will think you're a cake-decorating professional!

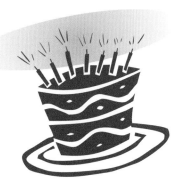

more WAX PAPER over →

FUNNEL SPICES INTO JARS • Filling narrow-mouthed spice jars can make a big mess on your kitchen counter. Roll a piece of wax paper into a funnel shape and pour spices into your jars without spilling a single mustard seed. In a pinch, you can even funnel liquids by using a couple of layers of wax paper offset so the seams in the layers don't line up.

SPEED KITCHEN CLEANUP • Wax paper can help keep all kinds of kitchen surfaces clean:

▓ Line vegetable and meat cold storage bins with a layer of wax paper. When it needs replacement, just scrunch it up and throw it in the garbage or, if it's not stained with meat juices, the compost pile.

▓ If your kitchen cupboards don't extend to the ceiling, a layer of wax paper on top will catch dust and grease particles. Every month or two, just fold it up, discard it, and put down a fresh layer.

▓ If you're worried about meat juices getting into the pores of your cutting board, cover it with three layers of wax paper before slicing raw meat and throw the paper out immediately. It beats disinfecting the cutting board with bleach!

PREVENT WAFFLES FROM STICKING • Having trouble extricating waffles from your waffle iron? Nonstick surfaces don't last forever. You can't fix the problem permanently, but if you just want to get it to work today, put a layer of wax paper in between the plates of your waffle iron for a few minutes while it heats up. The wax will be transferred to the plates, temporarily helping waffles pop out again.

KEEP CAST IRON RUST-FREE • Cast iron devotees agree that this superior cooking material is well worth a little extra effort to keep it in tip-top shape. To prevent rust from forming on cast iron between uses, rub a sheet of wax paper over your frying pan or casserole after washing, while it's still warm. Then place the sheet between the pot and the lid to store.

UNCORK BOTTLES WITH EASE

If you keep a bottle of cooking wine in your kitchen, you probably uncork it and recork it often before using it up. Instead of struggling with the cork each time, wrap some wax paper around the cork before reinserting it. It'll be easier to remove the next time, and the paper helps keep little bits of cork from getting into the wine.

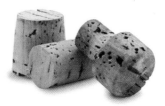

KEEP CANDLES FROM STAINING TABLE LINENS • Candles in colors that coordinate with your dining room linens make a lovely finishing touch to table settings, and it's helpful to store them all together. However, if you store the candles with table linens, the candle color can rub off on the linens. To avoid this, wrap colorful candles in plain wax paper before storage. And avoid paper with any kind of patterns, which can also stain linens.

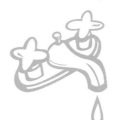

STOP WATER SPOTTING • Company's coming and you want every room in the house to look its best. To keep bathroom fixtures temporarily spotless, rub them with a sheet of wax paper after cleaning them. The wax that transfers will deflect water droplets like magic—at least until the next cleaning.

STORE DELICATE FABRICS • Treasured lace doilies and other linens handed down in your family can deteriorate quickly if not stored with care. A sheet of wax paper between each fabric piece will help block extraneous light and prevent transfer of dyes without trapping moisture.

GIVE YOUR CAR ANTENNA A SMOOTH RIDE • If you have a newer vehicle, your car antenna may retract each time you turn off the ignition, carrying grime with it that can eventually bring your antenna (and your reception) to a grinding halt. Every now and then, rub the antenna with a piece of wax paper to coat the shaft and help it repel dirt.

MAKE A SNOW SLIDE OR TOBOGGAN GO FASTER

Everyone knows, the more slippery the slide, the more fun it is! Keep kids swooshing on their behinds by balling up a large piece of wax paper and rubbing it all over their slide's runners.

Kids' Stuff

What kid wouldn't like homemade 'stained glass' art that takes only minutes to make? First, make crayon shavings using a vegetable peeler (keep each color separate). Put a paper towel or bag on the counter. Place a sheet of wax paper on top, sprinkle it with crayon shavings and cover with another layer of wax paper and paper towel. Press it for a few minutes using a warm iron and remove the paper towel layers. Cut your new see-through art into sun-catching medallions or colorful bookmarks using craft scissors to create a decorative edge.

PROTECT SURFACES FROM GLUE • Woodworkers know that there's enough glue in a wood joint if some squeezes out when they clamp the joint. They also know that excess glue will be a real pain to remove if it drips on the workbench, or worse, bonds the clamping blocks to the project. To prevent this, cover the bench with strips of wax paper and put pieces of wax paper between the clamping blocks and the project. The glue won't adhere to, or soak through, the wax.

MAKE EDUCATIONAL PLACEMATS • One way to make learning fun is with personalized placemats featuring maths facts or other lessons your child is trying to memorize. Take several flash cards and sandwich them between layers of wax paper cut to placemat size. Sandwich that between two layers of paper towels and press it all with a warm iron to 'laminate' the flash cards in place. Remove the paper towels before use.

$$2 + 5 = ?$$

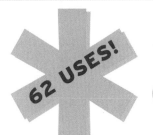

WD-40

around the house

TREAT YOUR SHOES • Spray WD-40 on new leather shoes before you start wearing them regularly. It will help prevent blisters by softening the leather and making the shoes more comfortable. Keep the shoes waterproof and shiny by spraying them periodically with WD-40 and buffing gently with a soft cloth. To give the old 'soft shoo' to squeaky shoes, spray some WD-40 at the spot where the sole and heel join and the squeaks will cease.

SEPARATE STUCK GLASSWARE • What can you do when you reach for a drinking glass and get two locked together, one stuck tightly inside the other? You don't want to risk breaking one or both by trying to pull them apart. Stuck glasses will separate with ease if you squirt some WD-40 on them, wait a few seconds for it to work its way between the glasses, then gently pull the glasses apart. Remember to wash the glasses thoroughly before you use them.

FREE STUCK LEGO BLOCKS • When a child's construction project hits a snag because some of the plastic blocks are stuck together, let WD-40 help get them unstuck. Spray a little on the blocks where they are locked together, wiggle them gently, and pull them apart. The lubricant in WD-40 will penetrate into the fine seam where the blocks are joined.inse and dry thoroughly.

TONE DOWN POLYURETHANE SHINE • A new coat of polyurethane can sometimes make a wooden floor look a little too shiny. To tone down the shine and cut the glare, spray some WD-40 on a soft cloth and wipe up the floor with it.

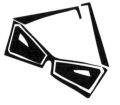

KEEP PUPPIES FROM CHEWING • Your new puppy is adorable, but will he ever stop chewing up the house? To keep puppies from chewing on telephone and television-cable lines, spray WD-40 on the lines. Puppies hate the smell.

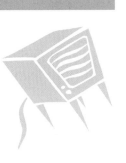

CAUTION: Do not spray WD-40 near an open flame or other heat source, near electrical currents, or battery terminals. And always disconnect appliances before spraying with the lubricant.

Do not place a WD-40 can in direct sunlight or on hot surfaces. Never store it in temperatures above 120°F (50°C) or puncture the pressurized can.

Use WD-40 in well-ventilated areas. Never swallow or inhale it (if swallowed, seek medical attention immediately).

REMOVE STRONG GLUE • You didn't wear protective gloves when using that super-glue and now some of it is super-stuck to your fingers! Don't panic. Just reach for the WD-40, spray some directly on the sticky fingers and rub your hands together until your fingers are no longer sticky. Use WD-40 to remove the glue from other unwanted surfaces as well.

GET OFF THAT STUCK RING • When pulling and tugging can't get that ring off your finger, reach for the WD-40. A short burst of WD-40 will get the ring to slide right off. Remember to wash your hands thoroughly afterwards, to clean off the lubricant.

FREE STUCK FINGERS • Use WD-40 to free a child's finger when it gets it stuck in a bottle. Just spray it on the finger, let it seep in, and pull the finger out. Be sure to wash the child's hand and the bottle afterwards.

LOOSEN ZIPPERS • Stubborn zippers on jackets, pants, backpacks, and sleeping bags will become compliant again after you spray them with WD-40. Just spray it on and pull the zipper up and down a few times to distribute the lubricant evenly over all the teeth. If you want to avoid getting the WD-40 on the fabric, spray it on a plastic lid, then pick it up and apply it with an artist's brush.

EXTERMINATE ROACHES AND REPEL INSECTS • Don't let cockroaches, insects, or spiders get the upper hand in your home. Try these tips:

■ Keep a can of WD-40 handy, and when you see a cockroach, spray a small amount directly on it for an instant kill.

■ To keep insects and spiders out of your home, spray WD-40 on windowsills and frames, screens, and door frames. Be careful not to inhale the fumes when you spray and do not do this at all if you have babies or small children at home.

CLEAN AND LUBRICATE GUITAR STRINGS

To clean, lubricate, and prevent corrosion on guitar strings, apply a small amount of WD-40 after each playing. Spray the WD-40 on a rag and wipe the rag over the strings rather than spraying directly on the strings—you don't want WD-40 to build up on the guitar neck or body.

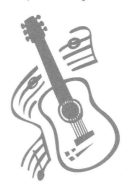

KEEP WOODEN TOOL HANDLES SPLINTER-FREE • No tools can last forever, but you can prolong the life of your wood-handled tools by preventing splintering. To keep wooden handles from splintering, rub a generous amount of WD-40 into the wood. It will shield the wood from moisture and other corrosive elements, keeping it smooth and splinter-free for the life of the tool.

UNSTICK WOBBLY SHOPPING-CART WHEELS • Attention supermarket shoppers: Keep a can of WD-40 handy whenever you go food shopping. When you get stuck with a sticky, wobbly-wheeled shopping cart, you can spray the wheels to reduce friction and wobbling. Less wobbling means faster shopping.

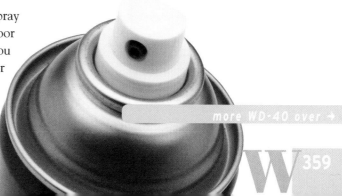

more WD-40 over →

DID YOU KNOW?

■ In 1953 Norm Larsen founded the Rocket Chemical Company in San Diego and, with two employees, set out to develop a rust-preventing solvent and degreaser for the aerospace industry. On the fortieth try, they succeeded in creating a 'water displacement' compound. The name WD-40 stands for 'Water Displacement—40th try'.

■ In 1958, a few years after WD-40's first industrial use, the company put it in aerosol cans and sold it for home use—inspired by employees who snuck cans out of the plant to use at home.

■ In 1962, when U.S. astronaut John Glenn circled the Earth in *Friendship VII*, the space capsule was coated with WD-40 and so was the Atlas missile used to boost it into space.

■ In 1969 Rocket Chemical renamed itself the WD-40 Company after the product.

REMOVE CHEWING GUM FROM HAIR • It's one of your worst nightmares: chewing gum tangled in a child's hair. You don't have to panic or run for the scissors. Simply spray the gummed-up hair with WD-40 and the gum will easily comb out. Make sure you are in a well-ventilated area when you spray and take care to avoid contact with the child's eyes.

BREAK IN A NEW BASEBALL GLOVE • Use WD-40 instead of neat's-foot oil to break in a new baseball glove. Spray the glove with WD-40, put a baseball in the palm and fold it sideways. Take a rubber band or belt and tie it around the folded glove. The WD-40 will help soften the leather and help it form around the baseball. Keep the glove tied up overnight, then wear it for a while so it will begin to fit the shape of your hand.

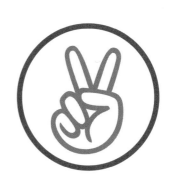

for cleaning things

REMOVE TOUGH SCUFF MARKS • Those tough black scuff marks on your kitchen floor won't be so tough anymore if you spray them with WD-40. Use WD-40 to help remove tar and scuff marks on all your hard-surfaced floors. It won't harm the surface, and you won't have to scrub nearly as much. Remember to open the windows if you are cleaning a lot of marks.

CLEAN DRIED GLUE ON SURFACES • Clean dried glue from virtually any hard surface with ease. Simply spray WD-40 onto the spot, wait at least 30 seconds, and wipe clean with a damp cloth.

DEGREASE YOUR HANDS • When you're finished working on the car and your hands are greasy and blackened with grime, use WD-40 to help get them clean. Spray a small amount of WD-40 into your hands and rub them together for a few seconds, then wipe with a paper towel and wash with soap and water. The grease and grime will wash right off.

REMOVE DECALS

You don't need a chisel or even a razor blade to remove old decals, bumper stickers, or cellophane tape. Just spray them with WD-40, wait about 30 seconds, and wipe them away.

REMOVE STICKERS FROM GLASS • What are manufacturers thinking when they put stickers on glass surfaces? Don't they know how hard they are to get off? When soap and water won't work and you don't want to ruin a fingernail or risk scratching the glass with a blade, try a little WD-40. Spray it on the sticker and glass, wait a few minutes, and use a plastic spatula or scraper to scrape the sticker off. The solvents in WD-40 cause the adhesive to lose its stickiness.

CLEAN TOILET BOWLS • You don't need a bald genie or a specialized product to clean ugly gunk and lime stains from your toilet bowl. Use WD-40 instead. Spray it into the bowl for a couple of seconds and swish with a nylon toilet brush. The solvents in the WD-40 will help dissolve the gunk and lime.

CLEAN YOUR FRIDGE

When soap and water can't get rid of old bits of food stuck in and around your refrigerator, it's time to reach for the WD-40. After clearing all foodstuffs from the areas to be treated, spray a small amount of WD-40 on each resistant spot, and wipe them away with a rag or sponge. Make sure you wash off all the WD-40 before returning food to the fridge.

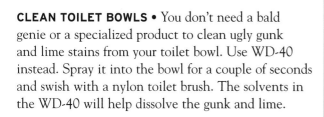

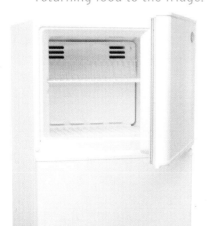

STAINS AWAY!

WIPE AWAY TEA STAINS • To remove tea stains from countertops, spray a little WD-40 on a sponge or damp cloth and wipe the stain away.

CLEAN CARPET STAINS • Don't let ink or other stains ruin your fine carpet. Spray the stain with WD-40, wait a minute or two, then use your regular carpet cleaner or gently cleanse with a sponge and warm, soapy water. Continue until the stain is completely gone.

GET TOMATO STAINS OFF CLOTHES • That homegrown tomato looked so inviting you couldn't resist. Now your shirt or blouse has a big, hard-to-remove tomato stain on it! To remove stains from fresh tomatoes or tomato sauce, spray some WD-40 directly on the spot, wait a couple of minutes, and wash as usual.

PRETREAT BLOODSTAINS AND OTHER STAINS • Oh no! Your child fell down and cut himself and there's blood all over his new shirt. After you tend to his wound, give that shirt some first aid, too! Pretreat bloodstains on fabric garments with WD-40. Spray some directly on the stain, wait a couple of minutes, and launder as usual. The WD-40 will help lift the stain so it comes out in the wash. Get to the stain while it's fresh. Once it sets, it will be harder to get out. Use WD-40 to pretreat other stubborn stains on clothing such as lipstick, dirt, grease, and ink.

more WD-40 over →

CLEAN UP A BLACKBOARD •

When it comes to cleaning and restoring a blackboard, WD-40 is the teacher's pet. Just spray it on and wipe with a clean cloth. The blackboard will look as clean and fresh as it did on the first day of school.

DID YOU KNOW?

A million cans of WD-40 are produced each week in the United States alone. The secret recipe is known only by a handful of people within the WD-40 Company. A lone "brew master" mixes the product at corporate headquarters in San Diego. The company refuses to reveal the ingredients, but will say, "WD-40 does not contain silicone, kerosene, water, wax, graphite, chlorofluorocarbons (CFCs) or any known cancer-causing agents." Good enough for most Americans: WD-40 can be found in 4 out of 5 American homes.

CONDITION LEATHER FURNITURE •

Keep your favorite leather recliner and other leather furniture in tip-top shape by softening and preserving it with WD-40. Just spray it on and buff with a soft cloth. The combination of ingredients in WD-40 will clean, penetrate, lubricate, and protect the leather.

REMOVE MARKER AND CRAYON MARKS • Have the kids used your wall as if it was a big coloring book? Don't worry, it's not the end of the world. Simply spray some WD-40 on the marks and wipe with a clean rag. WD-40 will not damage the paint or most wallpaper (test fabric or other special wall coverings first). It will also remove felt-tip pen and crayon marks from furniture and appliances.

in the backyard

REJUVENATE THE BARBECUE GRILL • To make a worn old barbecue grill look like new again, spray it liberally with WD-40, wait a few seconds, and scrub with a wire brush. Remember to use WD-40 only on a grill that is not in use and has cooled off.

RENEW FADED PLASTIC FURNITURE • Bring color and shine back to faded plastic patio furniture by simply spraying WD-40 directly onto the surface and wiping with a clean, dry cloth. You'll be surprised at the results.

SNOW PROBLEM

PREVENT SNOW BUILD UP ON WINDOWS • Does the weather forecast predict a big winter snowstorm? You can't stop the snow from falling, but you can prevent it from building up on your house windows. Just spray WD-40 on the outside of your windows before the snow starts and the snow won't stick.

KEEP A SHOVEL SNOW-FREE • Here is a simple tip to make shovelling snow quicker and less strenuous by keeping the snow from sticking to your shovel and weighing it down. Spray a thin layer of WD-40 on the shovel blade and the snow will slide right off.

PROTECT A BIRD FEEDER • To keep squirrels from taking over a bird feeder, spray a generous amount of WD-40 on top of the feeder. Those annoying critters will slide right off.

REMOVE CAT'S PAW MARKS • Your cat may seem like a member of the family most of the time, but that isn't what you are thinking about when you have to clean a trail of paw marks off your patio furniture or the hood of your car. To remove the paw marks, spray on some WD-40 and wipe them off with a clean rag.

KEEP ANIMALS FROM FLOWERBEDS • Animals just love to play in your garden, digging up your favorite plants you worked so hard to grow. What animals don't love is the smell of WD-40. To keep animal visitors out and your flowers looking beautiful, spray WD-40 evenly over the flowerbeds one or more times over the course of the season.

REPEL PIGEONS • Are local pigeons using your balcony more than you are? If pigeons and their feathers and droppings are keeping you from enjoying the view from your balcony, spray the entire area, including railings and furniture, with WD-40. The pigeons can't stand the smell and they'll fly the coop.

KEEP WASPS FROM BUILDING NESTS

Don't let wasps and yellow jackets ruin your spring and summer fun. Their favorite place to build nests is under eaves. Next spring, spray some WD-40 under all the eaves of your house. It will block them from building their nests there.

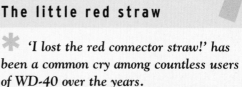

The little red straw

'I lost the red connector straw!' has been a common cry among countless users of WD-40 over the years.

In response, the company introduced a notched cap, designed to hold the straw in place across the top of the can when not in use. Because the straw exceeds the width of the can by quite a large margin, the notch may be of little use to those with limited storage space. To save space, store the straw by bending it inside the lip of the can or simply tape it to the side as it was when first purchased. A rubber band will also work well.

REMOVE DOGGIE-DOO FROM SHOES • Few things in life are more unpleasant than cleaning dog poo from the bottom of a shoe, but the task will be a lot easier if you have a can of WD-40 handy. Spray some on the affected sole and use an old toothbrush to clean the crevices, if there are any. Rinse with cold water and your shoes will be ready to hit the pavement again. Now, watch where you step!

KILL POISON IVY PLANTS • Don't let prickly weeds like poison ivy ruin your backyard or garden. Just spray some WD-40 on them and they'll wither and die off.

more WD-40 over →

in the great outdoors   ● ● ●

WD-40 AHOY!

PROTECT A BOAT FROM CORROSION • To protect a boat's finish from salt water and corrosion, spray WD-40 on the stern immediately after each use. The short time it takes will save you from having to replace parts, and it will keep your boat looking like it did on the day you bought it for a long time to come.

REMOVE BARNACLES ON BOATS • Removing barnacles from the bottom of a boat is a difficult and odious task but you can make it easier and less unpleasant with the help of some WD-40. Spray the area generously with WD-40, wait a few seconds and use a putty knife to scrape off the barnacles. Spray any remnants with WD-40 and scrape again. If necessary, use sandpaper to get rid of all of the remnants and corrosive glue still left by the barnacles.

WINTERPROOF BOOTS AND SHOES • Waterproof your winter boots and shoes by giving them a coat of WD-40. It acts as a barrier so water can't penetrate the material. Also use WD-40 to remove ugly salt stains from boots and shoes during the winter months. Just spray WD-40 on the stains and wipe with a clean rag. Your boots and shoes will look almost as good as new.

REMOVE OLD WAX • To remove old wax and dirt from skis and snowboards, spray the base sparingly with WD-40 before scraping with an acrylic scraper. Use a brass brush to further clean the base and remove any oxidized base material.

SPRAY ON FISHING LURES • Salmon fishermen often spray their lures with WD-40 because it attracts fish and disguises the human odor that can scare them off and keep them from biting. You can increase the catch on your next fishing trip by bringing a can of WD-40 along with you and spraying it on *your* lures or live bait before you cast. But first check local regulations to make sure the use of chemical-laced lures and bait is legal in your state.

UNTANGLE FISHING LINES • To loosen a tangled fishing line, spray it with WD-40 and use a pin to undo any small knots. Also use WD-40 to extend the life of curled (but not too old) fishing lines. Just take out the first 10 to 20 feet (3–6 m) of line and spray it with WD-40 the night before each trip.

CLEAN AND PROTECT GOLF CLUBS • Whether you're a duffer or a pro, you can protect and clean your clubs by spraying them with WD-40 after each use. Also use WD-40 to help loosen stuck-on spikes.

TIP

Don't overderdo the WD-40

※ *When you need to apply tiny amounts of WD-40 to a specific area, such as the electrical contacts on an electric guitar, an aerosol spray, releasing strong bursts of lubricant, is overkill.*

Instead, store some WD-40 in a clean nail-polish bottle (with cap brush) and brush on as needed.

REMOVE BURRS • To remove burrs from a horse's mane or tail without tearing its hair out (or having to cut any of its hair off!) just spray on some WD-40. You'll be able to slide the burrs right out. This will work for dogs and cats, too.

PROTECT HORSES' HOOVES • Winter horseback riding can be fun if you are warmly dressed but it can be downright painful to your horse if ice forms on the horseshoes. To prevent that from happening during cold winter rides, spray the bottom of the horse's hooves with WD-40 before you set out.

KEEP FLIES OFF COWS • If flies are tormenting your cows, just spray some WD-40 on the cows. Flies hate the smell and they'll stay clear. Take care not to spray any WD-40 in the cows' eyes, though.

DID YOU KNOW?

WD-40 is one of the few products with its own fan club. The official WD-40 Fan Club has more than 63,000 members and is growing. Over the years members have contributed thousands of unique and sometimes strange uses for the product. But according to the president and CEO of the WD-40 Company, the strangest use of all occurred in China. In Hong Kong some time ago a python was caught in the suspension of a public bus, so they used WD-40 to get the slippery offender out of there!

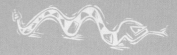

for your health

RELIEVE ARTHRITIS SYMPTOMS

For occasional joint pain or arthritis symptoms in the knees or other areas of the body, advocates swear by spraying WD-40 on the affected area and massaging it in, saying it provides temporary relief and makes movement easier. For severe, persistent pain, consult a health care professional.

CLEAN A HEARING AID • To give a hearing aid a good cleaning, use a cotton swab dipped in WD-40. Do not use WD-40 to try to loosen up the volume control (it will loosen it too much).

RELIEVE BEE-STING PAIN • For fast relief of pain from a bee, wasp, or hornet sting, reach for the WD-40 can and spray it directly on the bite site. It will take the "ouch" right out.

REMOVE STUCK PROSTHESES • If you wear a prosthetic device, you know how difficult it can be to remove at times, especially when no one is around to help. Next time you have a prosthesis stuck in place, spray some WD-40 at the junction where it attaches. The chemical solvents and lubricants in WD-40 will help make it easier to remove.

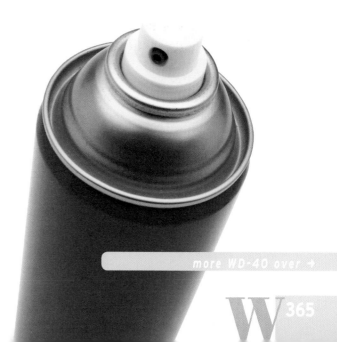

more WD-40 over →

in the garage

KEEP DEAD BUGS OFF A CAR GRILLE • It's bad enough that your car grille and hood get splattered with insects every time you go on a long road trip, but the worst part is that they're really hard to scrape off. To make it easier, just spray a bit of WD-40 on the grille and hood before you go for a drive and most of the insects will slide right off. The few that are left on the hood will be easy to wipe off later without damaging your car's finish.

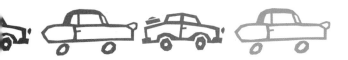

CLEAN AND RESTORE A LICENSE PLATE • To help restore a license plate that's beginning to rust, spray it with WD-40 and wipe with a clean rag. This will remove light surface rust and will also help prevent more rust from forming. It's an easy way to clean up lightly rusted plates and it won't leave a greasy feel.

COAT A TRUCK BED • For easy removal of a utility or truck-bed liner, spray the truck bed with WD-40 before you install the liner. When it comes time to remove it, the liner will slide right out.

CLEAN OIL SPOTS FROM A DRIVEWAY • If a leaky oil pan leaves a big ugly spot in the middle of your concrete driveway, get rid of the spot by spraying it with a generous amount of WD-40 and hose it down with water.

BRIGHT SPARKS

REMOVE STUCK SPARK PLUGS • To save time replacing spark plugs, spray WD-40 on stuck plugs to remove them quickly and easily.

REVIVE SPARK PLUGS • Can't get your car to start on a rainy or humid day? To get your engine purring, just spray some WD-40 on the spark-plug wires before you try starting it up again. WD-40 displaces water and keeps moisture away from the plugs.

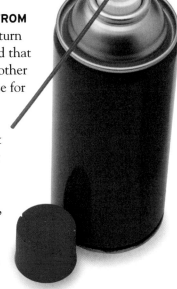

REMOVE 'PAINT RUB' FROM ANOTHER CAR • You return to your parked car to find that while you were gone, another vehicle got a bit too close for comfort. Luckily there's no dent, but now your car has a blotch of 'paint rub' on it from the other car. To remove those stains on your car and restore its original finish, spray the affected area with WD-40, wait a few seconds and wipe with a clean rag.

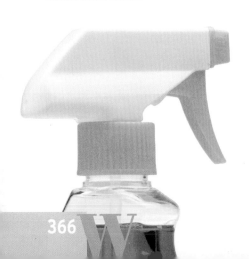

WINDOW CLEANER

REMOVE A STUCK RING • When a ring feels a little tight going on, it's likely to get stuck when it's time to get it off. Spray a bit of window cleaner on your finger for lubrication, and ease the ring off.

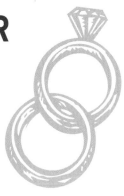

REDUCE SWELLING FROM BEE STINGS • Spritzing some window cleaner on a bee sting is a quick way to reduce the swelling and pain. But first make sure you remove any stinger. Flick it sideways to get it out—don't tweeze it out—then spray. Use only spray-on window cleaner that contains ammonia and never use a concentrated product. It is the small amount of ammonia that does the work, and beekeepers have known for years that a very dilute solution of ammonia helps relieve strings.

CLEAN YOUR JEWELRY • Use window cleaner to spruce up jewelry that is all metal or has crystalline gemstones, such as diamonds or rubies. Spray on the cleaner, then use an old toothbrush for cleaning. But don't do this if the piece has opaque stones such as opal or turquoise, or organic gems such as coral or pearl. The ammonia and detergents in the cleaner can discolor these porous surfaces.

REMOVE STUBBORN STAINS • If laundering with detergent isn't enough to get tough stains such as blood, grass, or tomato sauce out of a fabric, try a clear ammonia-based, spray-on window cleaner instead. (It's the ammonia in the window cleaner that does the trick, and you want uncolored cleaner to avoid staining the fabric.) Spray the stain with the window cleaner and let it sit for up to 15 minutes.

Blot with a clean rag, rinse with cool water, and launder again. Here are a few tips to remember:

▦ Do a test on a seam or other inconspicuous part of the garment to see if the color runs.

▦ Use cool water and don't put the garment in the dryer until the stain is completely gone.

▦ Don't use this on silk, wool, or their blends.

▦ If the fabric color seems changed after using window cleaner on it, moisten the fabric with white vinegar and rinse it with water. Acidic vinegar will neutralize alkaline ammonia.

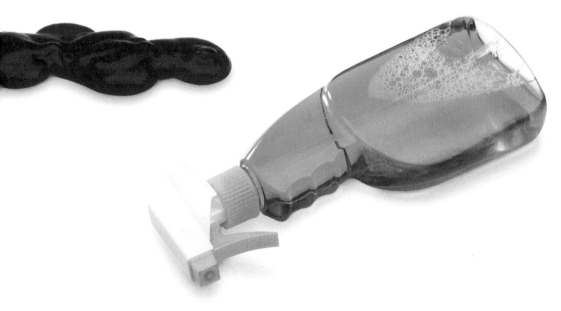

YOGURT

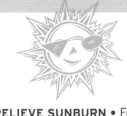

MAKE MOSS 'PAINT' FOR THE GARDEN • Wouldn't it be nice to simply paint some moss between the cracks of your stone walkway, on the sides of flowerpots or anywhere else you want it to grow? Well, you can. Just dump a cup of plain active-culture yogurt into your blender along with a handful of lawn moss and about a cup of water. Blend for about 30 seconds. Use a paintbrush to spread the mixture wherever you want moss to grow—as long as the spot is cool and shady. Mist the moss occasionally until it gets established.

MAKE A FACIAL MASK • You don't have to go to a spa to give your face a quick assist. Try these:

■ To cleanse your skin and tighten the pores, slather some plain yogurt on your face and let it sit for about 20 minutes, then rinse clean.

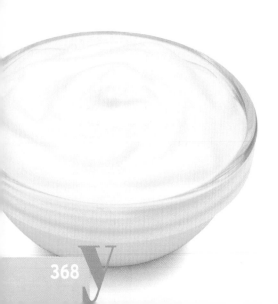

■ For a revitalizing face mask, mix 1 teaspoon (5 ml) plain yogurt with the juice from ¼ slice of orange, some of the orange pulp, and 1 teaspoon (5 ml) aloe vera. Leave on your face at least 5 minutes before rinsing thoroughly.

RELIEVE SUNBURN • For quick, temporary relief of mild sunburn, apply cold, plain yogurt. Yogurt adds much needed moisture and, at the same time, its coldness soothes. Rinse with cool water.

CURE DOG OR CAT FLATULENCE • If your pet has been a bit odoriferous lately, the problem may be a lack of the friendly digestive bacteria that prevent gas and diarrhea. The active culture in plain yogurt can help restore the beneficial bacteria. Add 2 teaspoons (10 ml) yogurt to the food of cats or small dogs weighing up to 14 pounds (6 kg), 1 tablespoon (15 ml) for medium-sized dogs 15 to 34 pounds (7–15 kg), 2 tablespoons (30 ml) for large dogs 35 to 84 pounds (16–38 kg), and 3 tablespoons (45 ml) for dogs larger than that.

MAKE PLAY FINGER PAINT

Ready for some messy rainy-day fun? Mix food coloring with yogurt to make finger paints and let the kids go wild. You can even turn it into a lesson about primary and secondary colors. For example, have the kids put a few drops of yellow food coloring and a few drops of red in the yogurt to make orange finger paint. Or mix red and blue to produce purple.

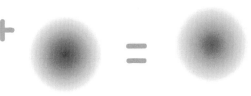

ZIPPERS

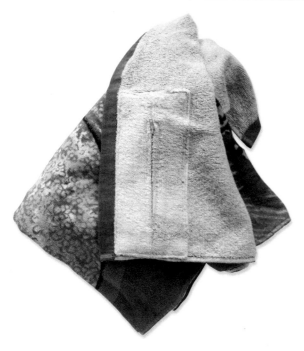

SECURE YOUR VALUABLES • Nothing ruins a holiday like reaching into your pocket and discovering it has been picked. To keep your wallet, passport, and other valuables safe, sew a zipper into the inside pocket of your jacket to keep items safely zipped inside.

MAKE A SOCK PUPPET • Create a happy sock puppet that will keep kids amused for hours. Just sew on buttons for the nose and eyes and some wool for hair, and use a small smiling upturned zipper to give the puppet an interesting mouth.

CREATE CONVERTIBLE PANTS • Here's a great idea for hikers and bikers who like to travel light. Cut the legs off a pair of jeans or other comfortable pants above the knee and reattach the legs with zippers. Zip off the legs when it gets warm and zip them back on for cool mornings and evenings. Besides lightening your load, you won't need to search for a place to change.

KEEP YOUR KEYS SAFE

Have you ever lost your car keys in the sand at the beach? Here's a great way to make sure it never happens again. Stitch a small zipped pocket—use matching terry toweling if you can—to one corner of the wrong side of your beach towel, just big enough for your keys, sunglasses, and maybe a few coins.

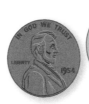
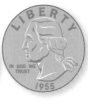

ZUCCHINI

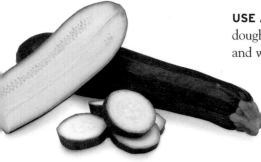

USE AS A ROLLING PIN • A large zucchini works well for rolling out dough for biscuits or a piecrust. The zucchini has just the right shape and weight, and the dough won't stick to its smooth skin.

USE AS MR. ZUCCHINI HEAD • When the kids get bored over the holidays, dust off that old Mr. Potato Head set with its ears, eyes, and glasses, and hand the kids a couple of large zucchini. The new vegetable is sure to renew their interest in the old toy.

INDEX

Note: **bold** page numbers refer to major headings.

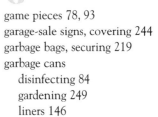